Transformations of Global Food Systems for Climate Change Resilience

Transformations of Global Food Systems for Climate Change Resilience: Addressing Food Security, Nutrition, and Health provides poignant case studies of climate change resilience frameworks for nutrition-focused transformations of agriculture and food systems, food security, food sovereignty, and population health of underserved and marginalized communities from across the globe. Each chapter is drawn from diverse cultural contexts and geographic areas, addressing local challenges of ongoing food and health system transformations and illustrating forms of resistance, resilience, and adaptations of food systems to climate change.

Fourteen chapters present global case studies, which directly address the United Nations Sustainable Development Goals and the Food and Agriculture Organization's global call to action for transforming agriculture, addressing food security and nutrition, and the health of populations impacted by climate change and public health issues. They also integrate reflections, insights, and experiences resulting from the COVID-19 pandemic.

This edited volume includes research on (1) enhancing food sovereignty and food security for underserved populations with a particular focus on Indigenous peoples; (2) improving locally contextualized definitions and measurements of climate change resilience, food security, hunger, nutrition, and health; (3) informing public health programs and policies for population health and nutrition; and (4) facilitating public and policy discourse on sustainable futures for community health and nutrition in the face of climate change and natural disasters, including ongoing and future pandemics or emergencies.

Within this book, readers will discover an array of approaches by the authors that exemplify the mutually engaged and reciprocal partnerships that are community-driven and support the positive transformation of the people with whom they work. By doing so, this book informs and drives a global sustainable future of scholarship and policy that is tied to the intersectionality and synergisms of climate change resilience, food security, food sovereignty, nutrition, and community health.

Transformations of Global Food Systems for Climate Change Resilience

Addressing Food Security, Nutrition, and Health

Edited by

Preety Gadhoke
Barrett P. Brenton
Solomon H. Katz

CRC Press
Taylor & Francis Group
Boca Raton London New York

CRC Press is an imprint of the
Taylor & Francis Group, an **informa** business

First edition published 2024
by CRC Press
6000 Broken Sound Parkway NW, Suite 300, Boca Raton, FL 33487-2742

and by CRC Press
4 Park Square, Milton Park, Abingdon, Oxon, OX14 4RN

CRC Press is an imprint of Taylor & Francis Group, LLC

Library of Congress Cataloging-in-Publication Data
Names: Gadhoke, Preety, editor. | Brenton, Barrett P., 1962–editor. |
Katz, Solomon H., 1939–editor.
Title: Transformations of global food systems for climate change resilience:
addressing food security, nutrition, and health / edited by Preety
Gadhoke, Barrett P. Brenton, and Solomon H. Katz.
Description: First edition. | Boca Raton, FL ; London : CRC Press, 2023. |
Includes bibliographical references and index. | Summary: Transformations of Global Food Systems for Climate Change Resilience: Addressing Food Security, Nutrition, and Health provides poignant case studies of climate change resilience frameworks for nutrition-focused transformations of agriculture and food systems, food security, food sovereignty, and population health of underserved and marginalized communities from across the globe. Each chapter is drawn from diverse cultural contexts and geographic areas, addressing local challenges of ongoing food and health system transformations. They illustrate forms of resistance, resilience, and adaptations of food systems to climate change. Fourteen chapters present global case studies directly address the United Nations sustainable development goals and the Food and Agriculture Organization's global call to action for transforming agriculture addressing food security and nutrition, and the health of populations impacted by climate change and public health issues. health—Provided by publisher.
Identifiers: LCCN 2023002200 (print) | LCCN 2023002201 (ebook) |
ISBN 9780367857622 (paperback) | ISBN 9781003014942 (ebook)
Subjects: LCSH: Food security—Climatic factors. | Public health—Climate
factors. | Nutrition policy—Climate factors.
Classification: LCC HD9000.5 .T7353 2023 (print) | LCC HD9000.5 (ebook) |
DDC 338.1/9—dc23/eng/20230616
LC record available at https://lccn.loc.gov/2023002200
LC ebook record available at https://lccn.loc.gov/2023002201

ISBN: 9780367857622 (pbk)
ISBN: 9781003014942 (ebk)

DOI: 10.1201/9781003014942

Typeset in Times
by codeMantra

Contents

Acknowledgments

It is with great respect that we honor the inspiration and vision of Solomon H. Katz for the initial conceptualization of this volume emerging out of his years of leadership of the American Anthropological Association's Presidential Task Force on World Food Problems. He has dedicated a steadfast lifelong career to integrating the voices of anthropologists and communities through his rights-based approach to food systems justice integrating health and nutrition for climate change resilience. His work has encouraged generations of students, colleagues, and communities who have had him as a teacher, mentor, scholar, and friend.

We acknowledge the patience and understanding of our contributors who forged ahead with their work amidst all of the challenges and loss faced during the COVID-19 pandemic. We express our deepest gratitude for the resilience and strength shown by all the contributors and communities in which they work. This collection of chapters exemplifies an impressive array of anthropologists who share the importance of taking action-oriented and applied approaches to mutual engagement with the people with whom they work. Their community-driven recommendations are strongly tied to the cultures, identities, and spaces upon which those partnerships are built and sustained.

A final special thanks to Derek Tepe and Pablo Sanchez for their editorial assistance.

Editors

Preety Gadhoke, PhD, MPH, was, at the beginning of this project, an Associate Professor in the College of Pharmacy and Health Sciences at St. John's University in New York City. She is currently an independent scholar with expertise in interdisciplinary, community-based, multilevel programs and policies that address social determinants of health and health equity for marginalized populations. She has worked on public health programs with Indigenous and urban communities in North America (Native Americans/Alaska Natives, Baltimore, New York, Chicago), South America (Ecuador), Asia (Thailand), and Africa (Ghana, Nigeria, Mozambique). She is the recipient of the 2020 Fulbright Global Research Fellowship and 2019 Catholic Relief Services Global Health Research Award. In her academic career, she has served the scientific community with the American Anthropology Association (AAA), Agriculture, Food, and Human Values Society, and Society for Applied Anthropology, American Public Health Association, and an appointed member of AAA's Presidential Task Force on World Food Problems. At St. John's University, she served as an Interim Director of the Master of Public Health Program and mentor for the Ozanam Scholars program, McNair Scholars program, Master of Arts degree program in Global Development and Social Justice, and Senior Fellow, Vincentian Center for Church and Society. She is extensively published in public health and anthropology, presented numerous papers at international and national scientific conferences, and served as a reviewer for multiple journals. She brings cross-cutting perspectives to academia from multilateral, governmental, and industry work experiences. Her passion about addressing the social ecology of food systems, nutrition, and disease prevention stems from her early memories of health disparities that she witnessed as a child within her East and West Indian communities. She earned her PhD in International Health from The Johns Hopkins Bloomberg School of Public Health, MPH in Health Policy and Management from Emory University Rollins School of Public Health, and a BA in Biology and Sociology/Anthropology at Knox College.

Barrett P. Brenton, PhD, currently serves as a Faculty Engagement Associate for Binghamton University's Center for Civic Engagement where he facilitates linking faculty with community-engaged teaching and research opportunities locally and abroad. He is also an Affiliated Senior Research Scholar with the Binghamton University Anthropology Department. He is a retired Professor of Anthropology from St. John's University, New York, where he served as the Director of the Center for Global Development and MA in Global Development and Social Justice; Coordinator of the Anthropology program; Faculty Advisor for the Ozanam Scholars Social Justice program; and Senior Fellow, Vincentian Center for Church and Society. Previously, he served as President of the Society for the Anthropology of Food and Nutrition, and of the Northeastern Anthropological Association; former coeditor of the international journal *Ecology of Food and Nutrition*; elected to the status of Fellow of the Society for Applied Anthropology; and appointed as a member of the AAA's Presidential Task Force on World Food Problems. As a specialist on the anthropology of sustainable food systems, nutrition, health, climate change, and environmental justice, his cross-cultural and applied fieldwork experience has focused on engagement with Indigenous communities in North America, South America, and sub-Saharan Africa, and in urban NYC and Upstate NY rural underserved communities. In addition to numerous papers presented at national and international conferences, he has an extensive publication record in the areas of food security, nutrition, health disparities, and sustainable global development. His commitment to creating sustainable and resilient food systems to climate change through food justice and food sovereignty advocacy stems from his experience of working and growing up in rural farming communities in Iowa and Nebraska. He earned his PhD in Biocultural Anthropology from the University of Massachusetts–Amherst with a focus on nutritional/medical anthropology and BA in Anthropology from the University of Nebraska–Lincoln.

Solomon H. Katz, PhD, is Director of the Krogman Center for Research in Child Growth and Development, Professor of Physical Anthropology, and Professor Emeritus of Orthodontics at the University of Pennsylvania. He has written, presented, and organized symposia resulting in over 200 major papers, books, and chapters lined to global field studies on diet and physical and mental health, neuroendocrinology, epidemiology of health problems in children, and the evolution of cuisine and nutrition practices, molecular biology and genetics, and cybernetics and biocultural evolution. He has also been involved in hundreds of newspaper, magazine, radio, and TV reports concerned with translating science to the public. He is the recipient of many awards and grants from the National Institutes of Health, National Science Foundation, MacArthur Foundation, Smithsonian Institution, Kellogg Foundation, and John Templeton Foundation. He is an elected fellow and has served as an officer and president at many professional organizations. He serves as Chair of the American Anthropological Association (AAA) Task Force on World Food Problems that addresses contemporary global food resources and security. He also serves as president of the "World Food Observatory," dedicated to promoting education, research, and enlightenment on the history, understanding, beliefs, values, and appreciation of food, nutrition, and diet throughout the world. Previously, Dr. Katz served as the Founder and Chairman of the AAA Task Force on African Famine. He also chaired the task force that redefined the UNESCO statement on race for the American Association of Physical Anthropologists and the International Union of Anthropological and Ethnological Sciences, a division of UNESCO. He was Series Editor of "Food and Nutrition in History and Anthropology" Gordon and Breach Publishers (with a dozen books in the series) and was Editor-in-Chief of the three-volume "Encyclopedia of Food and Culture" published by Scribners (Gale), which was awarded six major national and international awards and prizes.

Contributors

Cora Bender, University of Siegen, Germany

Barrett P. Brenton, Binghamton University, USA

Don Callaway, Independent Consultant, USA

Anna Batet Figueras, Rovira i Virgili University, Spain

Preety Gadhoke, Independent Consultant, USA

Adriana Garriga-Lopez, Kalamazoo College, USA

Cerian Gibbes, University of Colorado, USA

Jacquelyn N. Heuer, University of South Florida, USA

Robert K. Hitchcock, University of New Mexico, USA

Allison L. Hopkins, Texas A&M University, USA

Kara Hoving, The American University in Cairo, Egypt

Armando F. Inurreta Díaz, Texas A&M University, USA

Martina Jaskolski, The American University in Cairo, Egypt

Juan J. Jiménez-Osornio, Universidad Autonoma de Yucatan, Mexico

Shir Lerman Ginzburg, University of Connecticut – Health, USA

Jennifer Marshman, Wilfrid Laurier University, Canada

Casandra Owens, Texas A&M University, USA

Diana Pastrana Cervantes, Rosario del Universidad Autonoma de Yucatan, Mexico

Marsha Quinlan, Washington State University, USA

Dalia Rawandoozi, Texas A&M University, USA

Katia G. Rodríguez Ruz, Universidad Autonoma de Yucatan, Mexico

Mahmoud Shaltout, The American University in Cairo, Egypt

Amy E. Snively-Martinez, Wenatchee Valley College, USA

Marylynn Steckley, Carleton University, Canada

Joshua Steckley, University of Toronto, Canada

Devon Wilson, Devon, Project Harvest, USA

1 Addressing Food Security, Nutrition, and Health of Local Communities for Climate Change Resilience

Barrett P. Brenton and Preety Gadhoke

CONTENTS

INTRODUCTION TO THE VOLUME

In this timely anthology, we share poignant case studies that have touched on climate change resilience frameworks for nutrition-focused transformations of agriculture and food systems, food security, food sovereignty, and population health of underserved and marginalized communities from across the globe. Each chapter is drawn from diverse cultural contexts and geographic areas, addressing local challenges of ongoing food and health system transformations. They illustrate forms of resistance, resilience, and adaptations of food systems to climate change. Since this work was being written and produced during the ongoing COVID-19 pandemic, as editors, we made a special request to our contributors to add their reflections, insights, and experiences related to the pandemic. Another thread of the chapters was to ask the contributors to reflect on implications of their research tied to the United Nations Sustainable Development Goals (UN SDGs). Therefore, overall, this collection provides a diverse range of readers with a unique contribution to the literature in the field to date on the intersectionality of climate change resilience, food security, food sovereignty, nutrition, and health.

DOI: 10.1201/9781003014942-1

This edited volume includes research on (1) enhancing food sovereignty and food security for underserved populations, with a particular focus on Indigenous peoples; (2) improving locally contextualized definitions and measurements of climate change resilience, food security, hunger, nutrition, and health; (3) informing public health programs and policies for population health and nutrition; and (4) facilitating public and policy discourse on sustainable futures for community health and nutrition in the face of climate change and natural disasters, including ongoing and future pandemics or emergencies.

In response to the 2021 and 2020 United Nations Food and Agriculture Organization's (FAO) calls to action, each chapter speaks to the unique role of anthropologists in taking a global, collaborative, and interdisciplinary response to addressing the UN SDGs to eliminate global hunger and poverty crises and achieve good health and wellbeing for all. After a decade of improvements in food security, hunger, and undernutrition, there is an alarming rise in hunger among global populations living in poverty. Weather cycles, climate change, internal conflicts, and forced migrations exacerbate food insecurity and hunger, subsequently leading to allostatic stress, anxiety, depression, and social alienation, on the one hand, and disordered eating patterns as well as inadequate infant and child feeding, on the other hand. This complex pathway of foodways and public access to these foodways leads to a double burden of undernutrition and overweight/obesity, increasing the risk of diet-related stunting and wasting in children, as well as an increased risk of noncommunicable chronic diseases, such as diabetes and cardiovascular disease. These food insecurity-health disparity synergisms can have protracted consequences, especially for women and children, across their lifespan and for future generations. The UN mission to "leave no one behind" and achieve the UN SDGs by 2030 requires an urgent need for large-scale funding, partnerships, risk reduction, and climate change adoption programs and policies.

This edited volume of 14 chapters is truly unique in being multi-, inter-, and transdisciplinary by having contributors with an array of backgrounds, including anthropology, agriculture, ethnobiology, environmental and natural resources, geography and planning, global health, international development, nutrition, and community health. This work is intended as a highly useful resource for practitioners and policy makers, academics, and students who are interested in the sociocultural and political-economic impacts that transformations of global food systems have for climate change resilience while addressing the challenges of food security, nutrition, and health. It is appropriate for use in classrooms at the undergraduate and graduate levels to address the intersectional nature of climate change resilience, food security and nutrition, and health, including the impact of the COVID-19 pandemic. It is also relevant for policy makers, decision-makers, health officials, opinion leaders, advocates, lawyers, and environmentalists across the globe.

OVERVIEW OF CHAPTERS

Case studies in the following chapters are presented from across the globe, including Sub-Saharan Africa, Native North America, Latin America and the Caribbean, North Africa and the Middle East, North America, and Asia–Pacific. They directly address the UN SDGs and the FAO's global call to action for transforming agriculture to address food security and nutrition, and the health of populations that are impacted by climate change and public health emergencies. The impact of the COVID-19 pandemic is also noted. What follows is a brief review of each chapter organized by geographic area.

SUB-SAHARAN AFRICA

Hitchcock, in Chapter 2, "Climate Change Resilient Livelihoods and Adaptive Strategies among the Ju/'hoansi San of Nyae Nyae, Namibia," discusses ongoing challenges faced by Indigenous San communities from a deep historical perspective. A focus on the ongoing drought in the region provides critical insights into the importance of coping mechanisms that tap into Indigenous knowledge and traditional support networks.

NATIVE NORTH AMERICA

Bender, in Chapter 3, "Tribal Sovereignty and the Transformation of Food: Strategies and Practices in Upper Midwest Indigenous Communities," provides a comprehensive overview of conceptualizing various forms of sovereignty (Food (In)Security vs. Food Sovereignty) and key resilience frameworks for Indigenous health and nutrition in the United States. Their ethnographic work on food systems among an Upper Midwest Indigenous community highlights a myriad of strategies (e.g., wild rice – *Manoomin*) they use to navigate the constantly changing conditions of health, nutrition, and food insecurity in the context of climate change.

Heuer, in Chapter 4, "'How Decolonized Are We?' The Colonial Legacy of Commodity Foods and Food Insecurity Expressed by the Voices of Southwestern Native American Chefs," gives revealing insights from the U.S. Southwest into decolonizing commodity foods, their impact on Indigenous diet, health, and food insecurity, and current movements through forms of food sovereignty and resilience by Indigenous chefs.

Callaway, in Chapter 5, "Food Insecurity and Resilience in a Rapidly Warming Arctic," reports on surveys of key Inupiat (Alaskan Native) respondents who cited climate change and related changes in environmental conditions as a major threat to subsistence harvests and food security. A major obstacle to substituting traditional resilient adaptations with store-bought foods included low income, high cost of living, and transportation costs.

LATIN AMERICA AND THE CARIBBEAN

M. Steckley and J. Steckley, in Chapter 6, "Food Sovereignty for Food Security, Nutrition, and Climate Resilience: How Food Security Has Failed Haiti, and Why Peasants Want Food Sovereignty," discuss how Haiti's contemporary food security and climate vulnerability are rooted in rural development plans that have prioritized economic growth, running counter to building climate resilience, and disembodying connections between food, land, and the environment from people, nutrition, and health. They argue for centering peasant perspectives and food sovereignty in the post-earthquake period as key to rural development policy

Snively-Martinez and Quinlan, in Chapter 7, "Constraints on Family Poultry Systems in Guatemala," address how smallholder poultry-rearing families are adjusting to changing social and physical environment constraints in the context of climate change, poultry disease and antibiotic use, and poultry and livestock treatment. As women are the primary poultry health care providers in Guatemala, they argue that it is necessary to target health education through culturally appropriate messages to poultry care and human health in their villages.

Wilson, in Chapter 8, "Community-Led Change: Building Food Security, Gender Equity, and Climate Change Resilience in the Dry Corridor of Guatemala," presents multiple challenges to rural communities in an increasingly unpredictable world of climate change and food security. Working with one of Guatemala's Indigenous Maya groups, Wilson describes work with participants in "Project Harvest." The program grows family vegetable gardens to supplement food stores, diversify nutrition, and earn additional income with locally driven actions by a network of female community leaders and project promoters, to facilitate gender-equal ideas that respond to climate-based food shocks.

Hopkins et al., in Chapter 9, "Food Security and the Viability of Yucatec Maya Sustainable Traditional Subsistence Strategies," present results of a team-based participatory research process with Yucatec Maya communities in Mexico. In their fieldwork, they found that perceived food insecurity and lack of sovereignty by the participants were coupled with declines in agricultural production understood to be caused primarily by climate change. Many families are coping with this increased vulnerability by incorporating low-wage employment in regional urban centers into the mix of traditional livelihood strategies.

Figueras, in Chapter 10, "Agrochemicals, Health, and Environment in the Coast of Oaxaca: The Role of Agriculture in Climate Change," focuses on perceptions of food risk related to agrochemicals used by farmers in Oaxaca, Mexico. Figueras's case study examines how chemical pollution is part of social representations of risk and food security and suggests that alternative models to the industrial agricultural system are needed for combating the effects of climate change and impacts on health and food insecurity.

Garrigo-Lopez and Ginzburg, in Chapter 11, "Decolonizing Puerto Rico's Foodscape," critically examine the relationship between food sovereignty and colonialism in the Puerto Rican archipelago. They describe the contexts of building food sovereignty that are happening in the so-called Free Associated State of Puerto Rico and consider the connections between food sovereignty and decolonization, and the limitations to food sovereignty and food justice within this context. They argue that the most significant step that could be taken to improve factors of structural inequity such as poverty, food insecurity, and unemployment would be to end U.S. colonialism in Puerto Rico through a process of decolonization and self-determination for Puerto Ricans.

NORTH AFRICA AND THE MIDDLE EAST

Shaltout, Jaskolski, and Hoving, in Chapter 12, "Rooftop Farming: A Sustainable Food Production Initiative in Cairo, Egypt," discuss key health and climate challenges including agricultural land loss, rapid urbanization, food and water insecurity, obesity, and economic inequality facing a megacity in Egypt. They detail efforts made to create sustainable communities and address these issues within informal settlements, through the creation of green rooftops, and examine two different approaches to produce food, Cairo's abundant flat roof space – a community-based urban agriculture model and a commercial, healthy food production model.

NORTH AMERICA

Marshman, in Chapter 13, "The Bee City Movement in Canada," argues that food production, ecosystem resilience, and urban health are inextricably linked through the services provided by pollinators. Marshman's case study focuses on the Bee City movement in 32 locations throughout Ontario, Canada, as a conservation strategy that brings together municipal leadership with urban citizens. By embedding these efforts at the municipal level, the Bee City movement facilitates public and policy discourse through the primary criteria of habitat creation, education, and celebration that can be applied to the context of climate change and food security.

ASIA–PACIFIC

Gadhoke, in Chapter 14, "Walking the Middle Path of Food Sovereignty, Food Security, Nutrition, and Health in Chiang Mai Province, Thailand," details how food sovereignty is informed by the philosophy of sufficiency economy and a rich history of Thai migration and cultures. Through their ethnographic fieldwork with Indigenous Hmong and Karen farmers and community leaders in four villages, key lessons emerged, including learning from, being sensitive to the changes in, living off of, and caring for the forest, and transference of local Indigenous, intergenerational knowledge. These illustrative case studies show how local food systems can not only increase ownership in villages among poor households but also lead to empowerment for the health and nutrition of each community.

SUMMARY

Overall, it is our hope that the reader will find in each chapter an array of diverse approaches and case studies by the authors that exemplify the mutually engaged and reciprocal partnerships that are community driven and support the positive transformation of the people with whom they work. By doing so, this edited volume informs and drives a sustainable future of scholarship and policy that is tied to the intersectionality and synergisms of climate change resilience, food security, food sovereignty, nutrition, and community health.

2 Climate Change Resilient Livelihoods and Adaptive Strategies among the Ju/'hoansi San of Nyae Nyae, Namibia

Robert K. Hitchcock

CONTENTS

INTRODUCTION

The Ju/'hoansi San of the northwestern Kalahari Desert region in southern Africa have long been seen as a people who are resilient and who are able to adapt strategically to social, economic, and environmental changes (Marshall 1976; Yellen 1977; Lee 1979, 2013, 2016). Resilience, for our purposes here, is the persistence of relationships within a system. It is a measure of the ability of these systems to absorb changes of state variables, driving variables, and parameters, and still persist (Holling 1973, 17). Adaptation is the key mechanism of resilience (Gunderson and Holling 2002, 28). The Ju/'hoansi have responded to shocks to the environment where they live in innovative ways, drawing on age-old Indigenous knowledge, combined with local scientific knowledge.

This chapter will use the United Nations Sustainable Development Goals (SDGs) as a means of analyzing the Ju/'hoansi and their activities. The 17 SDGs and the 169 targets were contained in a United Nations document adopted by the 194 countries of the world on September 25, 2015. This document, titled *Transforming Our World:*

DOI: 10.1201/9781003014942-2

The 2030 Agenda for Sustainable Development (United Nations 2015), provided a detailed list of SDGs which the countries of the world are supposed to achieve by the year 2030. These goals include ending poverty and hunger, promoting health and well-being of all people, reducing inequalities, protecting the earth and its biodiversity, and taking urgent action to deal with climate change (United Nations 2015, 3; Dodds, Donoghue, and Roesch 2016). Particular emphasis is placed on those SDGs that affect Indigenous people, including SDG 1 (No Poverty), SDG 2 (Eliminate Hunger), SDG 3 (Good Health and Well-being), SDG 10 (Reducing Inequalities), SDG 13 (Climate Change Action), and SDG 15 (Protecting the Land). Implementation of the SDGs will ensure that human rights for all are achieved (Kaltenborn, Krajewski, and Kuhn 2020). Given that the Ju/'hoansi and other Namibians are facing social, economic, and environmental difficulties, they will need to follow recommendations made by the Food and Agriculture Organization (FAO 2018, 2019) to promote climate-resilient strategies and to protect themselves from economic downturns. This is particularly important, given that the progress of achieving many of the SDGs between 2015 and 2019 has slowed (United Nations Social and Economic Council 2019).

The research upon which much of this chapter is based took place in Namibia beginning in 1987 but especially over the past five years (2015–2020). The methods employed in this study were as follows: ethnographic interviews were done with groups and individuals, including Ju/'hoansi, nongovernment organization personnel, and government officials. Both qualitative and quantitative methods of analysis were applied. In addition, participant observation was employed. I also reviewed government policy documents, carried out archival research, recorded household assets and seeds and food in storage, kept a photographic record, carried out ethnoarcheological mapping of residential, agricultural, and special purpose sites, and analyzed aerial photography and space imagery of the Nyae Nyae area. Careful attention was paid to the principles of free, prior, and informed consent (FPIC) as outlined in the *United Nations Declaration on the Rights of Indigenous Peoples* (United Nations 2007).

The Ju/'hoansi, who number some 12,000 people in northeastern Namibia and northwestern Botswana, have adapted to a variety of changes, both natural and social, that have occurred over the past two centuries (Biesele and Hitchcock 2013; Lee 2013). These changes include a sizable number of droughts, the most recent of which was declared by the president of Namibia in May 2019. Rising temperatures and patchy rainfall resulted in livestock and crop losses in many parts of Namibia including Nyae Nyae. In some cases, shocks to the environmental and social systems of the Ju/'hoansi include a combination of drought and the outbreaks of livestock disease, as occurred, for example, in 1896–1897 when rinderpest caused the destruction of much of the wildlife and livestock populations of South West Africa and Bechuanaland (now Botswana) (Van Onselen 1972; Wilmsen 1989, 125, 140). There were other shocks to the Ju/'hoansi as a result of a combination of drought and livestock disease in the 1930s, 1940s, 1950s, 1960s, and 1970s (Hitchcock 2002).

There were contacts and conflicts between hunter–gatherers and pastoralists in the 19th and 20th centuries (Gordon and Douglas 2000). The establishment of the German colonial state in South West Africa in 1884 led to expansions of German settlers in various parts of Namibia, especially in what were to become commercial farming areas in the central and southern parts of the country (Guenther 2005;

Wallace and Kinahan 2011). The twentieth century saw significant efforts at land reform by the German and later South West African colonial states which reduced the amount of land available to hunter–gatherer, pastoralist, and agro-pastoralists populations by over 50% (Werner 1991). Historical factors that contributed to the vulnerability of the Ju/'hoansi to climate change were (1) a reduction of their land and resource base, (2) the relocation of other San from Angola and Caprivi by the South African Defense Force and South West African administration in the 1970s and 1980s (Hitchcock 2019a), and (3) incursions of pastoralists and their livestock herds in 2009.

Contacts between anthropologists and the Ju/'hoansi began in 1950–1951 (Marshall 1976, 1–11). The baseline data provided by the Marshalls (Marshall 1976) and their colleagues have been especially useful in providing a diverse set of information against which changes can be measured. The Ju/'hoansi also provide a superb case of diachronic multidisciplinary research. During and after the Marshall family visits (1951–1958), the South West African administration opted to establish an administrative center at Tsumkwe in what at that time was known as Bushmanland (now Nyae Nyae) and to encourage the Ju/'hoansi to settle there (Thomas and Shaw 2010, 279–281, 295–299). By 1978, virtually all of the dispersed Ju/'hoan communities had emptied and the Ju/'hoansi had moved into Tsumkwe, a process which had significant impacts on their well-being (Marshall and Ritchie 1984). The liberation struggle between the South West African Peoples Organization (SWAPO) and the Southwest African Territorial Force (SWATF) and the South African Defense Force (SADF) affected the people in the Nyae Nyae area and nearby Na Jaqna, particularly after 1978 (Hitchcock 2019a). San were incorporated into the war effort on all sides, though the Ju/'hoansi generally were not directly involved in the fighting.

During the struggle between the liberation forces in Namibia and the South African Defense Force, military bases were established in what at the time was Western Bushmanland (now N≠a Jaqna). The diet of the !Xun and Khwe soldiers and their families on the military bases was based on maize meal, flour, milk, sugar, and the occasional tin of canned beef. Wages of soldiers were used to purchase food, tea, tobacco, and alcohol from the military stores. There were high rates of domestic abuse, much of it related to alcohol consumption, in the army camps (Marshall and Ritchie 1984, 99). The departure of the South African military in 1989 resulted in a substantial reduction in wage income and a rise in unemployment in N≠a Jaqna. Demographic data collected by Marshall and Ritchie (1984, 47–53) revealed that there were more deaths than births among the Ju/'hoansi in the early 1980s. There was a high rate of infant mortality, approximately 75% of births (Marshall and Ritchie 1984, 53). Health challenges affecting the Ju/'hoansi and their neighbors in the early 1980s included tuberculosis, sexually transmitted diseases, malaria, and anemia. Undernutrition and alcohol consumption contributed to the poor health conditions that prevailed in the army camps.

At one time, the Ju/'hoansi land covered a 70,000–80,000 km^2 area in the borderland region of northwestern Botswana and northeastern Namibia. Over time, the land belonging to the Ju/'hoansi was reduced significantly as a result of government decisions and the expansion of other groups into their area. In the early 1980s, the government of South West Africa sought to turn the Nyae Nyae area into a game reserve and have the Ju/'hoansi live on the peripheries, entering the game reserve only as guides and cultural objects for tourists (Marshall 2003). Thanks to the lobbying of the Ju/'hoansi and their supporters, including anthropologists John Marshall and Claire Ritchie, the government reversed its decision about establishing a game reserve in Nyae Nyae in 1984 (Biesele and Hitchcock 2013, xxiii, 13–14).

An outgrowth of the work of Marshall and Ritchie was the establishment of a community-based organization, the Ju/wa Bushman Development Foundation (JBDF), which provided development assistance to the Ju/'hoansi in 1981. Tools, seeds, water points, livestock, and equipment were provided to communities willing to move out of the Tsumkwe administrative settlement to decentralized villages which were in their traditional territories. Some of the earliest moves into decentralized communities occurred in 1982–1983, when three villages were established (Marshall and Ritchie 1984, 123–157).

By 2020, there were some 42 villages distributed across a sizable area of nearly 9,000 km^2. The Ju/'hoansi were able to expand their control over local-level wildlife resources and tourism as a result of Namibian government conservation legislation passed in the mid-1990s. Their access to grazing, firewood, and other wild plant resources was expanded with the passage of a revised forest act in 2005 and the setting up of a community forest in Nyae Nyae in 2013 (Republic of Namibia 2005; Hazam 2017). The steps taken by the Ju/'hoansi correspond to SDG 15 (conservancy, restoration, and sustainable use, SDG 15.2 and 15.3 halting deforestation and combating desertification) and 15.7 (taking action to end wildlife poaching and trafficking). In the latter case, the Ju/'hoansi are collaborating with the Nyae Nyae Conservancy, the World Wildlife Fund–US, the local safari hunter, and the Ministry of Environment, Forestry and Tourism (MEFT) in work aimed at monitoring the area and, in some cases, tracking down potential poachers in Nyae Nyae (Nyae Nyae Conservancy 2019; Hitchcock 2019b).

THE NATURAL ENVIRONMENT IN NYAE NYAE

The Nyae Nyae study area lies in the northern Kalahari Desert, on the border with Botswana (see Figure 2.1). This part of the Kalahari is classified as tree-bush savanna, with a sandy substrate and east-west trending *alab* sand dunes that today are fixed with vegetation (Yellen 1977, 14–16; Yellen and Lee 1976, 33–36). Between the dunes are low areas where rainwater accumulates that are known locally as *molapos.* There are three major fossil river valleys in the Nyae Nyae-Dobe-/DuDa region (see Figure 2.2). The fossil river valleys flow in wetter times in the past contained stone that was used for tool manufacturing and shrubs and trees that were used to make bows, arrows, spears, and carrying nets (Yellen 1977).

An important feature of the northern Kalahari, which differs from many other parts of the Kalahari, is the presence of low-lying playa features, known as pans, where rainwater accumulates during the rainy season. Some 16 pans provide permanent water to the residents of the region (Marshall 1976, 64). There are many areas, however, that lack permanent water holes. In the past, mobility was geared in part toward the distribution of pans on the landscape. Ju/'hoansi would reside by the water holes during the dry season and would disperse in the wet season to places with other

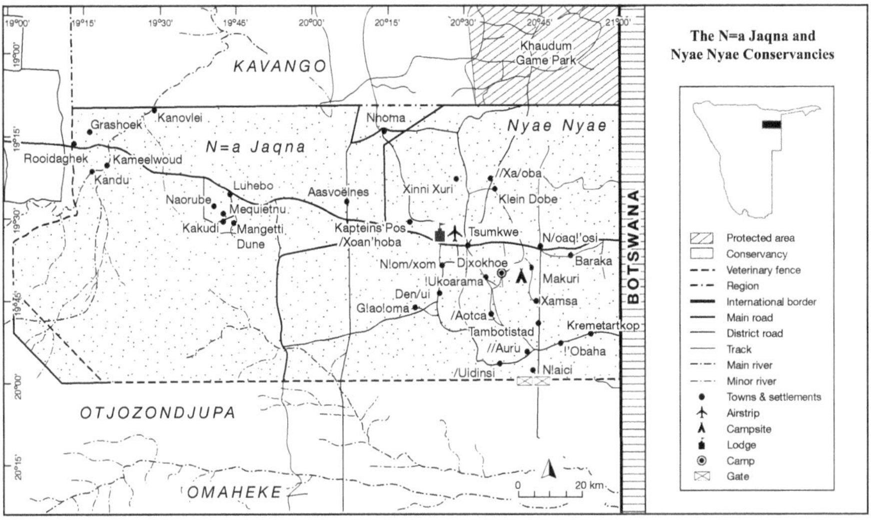

FIGURE 2.1 Map of Na Jaqna and Nyae Nyae Regions in Namibia

kinds of water sources (e.g., springs, holes in trees) and to patches of valuable plant resources and areas where antelopes and other wild animal species congregate (Lee 1979).

Beginning in the 1950s, boreholes and wells were established in Ju/'hoan areas, particularly in Nyae Nyae and the Omaheke Region to the south where sizable numbers of Ju/'hoansi reside on commercial farms (Hartung and Marshall 1988; Suzman 1999; Sylvain 1999; Lindholm 2006; Dirkx and Thiem 2014). These boreholes, at least in Nyae Nyae, were mainly for wildlife use and people were not allowed to obtain water there until the early 1980s. In the Omaheke Region, nearly all of the boreholes were on private farms except for those on three resettlement sites such as Skoonheid. By 2020, there were over 100 functioning water points in the Nyae Nyae region.

The Kalahari is not so much a desert as it is a savanna ecosystem, with extensive tracts of grazing for wild and domestic animals (Mendelsohn et al. 2009; Thomas and Shaw 2010). In the Kalahari, there are two primary climatic mechanisms involving atmospheric circulation, which are dominated by the Kalahari high anticyclone. The north and northwest parts of the Kalahari lie in the intertropical convergence zone (ITCZ), which generates rain in the wet season, whereas the continental trade winds influence the dry season (Thomas and Shaw 2010, 87–92). Drought events are correlated to some extent with the El Niño Southern Oscillation (ENSO) from the Indian Ocean and ultimately the Pacific Ocean, as was seen, for example, in the 2015–2016 severe drought (Baudoin et al. 2017; Mayaud, Bailey, and Wiggs 2017). ENSO also affected drought and flood cycles and adaptive strategies employed during the Iron Age of southern Africa (Huffman 2009, 2010; Hannaford and Nash 2016). Recent analyses have linked Indian Ocean conditions to droughts, floods, hunger, and famine in eastern and southern Africa (Voosen 2020, 228).

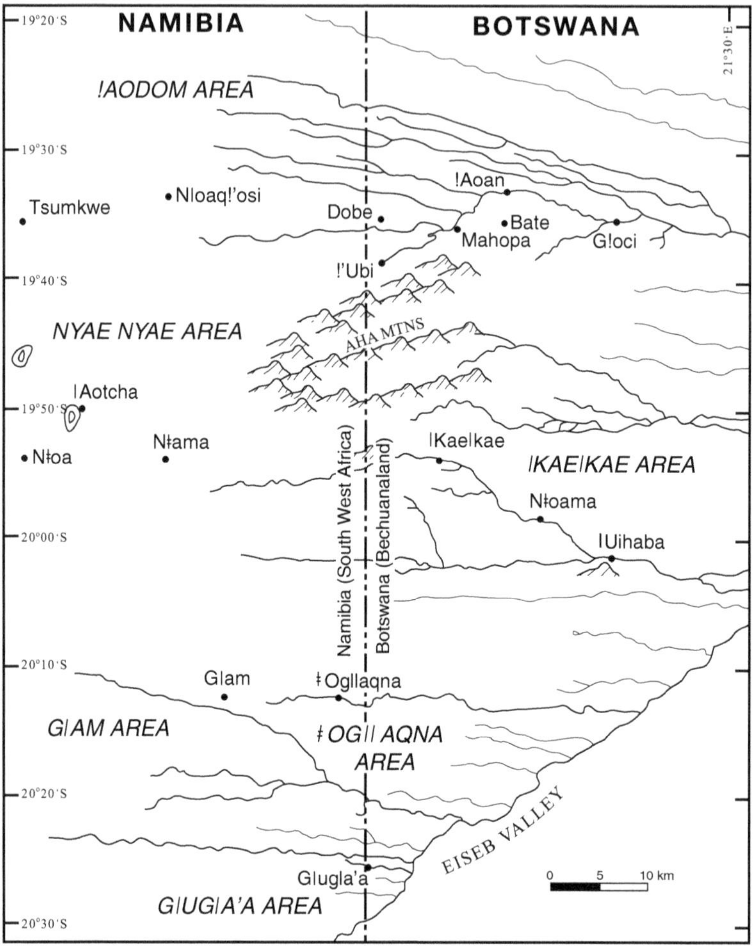

FIGURE 2.2 Nyae Nyae and Dobe-Kae Kae Region

The northern Kalahari has a mean annual rainfall of 300–600 mm, with rain falling mainly between November and April. Rainfall can be highly variable in space and time, with some areas experiencing insufficient rainfall and drought as often as three out of five years. In the summer, day temperatures may soar over 40°C, while winter days generally are sunny with night temperatures often falling below freezing. The dry season sometimes lasts eight months or more, and the wet season typically lasts from four to five months, depending on location (Mendelsohn et al. 2009; Thomas and Shaw 2010). The later dry season (e.g., October) can be particularly stressful for human, wild animal, and plant populations alike. Stories were told by elderly Ju/'hoansi of what it was like to experience the severe droughts of the early 1930s, 1947, and the early 1960s (Hitchcock, field data, 1987, 1992, 1995, 1999, 2014–2019).

Climate change in the northern Kalahari may increase the likelihood of reactivation of the Kalahari sands. Grazing of these lands, by reducing vegetation cover and breaking up soil crusts, will also increase the likelihood of increased wind erosion and dust emission, causing some breathing and other health difficulties for some local people. The health of the Nyae Nyae community members could be characterized as moderate, with difficulties including undernutrition, tuberculosis, scabies, parasites, and a low percentage of the population having HIV/AIDS. Overall, health and well-being of the Ju/'hoansi clearly need improvement, in line with SDG 3, particularly in response to the ongoing COVID-19 pandemic.

Landscapes in the undulating plains of the northwestern Kalahari were not homogeneous; rather, they were heterogeneous, and people utilized them differentially, depending on a whole series of factors, including season, natural resource type and density, group size and composition, the health and nutritional status of the population, the presence of predators and other dangerous animals, and technology available to the population. Climate change has caused shifts in the ways that landscapes are used, as has the expansion of development projects and infrastructure in the Nyae Nyae and nearby areas (Reid et al. 2007; Cole 2018; Nyae Nyae Conservancy 2019; Hitchcock 2020). Recently, in April–May 2020, the coronavirus pandemic led to a lockdown in Namibia, which had impacts on the distribution of food and medical assistance in the country, including in areas where San are residing, the Nyae Nyae region being one of them, which had been experiencing both drought and floods in 2019–2020.

THE SOCIAL ENVIRONMENT OF THE NYAE NYAE REGION

A significant event in the history of Nyae Nyae was the establishment of a nongovernment organization, later called the Nyae Nyae Development Foundation of Namibia (NNDFN) in 1981 (Biesele and Hitchcock 2013; Cole 2018). This organization provided funding for an array of development projects in Nyae Nyae ranging from water development to capacity building and from agricultural and livestock assistance to providing help with land use planning (Cole 2018; Nyae Nyae Conservancy 2019). The NNDFN was present at the end of apartheid (separate development) in 1989 and the withdrawal of South African military forces. NNDFN members, along with Ju/'hoan representatives, attended the celebrations of the new nation of Namibia in 1990.

In June–July 1991, the Ju/'hoansi were present at the National Conference on Land Reform and the Land Question. At that meeting, Tsamkxao ≠Oma described in detail the Ju/'hoan land use and land management system, consisting of a set of territories, n!oresi, each of which was overseen and managed by a Ju/'hoan land manager, a n!ore kxao. Together, these territories made up the land of the Ju/'hoansi. The *kxa/ho*. a Ju/'hoan term that literally means "sand surface" and refers to all of the land inhabited traditionally by the Ju/'hoansi and all of its water, bush foods, game, grazing, wood, minerals, and other natural resources. This speech laid the foundations for a visit to Nyae Nyae of then President San Nujoma, who, along with his Land Minister, declared Nyae Nyae "the land of the Ju/'hoansi" (Biesele and Hitchcock 2013).

The Ju/'hoansi, who currently are suffering from a severe drought, said to be the worst in five decades, are employing a variety of adaptive strategies to cope with social, political, economic, and environmental change. They see the value of SDG 2.4 (ensure sustainable food production systems and implement resilience practices). These strategies include employing foraging as a buffering strategy (see Lee 2016), depending on NGOs and the state for food and goods under social safety net (SSN) programs. In addition to these strategies, support can come from doing a certain amount of out-migration for seeking employment in other parts of Namibia, as well as locally from well-to-do (mostly non-San) individuals in the area.

A particular concern of the Ju/'hoansi is around SDG 2.2 (malnutrition). Ju/'hoansi are currently expanding their diet to include plants that are considered "fallback foods." Diversification of the diet helps to reduce malnutrition in stressful times, with greater exploitation of high-value foods such as mongongo nut (*Schinziophyton rautanenii*) and morama beans (*Tylosema esculentum*) (Lee 2016). For additional information on the variety of some of the wild plant foods exploited by Ju/'hoansi in drought periods, see Table 2.1. Some of these species are highly nutritious and contain substantial amounts of carbohydrates, fats, vitamins, and proteins.

Some Ju/'hoan households are sinking deeper into debt, borrowing from owners of small general dealerships and *shebeens* (bars), of which there were over 40 in Nyae Nyae (Laws 2019; Hitchcock, field data, 2019; Leon Tsamkxao, personal communication, March 2020). There are greater socioeconomic disparities today in Nyae Nyae than was the case in the past. Sharing systems are narrowing, with some better-off households reducing their sharing with poorer households. At least some of these changes are due directly or indirectly to climate change.

What is now known as the Nyae Nyae Conservancy in the Otjozondjupa Region of Namibia consists primarily of Ju/'hoansi San who have been involved in work related to climate change adaptation and the diversification of livelihood strategies since the conservancy was established under Namibian government wildlife legislation in 1998 (Cole 2018). The Nyae Nyae area is 8,992 km^2 in extent and is located on the Botswana-Namibia border, north of the Red-Line Veterinary Cordon Fence, and west of the N≠a Jaqna Conservancy, the largest communal conservancy in Namibia, which is 9,003 km^2 in area. Anthropologists and development workers have promoted small-scale community-based development that includes agriculture, livestock, forestry, and income generation activities (Biesele and Hitchcock 2013).

Intensive gardening projects involving the provision or purchase of tools, seeds, gardening tools, pipes, pumps, and other materials, along with extension advice, began in the new millennium, roughly after 2010 (Hitchcock 2020). This work links well with SDG 2.3 (small-scale food producers) (United Nations 2015, 17–18). The development of water facility points (that is, boreholes) for both people and wildlife has been a key part of the strategy for enhancing the livelihoods and well-being of Ju/'hoansi (Rispel and Lendelvo 2016; Cole 2018).

In an effort to promote development and offset some of the livelihood risks faced by the Ju/'hoansi, the Nyae Nyae Development Foundation of Namibia has sought international support for projects involving capacity building, small-scale agriculture. This effort fits in well with SDG 2.A (capacity building through international cooperation). The work of the Nyae Nyae Development Foundation and its partners

TABLE 2.1
Nutritional Composition of Some Major Plant Food Resources Used by Ju/'hoansi in Nyae Nyae, Namibia and /Xai/Xai, Botswana

Species/Common Name (Grams per 100 Grams)	Plant Part	Protein	Fat	Carbohydrate	Water
Acanthosicyos naudiniana (gemsbok or Herero cucumber) *dcaà*	Tuber	1.3	0.04	6.2	74.7
Acanthosicyos naudiniana	Fruit	1.3	0.2	4.8	90.6
Bauhinia petersiana (wild coffee bean) *≠ángg≠oa*	Seed	25.2	18.1	31.4	6.8
Adansonia digitata (baobab) *≠'óm*	Fruit	2.68	0.52	78.52	12.4
Citrullus lanatus (tsama melon) *tamah*	Flesh	0.1	0.02	0.9	94.2
Citrullus lanatus *Tamah*	Seed	17.9	20.2	12.5	5.7
Cucumis kalahariensis hu'uru	Tuber	1.1	0.2	8.9	88.7
Grewia flava (wild currant bush) *n/àang*	Seed (dried flesh)	4.6	0.2	82.1	--
Grewia retinervis (Kalahari raisin) *g!oà*	Fruit	6.3	2.7	42.9	6.9
Schinziophyton rautanenii mongongo *//'xa*	Nut	28.8	57.3	2.7	4.8
Terfezia pfeilii (Kalahari truffle) *Dcodcoó*	Fresh	2.5	3.3	5.2	80.1
Terfezia pfeilii *Dcodcoó*	Dried	24.6	17.0	34.1	--
Tylosema esculentum (morama bean) *dshìn*	Seed	32.9	37.8	20.5	3.7
Tylosema esculentum *Dshìn*	Tuber	0.7	0.1	6.0	90.5

Note: Data obtained from Tanaka (1980:56, 71, Tables 8 and 12); Arnold, Wells, and Wehmeyer (1985, 78–80, Table 6.1); Wehmeyer, Lee and Whiting (1969, 1530); Marshall (1976, 108–123); Lee (1979, 158–204); Leffers (2003).

includes diversification of crops grown, crop rotation, use of drought-resistant crops (e.g., sweet potato, *Ipomoea batatas* L.), and conservation tillage (limiting the breaking up the ground surface). In Nyae Nyae, conservation agriculture strategies built on the principles of permaculture are being employed. These strategies include crop rotation, addition of soil nutrients, addition of ground cover and trees for shade, green mulching, and compost. In addition, in Nyae Nyae, mixed agriculture-livestock production systems, water provision and protection, and fencing of fields to prevent encroachment by elephants, antelopes, and other animals are being implemented (Nyae Nyae Development Foundation of Namibia 2011, 2015).

Some 90 fields and gardens existed in Nyae Nyae where at least 23 species of domestic crops were grown by Ju/'hoansi in 2019 (Hitchcock 2020). Many of these gardens, particularly those with irrigation, were doing relatively well in 2019, but crop failures in dryland fields were a constraint for some Ju/'hoan households. Careful management of fire and small-scale patch burning practices around villages and high-value resources are employed to mitigate large burn-offs (see Nyae Nyae Conservancy 2019). Tree planting helps retain water and provides food and fiber for community members. Rainwater harvesting techniques are being experimented with in order to extend the reach of villagers into more remote areas, mimicking the mobility strategies of preresidentially stationary mobile groups. The expansion in the numbers of locations of the Nyae Nyae villages poses some challenges for the Nyae Nyae Conservancy and the NNDFN as well as the Ju/'hoan Traditional Authority, since investments need to be made in the water and other infrastructure in the new villages. Government agencies are contributing to these efforts but not as effective as they might be. The Ju/'hoansi are emphasizing SDG 15.9 (Integrate Ecosystem and Diversity Values in National Planning) and SDG 15.B (Mobilize Significant Resources).

Wild plant food dependence continues to exist, primarily as a kind of buffering strategy, among many San in the northwest Kalahari Desert region (Lee 2016). In Nyae Nyae area, nearly all villages exploited wild plant foods and utilized "fallback foods" such as gum from *Vachellia* (formerly *Acacia*) trees such as *Vachellia mellifera* (blackthorn). Some of the wild plant foods consumed by Ju/'hoan San today include Grewia berries, (e.g., *Grewia flava*), baobab fruits (*Adansonia digitata*), sour plum (*Ximenia caffra*), and melons (e.g., *Citrullus lanatus*) (Wehmeyer, Lee, and Whiting 1969; Cole 2014, 71–80). A sizable proportion of the Ju/'hoansi, some 90% in 2019, were receiving drought relief food from the government and from faith-based groups. These social safety net programs distribute commodities such as 25 kg bags of maize, tinned meat or fish, beans, sugar, and vegetable oil. The social safety net programs and development programs being implemented by government, non-government organizations, and faith-based institutions in Nyae Nyae will help to meet SDG 2 (Elimination of Malnutrition) and SDG 3 (Improving Health). One way that such goals can be achieved is for the Nyae Nyae Conservancy and its partners to carry out a household income and expenditure survey and a nutritional assessment in order to establish a baseline against which to measure a change in nutrition and health status of the Ju/'hoansi.

CHALLENGES FACING THE JU/'HOANSI

Severe challenges facing the Ju/'hoansi at present include drought (in Ju/'hoan, /káu), incursions of pastoralists who are competing for grazing and water, the presence of large numbers of elephants (*Loxodonta africana*) which sometimes destroy water points and gardens, and to a limited extent, tourist saturation, especially in particular villages such as //Ao//oba (Hitchcock 2019b). The degree of dependence on wild foods has generally declined, especially mongongo nuts (*Schinziophyton rautanenii*), in part, reportedly, because the processing time for these nuts is substantial (Marshall 1976, 114–116; Lee 1979, 182–204). Talks around the fire at night among the Ju/'hoansi focus on a variety of issues, not least of which is the presence of sizable numbers of herders and their livestock in Nyae Nyae and the social and ecological implications of this presence (Wiessner 2014). Some Ju/'hoansi noted in interviews that there were problems of overgrazing in Nyae Nyae in areas where there are large numbers of livestock (see WIMSA 2009).

One way that the Ju/'hoansi are responding to these changes is increased engagement in the exploitation of Devil's Claw (*Harpagophytum procumbens*), which generates N$25–N$30 for a full day of labor. Devil's Claw is a tuber with medicinal qualities that has a large international market, especially in Europe where it is used for rheumatoid arthritis and kidney disease (Cole 2014, 33–57; Stewart and Cole 2005). It was estimated that European consumers purchased over 4,500,000 euros in 2018 (Dave Cole, personal communication, 2019). The Devil's Claw harvesting, which is done on a seasonal basis, sometimes interferes with agriculture and livestock production and domestic tasks, including childcare, in the villages (Polly Wiessner, personal communication, 2020). As a result, hunger is on the increase in some of the villages that are heavily dependent on Devil's Claw production, in spite of government, faith-based, and NGO-sponsored commodity and cash provision programs (Kalahari Peoples Fund 2019; Hitchcock 2020). It should be noted that the Devil's Claw harvest in 2019 generated over a million Namibian dollars for some 500 harvesters (Nyae Nyae Development Foundation of Namibia, personal communication, 2020). When the families were out harvesting, they had to pay people to bring them food and water, reducing the cash they received. Most of them attempted to buffer themselves by a local-level gathering of wild plants and trapping of birds such as guinea fowl (*Numidus meleagris*) and small animals.

It is interesting to note that the Ju/'hoansi, unlike many other Indigenous and minority people in Africa, are not engaging in climate-related migration (CRM) (International Organization for Migration 2019). This differs somewhat from their neighbors the Herero, part of whose justification for their incursion into Nyae Nyae in 2009 was that they were experiencing overgrazing and climate-related ecological transformations in the area where they were residing, /Gam, to the south of Nyae Nyae (Hays 2009; WGIMSA 2009; Hitchcock 2020). Some Ju/'hoansi were involuntarily relocated from the Khaudum National Park when it was established in 2007 who moved to Nhoma, northwest of Tsumkwe (Biesele and Hitchcock 2013, 17, 40–41). There were Ju/'hoansi who left Botswana during the outbreak of contagious bovine pleuropneumonia (CBPP, Lung Sickness) in 1995–1996 and moved into Namibia (Hitchcock 2002).

A dozen or so Ju/'hoan households opted to move to Grootfontein, to tourist lodges in the area near Otjiwarongo, south and west of Nyae Nyae, and to the Omaheke to the south, but generally, these moves have lasted only a few months, with people almost always returning to their home villages in Nyae Nyae (Hitchcock 2019b). While they were away from home, some of them sent remittances to their relatives in the Nyae Nyae villages. There are nutritional and health implications for villagers who remain at home, since they do not have the support of tourism-related migrants who otherwise would be at home contributing wild plant and animal foods and labor (e.g., childcare) to the community. Some of the individuals who have left the villages are traditional healers who would otherwise be involved with helping to treat local people who are sick.

A key strategy that Ju/'hoansi have used to adapt to drought periods is through the sharing of high-value goods, such as necklaces and bracelets made of ostrich (*Struthio camelus*) eggshell over extensive areas, estimated to cover as much as 70,000–80,000 km^2 in area. This delayed exchange system, known as *hxaro* (*xaro*), created alliances that allowed *hxaro* partners to take advantage of visitation rights to communities with whom they had social ties (Wiessner 2002). It appears that there have been changes in the extent to which Ju/'hoansi are taking advantage of the options to move to other areas where they have *hxaro* links, possibly because many of them have substantial investments and possessions in the villages in which they reside. One of the responses of the Ju/'hoansi to the drought conditions in recent years has been to sell off their heirlooms, which has contributed to changes in the *hxaro* system (Osborn and Hitchcock 2019; Polly Wiessner, personal communication, 2020). The items being sold include ostrich eggshell bead necklaces, bracelets, and leather bags with beads, generating as much as N$200 to N$2,000 per item. Much of the money earned is spent on food, clothing, blankets, and other household goods.

In the past two years, there has been a reduction in the availability of highly sought-after foods such as maize meal, in part because of increased prices in towns. As a result, Ju/'hoansi are turning to local general dealers and itinerant salespeople to obtain bags of maize meal, a process which is leading to increased indebtedness, especially to the owners of the stores in Tsumkwe. The Nyae Nyae Development Foundation and the Nyae Nyae Conservancy have sought to mitigate some of these problems by expanding their development-related activities (see Nyae Nyae Conservancy 2019). The Nyae Nyae Conservancy has provided annual benefit distributions of cash in December of each year. These annual cash payouts have sometimes been used by local stakeholder households to pay off some of their debts. Wild animal protein is made available to the Ju/'hoansi in Nyae Nyae through the activities of the safari hunting company that has the Nyae Nyae lease; meat from the kills by safari clients is distributed to Nyae Nyae residents, though some people say that they prefer not to eat elephant meat. This is not so much because of a food taboo as it is the taste.

The tensions between Ju/'hoansi and the outsiders who have migrated into Tsumkwe and who are illegally grazing livestock on conservancy land have increased, particularly after the filing of a legal case targeting six illegal immigrants in 2016. The case was heard in the Namibia High Court in October 2019 but thus far no judgment has been issued (Hitchcock 2020). In the meantime, additional people have moved into Tsumkwe, and population density in the municipality is increasing. Residents of Tsumkwe have called for a more flexible and effective risk management system to be put in place at the local and regional levels. They have also called for new elections to be held in Tsumkwe to replace the long-standing mayor, who has been said to be supportive of the positions of the immigrants. The immigrants, who originally were Herero pastoralists, now include Damara, Ovambo, and Kavango coming from western, northern, and eastern Namibia. The numbers of immigrants have yet to be calculated, but it is estimated to be several hundred in the past two years. Some of them are engaged in the sale of *katjipembe* (*g//kaa*), a local alcohol, to local communities, which has worsened the nutritional and domestic abuse situations.

It is important to note that the Ju/'hoansi have sought international, national, and local-level support for their legal efforts to address issues of illegal grazing, in line with SDG 15.7 and SDG 15.A–15.C. The Ju/'hoansi are pushing the government and the high court to address the issue of illegal grazing and to implement decisions made by the high court in an equitable way.

NUTRITION, HEALTH, WELL-BEING, AND INDIGENOUS LIVELIHOODS

The Ju/'hoansi today have a diversified livelihood system. There is significant variation in the 38 villages in Nyae Nyae in nutrition and food security. Some villages are well-off, with gardens and herds of livestock providing a portion of household subsistence. Others are experiencing significant food insecurity. Approximately 70 people have formal sector jobs in Nyae Nyae with the government, the Nyae Nyae Conservancy, the safari hunter, small general dealerships, Tsumkwe Lodge, or faith-based institutions for which they receive cash, usually on a monthly basis. They use the cash to purchase food, clothing, and household goods. During the 2019–2020 drought, cash incomes have declined, which have affected household well-being. Food prices have increased, as have costs for transport (e.g., to Mangetti Dune, where there is a hospital, and to Grootfontein where people shop and visit relatives in the hospital there). SDG 2.3, and SDG 2.A–2.C relate to food prices and commodity markets. Both incomes and agricultural productivity are in need of expansion, in line with SDG 2.3. Also in line with SDG 2.5 there is a significant need for maintenance of genetic diversity in seeds, cultivated plants, domestic animals, and wild species.

Undernutrition is a problem for individuals, households, and in some cases whole communities in Nyae Nyae. This is the case, for example, in remote communities which are not visited very often by the Nyae Nyae Conservancy or government personnel of the Ministry of Agriculture, Water and Forestry that are in need of having their water facilities repaired. A few Ju/'hoansi noted that their nutritional and health statuses were better in the past than they are today (see Ingstad and Fugelli 2006 for similar comments by San in Botswana). Health problems include malaria, tuberculosis, parasites, and a low rate of HIV/AIDS (Lee and Susser 2006). Social safety net programs offset some of the nutritional deficiencies that exist in Nyae Nyae, but these programs are variable in their implementation, with people not being provided with commodities regularly.

Health needs assessments reveal that tuberculosis is a major problem, including drug-resistant TB, and there is a need for a more effective TB treatment program in Nyae Nyae. The Nyae Nyae Development Foundation of Namibia and its partners have developed an effective program to address and mitigate climate change impacts, in line with SDG 13.1. Climate change awareness programs are being conducted with the communities in Nyae Nyae and with the Nyae Nyae Conservancy. These programs and the activities related to them seek to achieve SDG 15, which is "to protect, restore, and promote sustainable use of terrestrial ecosystems, sustainable manage forests, combat desertification and half and reverse land degradation and halt biodiversity loss" (United Nations 2015, 27). Attention has been paid to the protection and prevention of the extinction of endangered and threatened plant and animal species, in line with SDG 15.5. These efforts could be enhanced in coordination with the various stakeholders operating in Nyae Nyae. In order to achieve these goals, there must be greater transparency and access to information for all concerned in Nyae Nyae.

The Nyae Nyae people are pushing for the achievement of SDG 16, seeking to promote peaceful and inclusive societies for sustainable development. Given some of the tensions with outsiders who have entered Nyae Nyae, the Ju/'hoansi want to significantly reduce violence, in line with SDG 16.1.

According to the Ju/'hoansi, enhanced education is a key to the well-being of children and adults in Nyae Nyae. This is in line with SDF 4, ensuring inclusive and equitable quality education and promotion of lifelong learning opportunities for all (United Nations 2015, 19–20).

And last but not least, the Ju/'hoansi want to see the achievement of SDG 1, ending poverty in all its forms everywhere. Relatively few Ju/'hoansi households have incomes that are above US$75.00 per month (US$1.25/day, US$900/year). This is particularly true for female-headed households and poor households with large numbers of children. Ju/'hoansi would like to see the achievement of SDG 1.5, building of the resilience of the poor and the vulnerable and a reduction of their vulnerability to climate-related and other social, economic, and environmental shocks.

CONCLUSIONS

The effects of climate change on past and indeed future Namibian and other societies cannot be understated. There are multiple drivers involved in climate change processes, which affect human food availability and livelihoods. When droughts and other environmental challenges hit, the people at the bottom of the socioeconomic ladder tend to be squeezed, and they have to compete with other people for resources and economic opportunities (Devitt 1977). Nutritional stress occurs among some drought-afflicted groups, especially among more vulnerable members of the population including the elderly, pregnant and lactating women, children, the ultra-poor, and those who are physically incapacitated (World Bank 2015; United Nations, Human Security Unit 2016, 2018). The social and economic impacts of climate change on the Namibian economy and the societies residing in Namibia are definitely significant (see Reid et al. 2007).

From Kalahari ethnography, we know that food shortages were common at various times, and that food storage and sharing were central to survival during disasters and climate change. One question is what will happen to Kalahari dune fields in the twenty-first century? There are 2.5 million square kilometers of dunes in southern Africa, most of them deposited by wind during the Pleistocene and Quaternary. Currently, most dunes, like those in the Nyae Nyae and Dobe-/Kae/Kae regions, are vegetated and used for foraging and grazing (Yellen and Lee 1976; Thomas and Shaw 2010, 141–157). With overgrazing and drought, there has been an expansion in dust in the atmosphere, causing some breathing difficulties for Ju/'hoansi who have asthma and tuberculosis.

Foraging strategies and Indigenous knowledge of the Kalahari landscapes are sophisticated and well-developed among the Ju/'hoansi. It should be stressed that navigating one's way across the Kalahari is not easy, and local people employ a combination of strategies in order to do so. It is especially difficult to figure out where one is on the landscape in the late dry season (known as *!ga,* September–October), a time when it is also hard to travel due to thirst and hunger. Ju/'hoansi in the northwestern Kalahari say that they use the Tsodilo Hills as a kind of navigational device as they tower some 385 m above the surrounding plains. Some of the Ju/'hoansi, !Xun, and Khwe in Nyae Nyae and N≠a Jaqna use the Aha Hills in Botswana for way-finding purposes (Leon Tsamkxao, Tsamkxao Ciqae, personal communications, June 2019).

Sub-surface water availability in some parts of the Nyae Nyae region has decreased in some areas, in part because of higher extraction rates for people, domestic stock, and irrigation and likely also a result of aridification due to climate change. This decline in the water table has resulted in increased competition between better-off and poorer households. The Nyae Nyae Development Foundation and the Tradition and Transitions Fund have expanded their water protection efforts and have sought to expand the use of drought-resistant crops in the gardens and fields of Nyae Nyae communities (Nyae Nyae Conservancy 2019; Hitchcock 2020). These efforts are costly and tend to increase the dependency of local communities on outside sources of support.

The Indigenous and minority peoples of the Kalahari, like those in other savannas and deserts of the world, are on the frontline of global climate shifts. In response to the challenges of climate change, many Ju/'hoansi have opted to diversify their livelihoods, pursue strategies that incorporate income generation, engage in both formal and informal sector employment, and depending on the state, something that is not easy given the economic downturn that Namibia has experienced in recent years (Republic of Namibia 2019). At the same time, the Ju/'hoansi are tapping into traditional social systems of reciprocity, sharing, and cooperation to support these strategies. Today, the Ju/'hoansi, along with their neighbors, are seeking to address food security, nutrition, and health issues and to promote climate change resilient livelihoods. They are hopeful that their Indigenous knowledge and willingness to cooperate with each other and with outsiders, combined with new technologies and adaptive strategies, will ensure their long-term well-being.

RECOMMENDATIONS

In light of the experience of the Ju/'hoansi over time, a number of recommendations can be made which are in line with the SDGs. First, greater emphasis needs to be placed on poverty alleviation in Nyae Nyae, in line with SDG 1. There should be equal access to economic resources and basic services, in line with SDG 2.5. Second, reduction of hunger, improvements in food security and nutrition, and greater promotion of sustainable agriculture, in line with SDG 2, are necessary. Third, there must be greater emphasis on the expansion of water infrastructure and maintenance, including the use of portable rainwater harvesters in dry areas, in line with SDG 2a and SDG 6. Fourth, significant health improvements need to be made in Nyae Nyae, in line with SDG 3, including addressing both epidemic and endemic disease, enhancing health and safety measures, improving reproductive health, and making health information more widely available, including that relating to coronavirus.

Fifth, expansion of primary and secondary school access, in line with SDG 4, is necessary. This should include efforts to provide culturally relevant education and vocational skills training for men, women and children, in line with SDG 4.4 and 4.5. Sixth, programs aimed at gender equity and empowerment of women and girls, in line with SDG 5, should be implemented more widely in Nyae Nyae.

While improvements in access to energy systems such as solar power and windmills have been made in Nyae Nyae, there is a need to ensure that there is greater equity in access to systems of energy (SDG 7). Greater emphasis needs to be placed on the promotion of formal and informal sector job growth in Nyae Nyae (SDG 8). Efforts need to be made to reduce the debt burden of Ju/'hoan households, in line with SDG 1 and SDG 8. Virtually all Ju/'hoansi would agree that there is a need to take urgent action to combat climate change and its impacts (SDG 13). It is important that the Ju/'hoansi and their neighbors engage in efforts to combat desertification, deforestation, biodiversity loss, and trafficking high-value wild plant and animal products (SDG 15).

As of 1 June 2020, Namibia has few confirmed cases of coronavirus (23), 14 people have recovered, and there have been no deaths. None of the Ju/'hoansi has yet contracted coronavirus or COVID 19. The main impact has been that some people have left Tsumkwe to return to their villages, and they have been provided with information in the Ju/'hoan language about social distancing, hand washing, and social care by the Kalahari Peoples Fund and the government of Namibia's COVID 19 Task Force. The Tsumkwe COVID-19 Constituency Committee has been criss-crossing the Nyae Nyae area providing health-related information. Members of this committee have noted that in a few cases, social distancing is not being practiced very much in some of the communities. One area where there appears to be an impact, due to the lockdown, food and other commodities were not delivered to the Ju/'hoansi and other communities in Nyae Nyae and Na≠a Jaqna, leaving some people hungry, and the nutritional situation there has deteriorated. The near-complete reduction in safari and other tourist visits to the two conservancies in April, May, and June 2020 has resulted in a loss of income, jobs, and meat available to local communities. Devil's Claw harvesting, an important source of income, had not begun as of June 2020.

One major difference between the Ju/'hoan social distance and that of the Tsimané in the Amazonian part of Bolivia (see Kaplan et al. 2020) is that the Ju/'hoansi do not have the medical infrastructure and medical assistance in Nyae that some Tsimané do. SDG 3.3 says that "By 2030, end the epidemics of AIDS, tuberculosis, malaria, and neglected tropical diseases, and combat hepatitis, water-borne diseases and other communicable diseases" (United Nations 2015, 18). Given the extreme danger from coronavirus, the Ju/'hoansi are hoping that there will be an acceleration of health assistance, testing, and an expansion in the availability of soap, hand sanitizer, and personal protective equipment (PPE) for personnel involved with health delivery. There are important lessons to be learned from the responses of Indigenous people such as the Ju/'hoansi, Navajo, Tsimané, and the Yanomamo to the coronavirus pandemic.

Conflict resolution involving land and resource access is crucial in Nyae, where the numbers of communities and of people from outside of the area are expanding. Promoting peace and justice and fairness for all is crucial (SDG 16). One way to do this is to ensure responsive, inclusive, participatory, and representative decision-making at all levels (SDG 16.7). Finally, given the severity of the crisis involving coronavirus, ensuring access to information, especially that involving health, nutrition, and social well-being, is crucial (SDG 16.10).

ACKNOWLEDGMENTS

Support of some of the research upon which this paper is based was provided by the U.S. National Science Foundation (Grant BCS 1122932), Brot für die Welt (Project no. 2013 0148 G), the Millennium Challenge-Account-Namibia (MCA-N) (Grant no. MCC-08–011-1AA-94), and the U.S Department of State (Namibia) (Grant no. SWA80018GR0028). I wish to thank the Nyae Nyae Conservancy, the Nyae Nyae Development Foundation of Namibia, the Ju/'hoansi Traditional Authority, the Legal Assistance Center of Namibia, and the people of Nyae Nyae for the assistance and advice that they provided. Preety Gadhoke, Barry Brenton, Solomon Katz, Hileni Amutenya, Ben Begbie-Clench, Megan Biesele, Tsamkxao Ciqae, Dave Cole, Lara Diez, Judy Frost, Jennifer Hays, Gabriel (Gabes) Hipandulwa, Steve/Kunta, Job Morris, Willem Odendaal, Tsamkxao≠Oma, Alan Osborn, Maria Sapignoli, Axel Thoma, Leon Tsamkxao, Wendy Viall, and Melinda Kelly made useful comments on this paper, and I thank them for their help. The people of Nyae Nyae very graciously responded to my questions and provided many useful insights on the impacts of climate change.

REFERENCES

T.H. Arnold, M.J. Wells, A.S. Wehmeyer (1985). Khoisan food plants: taxa with potential for future economic exploitation. In *Plants for Arid Lands*, G.E. Wickens, J.R. Goodin, D.V. Field eds. Pp. 69–86. Springer.

Baudoin, Marie-Ange, Coleen Vogel, Kirsty Nortje, and Myra Naik (2017) Living with Drought in South Africa: Lessons Learnt from the Recent El Niño Drought Period. *International Journal of Disaster Risk Reduction* 23: 128–137.

Biesele, Megan and Robert K. Hitchcock (2013) *The Ju/'hoan San of Nyae Nyae and Namibian Independence: Development, Democracy, and Indigenous Voices in Southern Africa.* Paperback Edition. New York: Berghahn Books.

Cole, Dave (2014) *Indigenous Plant Products in Namibia.* Windhoek: Venture Publications.

Cole, Dave (2018) *Water, Land and a Voice: the Nyae Nyae Development Foundation of Namibia. 36 Years of Support to the Ju/'hoan San Living in Namibia.* Windhoek: Nyae Nyae Development Foundation of Namibia.

Devitt, Paul (1977) Coping with Drought in the Kalahari. In *Coping with Drought in Africa 2*, Dalby, David, R. J. Harrison Church, and Fatima Bezzaz, eds. Pp. 186–200. London: International African Institute.

Dirkx, Erik and Maarit Thiem (2014) Omahake Region. In *Scraping the Pot': San in Namibia Two Decades after Independence*, Dieckmann, Ute, Maarit Thiem, Eric Dirkx, and Jennifer Hays, eds. Pp. 39–92. Windhoek: Legal Assistance Centre and Desert Research. Foundation of Namibia.

Dodds, Felix, Davi Donoghue, and Leiva Roesch Roesch (2016) *Negotiating the Sustainable Development Goals: A Transformational Agenda for an Insecure World.* London: Routledge.

Food and Agriculture Organization (2018) *The State of Food Security and Nutrition in the World 2018: Building Climate Resilience for Food Security and Nutrition.* Rome: Food and Agriculture Organization (FAO).

Food and Agriculture Organization (2019) *The State of Food Security and Nutrition in the World 2019: Safeguarding Against Economic Slowdowns and Downturns*. Rome: Food and Agriculture Organization (FAO).

Gordon, Robert J., and Stuart Sholto Douglas (2000) *The Bushman Myth: The Making of a Namibian Underclass*. Second Edition. Boulder, CO: Westview Press.

Guenther, Mathias, ed. (2005) *Kalahari and Namib Bushmen in German South West Africa: Ethnographic Reports by Colonial Soldiers and Settlers*. Koln: Rudiger Koppe Verlag.

Gunderson, L., and C. S. Holling, eds. (2002) *Panarchy: Understanding Transformations in Human and Natural Systems*. Washington, DC: Island Press.

Hannaford, Matthew J., and Donald J. Nash (2016) Climate, History, Society Over the Last Millennium in Southeast Africa. *WIREs Climate Change* 7: 370–302.

Hartung, Charles and John Marshall (1988) *Ju/wa Farming in Eastern Bushmanland: Problems and Recommendations*. Windhoek: Ju/wa Bushman Development Foundation.

Hays, Jennifer (2009) The Invasion of Nyae Nyae: A Case Study in On-Going Aggression Against Hunter-Gatherers in Namibia. In *Forum Conference on Indigenous Peoples 2009: Violent Conflicts, Ceasefires, and Peace Accords Through the Lens of Indigenous Peoples*, R.K. Hitchcock, M. Myrvoll, T. Bleie, et al., eds. Report. Pp. 25–32. Tromso: Forum for Development Cooperation with Indigenous Peoples.

Hazam, John (2017) *Conservancies, Community Forests, and Land Issues from a Legal Perspective: Constraints and Opportunities*. Windhoek: Legal Assistance Centre.

Hitchcock, Robert K. (2002) Coping with Uncertainty: Adaptive Responses to Drought and Livestock Disease in the Northern Kalahari. In *Sustainable Livelihoods in Kalahari Environments*, Sporton, Deborah and David S. G. Thomas, eds. Pp. 169–192. Oxford: Oxford University Press.

Hitchcock, Robert K. (2019a) The Impacts of Conservation and Militarization on Indigenous Peoples: A Southern African San Perspective. *Human Nature* 30: 217–241.

Hitchcock, Robert K. (2019b) Ecotourism, Heritage Tourism and Community-Based Development in a Southern African Borderland. In *Bewildering Borders: The Economy of Conservation*, Zips, Werner, and Manuela Mairitsch-Zips, eds. Pp. 61–89. Münster: Lit Verlag Wien.

Hitchcock, Robert K. (2020) Domestic Crop Production among the Ju/'hoansi San of Nyae Nyae, Namibia: Ethnoarchaeological and Ethnographic Perspectives. In *Archaeology On the Threshold: Studies in the Processes of Change, Archaeology on the Edge(s): Transitions, Boundaries, Changes, and Causes*, Joseph Wardle K. Hitchcock, Matthew Schmader, and Pei-Lin Yu eds. Pp. 174–205. Gainesville: University Press of Florida.

Holling, C. S. (1973) Resilience and Stability of Ecological Systems. *Annual Review of Ecological Systems* 4: 1–23.

Huffman, Thomas N. (2009) A Cultural Proxy for Drought: Ritual Burning the Iron Age of Southern Africa. *Journal of Archaeological Science* 36: 991–1005.

Huffman, Thomas N. (2010) Intensive El Niño and the Iron Age of South-Eastern Africa. *Journal of Archaeological Science* 27: 2572–2586.

Ingstad, Benedicte and Per Fugelli (2006) 'Our Health Was Better in the Time of Queen Elizabeth': The Importance of Land to the Health Perception of the Botswana San. In *Updating the San: Image and Reality of an African People in the 21st Century*, Hitchcock, Robert K., Kazunobu Ikeya, Megan Biesele, and Richard B. Lee, eds. Pp. 61–79. Osaka, Japan: National Museum of Ethnology.

International Organization for Migration (IOM) (2019) Climate Change and Migration in Vulnerable Countries. Geneva: IOM.

Kalahari Peoples Fund (2019) *Kalahari Peoples Fund Year-End Report, 2019*. Austin, TX: Kalahari Peoples Fund.

Kaltenborn, Markus, Markus Krajewsi, and Heike Kuhn, eds. (2020) *Sustainable Development Goals and Human Rights*. Cham: Springer.

Kaplan, Hillard S., Benjamin C. Trumble, Jonathan Stieglitz, Roberta Mendez Mamany, Maguin Gutierrez Cayuba, Leonardina Maito Moye, Sarah Alami, Thomas Kraft, Raul Quispe Gutierrez, Juan Copajira Adrian, Randall C. Thompson, Gregory S. Thomas, David E. Michalik, Daniel Eid Rodriguez, Michael D. Gurven (2020) Voluntary Collective Isolation as a Best Response to COVID-19 for Indigenous Populations? A Case Study and Protocol from the Bolivian Amazon. *Lancet* 395: 1727–1734. https://doi.org/10.1016/S0140–6736(20)31104–1.

Laws, Megan (2019) All Things Being Equal: Uncertainty, Ambivalence, and Trust in a Namibian Conservancy. PhD dissertation, London: London School of Economics and Political Science.

Lee, Richard B. (1979) *The!Kung San: Men, Women, and Work in a Foraging Society*. Cambridge: Cambridge University Press.

Lee, Richard B. (2013) *The Dobe Ju/'hoansi*. Fourth Edition. Independence, KY: Cengage

Lee, Richard B. (2016) 'In the Bush the Food is Free": The Ju/'hoansi of Tsumkwe in the 21st Century. In *21st Century Hunting and Gathering*, Codding, Brian F., and Karen L. Kramer, eds. Pp. 62–87. Santa Fe, NM: School for Advanced Research Press and Albuquerque. University of New Mexico Press.

Lee, Richard B., and Ida Susser (2006) Confounding Conventional Wisdom: Gender, Poverty, and HIV/AIDS among the Ju/'hoansi. In *Updating the San: Image and Reality of an African People in the 21st Century*, Hitchcock, Robert K., Kazunobu Ikeya, Megan Biesele, and Richard B. Lee, eds. Senri Ethnological Studies 70. Osaka: National Museum of Ethnology.

Leffers, Arno (2003) *Gemsbok Bean & Kalahari Truffle: Traditional Plant Use by Ju/'hoansi in North-eastern Namibia*. Windhoek, Namibia: Gamsberg Macmillan.

Lindholm, Karl-Johan (2006) *Wells of Experience: A Pastoral Land-Use History of Omaheke, Namibia*. Studies in Global Archeology 9. Department of Archaeology and Ancient History. Uppsala: University of Uppsala.

Marshall, John (2003) *A Kalahari Family*. (film). Watertown, MA: Documentary Educational Resources.

Marshall, John and Claire Ritchie (1984) *Where Are the Ju/Wasi of Nyae Nyae? Changes in a Bushman Society: 1958–1981*. Communications No. 9, Center for African Area Studies, University of Cape Town. Cape Town, South Africa: University of Cape Town.

Marshall, Lorna (1976) *The!Kung of Nyae Nyae*. Cambridge: Harvard University Press.

Mayaud, Jerome R., Richard M. Bailey, and Giles F. Wiggs (2017) Modeled Responses of the Kalahari Desert to 21st Century Land Use Change. *Scientific Reports* 7: 387. https://doi.org/10.1038/54198–017–0434–0.

Mendelsohn, John, Alice Jarvis, Carole Roberts, and Tony Robertson (2009) *Atlas of Namibia: A Portrait of the Land and its People*. Third edition. Cape Town, South Africa: Sunbird Publishers.

Nyae Nyae Conservancy (2019) *Annual Report of Nyae Nyae Conservancy Management Committee, September 2019*. Tsumkwe: Nyae Nyae Conservancy.

Nyae Nyae Development Foundation of Namibia (2011) *Let's Act to Adapt: Dealing with Climate Change: A Community Information Toolkit on Adaptation*. Windhoek: Nyae Nyae Development Foundation of Namibia.

Nyae Nyae Development Foundation of Namibia (2015) *Dealing with Climate Change N≠a Jaqna and Nyae Nyae Conservancy and Community Forest*. Windhoek: Ministry of Environment and Tourism and Nyae Nyae Development Foundation of Namibia.

Osborn, Alan J., and Robert K. Hitchcock (2019) Information Sharing in Times of Scarcity: An Ethnographic and Archaeological Examination of Drought Strategies in the Kalahari Desert and the Central Plains of North America. In *Towards a Broader View of Hunter-Gatherer Sharing*, Lavi, Noa, and David Friesem, eds. Pp. 123–141. Cambridge: McDonald Institute for Archaeological Research.

Reid, Hannah, Linda Sahlen, Jesper Stage, and James MacGregor (2007) *The Economic Impact of Climate Change in Namibia: How Climate Change Will Affect the Contribution of Namibia's Natural Resources to Its Economy*. London: International Institute of Environment and Development.

Republic of Namibia (2005) Forest Amendment Act of 2005. Act No. 13 of 2005. Windhoek: Government of the Republic of Namibia.

Republic of Namibia (2019) *State of the Nation Address by His Excellency Dr. Hage C. Geingob, President of the Public of Namibia. 17 April 2019*. Windhoek: Republic of Namibia.

Rispel, Melanie, and Selma Lendelvo (2016) The Utilization of Water Points by Wildlife Species in Nyae Nyae Conservancy, Namibia. *Environment and Natural Resources Research* 6(4): 91–103.

Stewart, K. M., and David Cole (2005) The Commercial Harvest of Devil's Claw (Harpagophytum spp.) in Southern Africa: The Devil's in the Details. *Journal of Ethnopharmacology* 100: 225–236.

Suzman, James (1999) *"Things from the Bush": A Contemporary History of the Omaheke Bushmen*. Basel Namibia Studies Series 5. Basel, Switzerland: P. Schlettwein Publishing.

Sylvain, Renee (1999) 'We Work to Have Life': Ju/'hoan Women, Work and Survival in the Omaheke Region, Namibia. Ph.D. Dissertation, Toronto, Ontario, Canada: University of Toronto.

Tanaka, Jiro (1980) *The San, Hunter-Gatherers of the Kalahari. A Study in Ecological Anthropology*. David W. Hughes, Translator. Tokyo: Tokyo University Press.

Thomas, David S. G., and Paul A. Shaw (2010) *The Kalahari Environment*. Cambridge: Cambridge University Press.

United Nations (2007) United Nations Declaration on the Rights of Indigenous Peoples. New York: United Nations.

United Nations (2015) Transforming Our World: The 2030 Agenda for Sustainable Development. United Nations Document A/RES/70/1. New York: United Nations.

United Nations, Human Security Unit (2016) Human Security Handbook: An Integrated Approach for the Realization of the Sustainable Development Goals and the Priority Areas of the International Community and the United Nations System. New York: United Nations, Human Security Unit.

United Nations Social and Economic Council (2019) *Special Edition: Progress Towards the Sustainable Development Goals*. New York: United Nations Social and Economic Council.

Van Onselen, C. (1972) Reactions to Rinderpest in Southern Africa 1896–97. *Journal of African History* 13(3): 473–488.

Voosen, Paul (2020) The Hunger Forecast. *Science* 368: 226–229.

Wallace, Marion with John Kinahan (2011) *A History of Namibia: From the Beginning to 1990*. New York: Columbia University Press.

Wehmeyer, A. S., Richard B. Lee, and Marjorie Whiting (1969) The Nutrient Composition and Dietary Importance of Some Vegetable Foods Eaten by Kung Bushmen. *South Africa Tydskrif vir Geneeskunde* 95: 1529–1530.

Werner, Wolfgang (1991) A Brief History of Land Dispossession in Namibia. In *National Conference on Land Reform and the Land Question, Windhoek, 25 June –1 July, 1991, Volume 1: Research Papers, Addresses, and Consensus Document*, Pp. 43–59. Windhoek: Government of the Republic of Namibia.

Wiessner, Polly (2002) Hunting, Healing, and Hxaro Exchange: A Long-Term Perspective on Kung (Ju/'hoansi) Large Game Hunting. *Evolution and Human Behavior* 23: 407–436.

Wiessner, Polly (2014) Embers of Society: Firelight Talk among the Ju/'hoansi Bushmen. *Proceedings of the National Academy of Sciences* 111(39): 14027–14035.

Wilmsen, Edwin N. (1989) *Land Filled with Flies: A Political Economy of the Kalahari*. Chicago, IL: University of Chicago Press.
WIMSA (Working Group of Indigenous Minorities in Southern Africa) (2009) Briefing on Illegal Settlement and Grazing in the Nyae Nyae Conservancy. Windhoek: Working Group of Indigenous Minorities in Southern Africa.
World Bank (2015) *Botswana Poverty Assessment*. Washington, DC: World Bank.
World Bank (2018) *The State of Social Safety Nets 2018*. Washington, DC: World Bank.
Yellen, John E. (1977) *Archaeological Approaches to the Present: Models for Reconstructing the Past*. New York: Academic Press.
Yellen, John E. and Richard B. Lee (1976) The Dobe-Du/Da Environment: Background to a Hunting and Gathering Way of Life. In *Kalahari Hunter-Gatherers: Studies of the Kung San and Their Neighbors*, Lee, Richard B., and Irven DeVore, eds. Pp. 27–46. Cambridge, MA: Harvard University Press.

3 Tribal Sovereignty and the Transformation of Food

Strategies and Practices in Upper Midwest Indigenous Communities

Cora Bender

CONTENTS

INDIGENOUS PEOPLE, SUSTAINABILITY, AND CLIMATE CHANGE: AGAINST "VULNERABILITY"

The UNESCO publication "Weathering Uncertainty" (Nakashima et al. 2012) on the meaning of traditional knowledge for climate change assessment and adaptation points out that

> [it] has become common currency to argue that Indigenous peoples are particularly vulnerable to climate change due to their dependence upon resource-based livelihoods and the location of homelands in marginal habitats, such as polar regions, desert margins or high altitude areas.
>
> *(Nakashima et al. 2012, 39)*

DOI: 10.1201/9781003014942-3

Indeed, the latest research demonstrates how Indigenous peoples of Canada and the United States are affected by climate change in unique ways. At stake are issues of displacement and relocation (Maldonado et al. 2013), impacts on resources such as forests (Voggesser et al. 2013), water (Cozzetto et al. 2013; Dittmer 2013), culturally significant species and their protection (Grah and Beaulieu 2013), Indigenous health (Doyle et al. 2013), traditional tribal foods (Lynn et al. 2013), justice and responsibilities in cooperation between tribes and nontribal entities and actors (Whyte 2013), and many more.

However, the UNESCO publication continues pointing out that Indigenous people's livelihoods are also *resilient*, "because they rely upon multiple resources and a diversity of crops and crop varieties, whereas specialization on single resources and monocultures with high capital investment render 'modern' systems particularly vulnerable" (Nakashima et al. 2012, 39). Traditional Indigenous knowledge is increasingly recognized as a key source of knowledge for Western climate science and "valuable for adaptation to climate change" (Williams and Hardison 2013, 431). This is also reflected by the inclusion of Indigenous peoples in the United Nations Sustainability programs, most notably, the Sustainable Development Goals (SDGs), a program of seventeen goals established by the United Nations in 2015 as the core of the UN 2030 Agenda for Sustainable Development, which was adopted by General Assembly in September of 2015.[1] Designed to succeed the UN Millennium Development Goals, the SDGs promise to combat global hunger and poverty crises, achieve good health and wellbeing for all while reconciling capitalist economic growth with the need to tackle climate change. The SDGs have been criticized for the heavy involvement of large-scale private sector agents in the pre-2015 consultation process (Scheyvens et al. 2016; Pingeot 2014, 2016) and for a neglect to recognize Indigenous people not merely as recipients of benefits but as active participants in the setting and attaining of the goals and targets (Fredericks 2019, 189).

In what follows, I will critically discuss SDGs 2 (Zero Hunger) and 3 (Good Health and Wellbeing) against the issues of food and sovereignty in Upper Midwest Indigenous communities, focusing on the concepts of food insecurity vs. food sovereignty, and exploring present-day Anishinaabe (Ojibwe) food practices as a living tradition of smart survival, mixing regenerative strategies such as gathering and gardening with what is available to them in terms of federal and charity food assistance. My aim is to demonstrate the benefits but also the limits of the SDGs for Indigenous people. A short recommendations section at the end of the article urges to review and revise the SDGs through the lens of tribal sovereignty and abandon the language of "vulnerability" that haunts UN parlance.

In my view, it is important to realize that Indigenous resilience to climate change is not only based upon a preservation of their timeless traditional knowledge but also to their *tradition of change*, i.e., their capabilities to integrate new strategies, which have been put to the test by colonialism and its concomitant catastrophes (Reo and Parker 2013). Dispossession from their lands, sweeping pauperization, forced separation of families and the abduction of whole generations of children to boarding schools, and an overall serious decline in health and life expectancy are historical dimensions of experience for every native community in North America. These render the threats of climate change – i.e., dispossession, relocation, economic hardships – a little less surprising to native people as they appear to a nonnative majority of society in developed countries.

This becomes especially obvious in the present COVID-19 crisis. Even though the data provided by states and cities are insufficient, news commentators and medical experts agree that the Indian Country is suffering disproportionately during the corona pandemic (Centers for Disease Control and Prevention 2020; Healy 2021; Lakhani 2021). The Navajo Nation and the Mississippi Choctaw, for instance, suffered death rates twice and three times the rate of New York City, respectively (Hostetter and Klein 2020). Many Indigenous communities, however, approach the crisis not as something totally out of the ordinary, but as a "sharpening of the already present," as the Dakota scholar Kim TallBear put it (TallBear 2020), referencing previous Indigenous experience with environmental and health disruptions (Grossman 2021).

Traditionally dependent on resources of the land for their economies and more specifically for their food, native people learned throughout the nineteenth and twentieth centuries how to survive the damage and loss of their traditional livelihoods, and how to regroup and fight back. As many examples demonstrate, "Indigenous nations are among the most proactive and prepared communities in emergency planning and climate change adaptation, providing models for non-Native communities to follow" (Grossman 2021). To me, the single most important factor of this ability to survive the destruction directed at tribal communities is *tribal sovereignty*. Important court decisions concerning native treaty rights reaffirmed native sovereignty in the 1980s; the 2007 United Nations Declaration on the Rights of Indigenous Peoples (UNDRIP) proclaimed these globally:

> The right of self-determination, the right to exist as tribes and distinct peoples, the right of tribes to own their land and resources, the right to the enforcement of and respect for treaties, and protection and access to sacred sites are all proclaimed in the Declaration.
>
> *(Indian Law Resource Center n.d.)*

Two decades into the new millennium, native people are nowadays fighting, for example, at the frontlines of energy politics, talking back to multinational energy companies and national governments, reaching global audiences, and activating millions of supporters worldwide (Estes 2019; Estes et al. 2019).

The inclusion of Indigenous peoples as one of the "major groups" involved in the consultation process leading to the establishment of the United Nations Sustainable Development Goals (SDGs) in the context of the UN Agenda 2030 is an outcome reflective of Indigenous agency and activism on a global scale. In 2015, when SDGs were first established, many anthropologists agreed that the new framework differs from its predecessor, the Millennium Development Goals (MDGs). These only applied to so-called developing countries, eschewing a focus on the failures and insufficiencies of societies located in the Global South. In the perspective of the SDGs, by contrast, "we're all developing countries now," as British social anthropologist Henrietta Moore commented in *The Guardian*, pointing out how "abysmally" the UK and the US have fared on the goal of reducing inequality: "Consequently, we can hope to see an end to the so-called developed world lecturing the global south on how it should be aspiring to become just like us, with our outdated model of never-ending growth and unsustainable carbon footprints" (Moore 2015).

As one of the "major groups" involved in the SDG process, Indigenous people the world over could be expected to benefit from these principal policy shifts expressed in seventeen goals measured against success in 169 targets (see, for instance, Dhir 2016). In fact, even though Indigenous people are expressly mentioned in only six of these targets, many commentators emphasize that Indigenous people have a crucial role in implementing the 2030 Agenda (UN Permanent Forum on Indigenous Issues 2019). However, in 2020, the Indigenous Peoples Major Group for Sustainable Development issued a critical review stating that "[a]fter four years of SDG implementation, Indigenous peoples across the globe are not just left behind but pushed further behind." Serious problems faced by Indigenous people can be seen to be increasing instead of diminishing, among them wide-spread land- and resource-grabbing, poverty and hunger, destruction of cultural heritage, and rising inequality and lack of access to justice. In their 2016 paper, the Indigenous Peoples Major Group had already predicted that "the linear monetary measure of poverty," applied throughout the SDGs, can contribute to further impoverishing Indigenous peoples under the guise of the theme "leaving no one behind" (Indigenous Peoples Major Group for Sustainable Development 2020). In the 2020 report, it becomes clear that some SDG goals actually work *against* Indigenous people. For instance, Goal 7 (Clean and Affordable Energy) and Goal 8 (Decent Work) have to be reviewed against increasing cases of land grabs and human rights violations in connection with imposed renewable energy and other economic growth projects in Indigenous territories.

Generally, the SDGs have been criticized for their inadequate recognition of Indigenous peoples in the goals and targets, themselves, for a failure to disaggregate figures specifically pertaining to Indigenous people from country-level data, and for a neglect to recognize Indigenous people not merely as recipients of benefits but as active participants in the setting and attaining of the SDGs (Fredericks 2019, 189).

In order to overcome both the failures of the goal-setting as well as the lag of the United States in implementing the goals, Carla Fredericks suggests that the United States places a special focus on tribal nations as partners in "achieving the SDGs domestically": "Pragmatically speaking, particular focus on tribes is crucial for attainment of the SDGs of the United States" (Fredericks 2019, 186). This recommendation has to be seen against the backdrop of a peculiarly volatile "twist" the sustainability debate has taken on in the United States. The Global Goals "remain unfamiliar to many civil society, philanthropic, and government actors," even though these are working to alleviate the exact problems addressed by the SDGs: "they have rarely factored into national policy and funding" (Lieberman 2018). This is partly due to the fact that the Trump administration (2016–2020) was generally hostile to the United Nations and International Human Rights Bodies (Finoh 2020). But Trump's "America-First" Agenda was not the only roadblock to developing a U.S. approach to the Global Goals. As a reminder, the United States has not even ratified the International Covenant on Economic, Social and Cultural Rights, which recognize a lot of the rights to social security, education, and health that form the basis of the SDGs. Even for wealthy U.S. philanthropies, Global Goals are, in the eyes of Edmund Cain, the vice president of grant programs at the Hilton Foundation, "a hard sell" as 70% of all U.S. philanthropy by foundations is domestically focused (Lieberman 2018). Accordingly, for instance, in 2016, the U.S. Agency for International Development (USAID) homepage, while advertising the SDGs, made them appear as an international aid policy agenda, not something the U.S. could be in need of implementing domestically. A notable exception is the engagement of a number of bigger cities such as Los Angeles and New York. Here, mayors and administrations adopted SDGs and used them to develop their own "local goals" (Los Angeles mayor Eric Garcetti, see Pipa et al. 2020). As far as Tribal Nations in the United States are concerned, the fact that an appeal to "partner with them!" remains an unfulfilled political desideratum even in 2019, leaves room for debate and recommendations.

Seen in this perspective, as the UNESCO report mentioned, a number of technical terms used to describe the position of native people vis-à-vis the myriads of adversities, more specifically the notion of "vulnerability," do not make much sense. Equally, "resilience," when applied to native communities, can easily be misconstrued as a desirable functionality that outside agents executing welfare programs of the nation-state will somehow, "magically," elicit in what is otherwise seen as a dysfunctional native sociality. *Resilient* is what native people have proved themselves to be during hundreds of years of colonial onslaught against their cultures and ways of life. Hence, in the present chapter, I plead for a focus not on what native people *should* do or what they, supposedly, need, but for what we can learn from their practice, centering research attention on their translations, strategies, and embodiments.

INDIGENOUS PEOPLE AND FOOD: FOOD (IN)SECURITY VS. FOOD SOVEREIGNTY?

In 2006, the United States Department of Agriculture (USDA) announced that the term "food insecurity with hunger" would be removed from official statements, substituting it with the term "very low food security," because, according to USDA sociologist Mark Nord, "'hunger' is 'not a scientifically accurate term for the specific phenomenon being measured in the food security survey'" (Himmelgreen and Romero-Daza 2010, 96; see also Nord et al. 2007). At the time, this mandated euphemistic change in vocabulary was responded to by a global outpour of sarcastic media commentaries, protests, and debate in the academic community. Ten to fifteen years later, however, "food insecurity" has become an important term to address and describe the seemingly paradox looping effect between poverty and obesity, and by extension also between poverty and diabetes and other metabolic and cardiovascular diseases (Pan et al. 2012; Dhurandhar 2016; Dinour et al. 2007). Instead of addressing the economic source of hunger and food insecurity – capitalism – directly, it seems that many national governments have delegated the task of solving the crisis of mass undernutrition–overweight to those agencies who are seen by many as causing it, in the first place (Brett 2010). "Food security," originally developed "in the context of the UN-specialized agencies dealing with food and nutrition" (Windfuhr and Jonsén 2005),[2] has become the convenient catchword used by a coalition of

> multinational food corporations, an international network of research institutions and international agencies such as the World Bank, FAO and INFAD, and [a view] implemented by many national governments, that the only realistic path to future food security is through large-scale, high-tech, input-intensive, industrial agricultural methods combined with a global system of procurement and distribution managed by capitalist enterprise.
>
> *(MacRae 2016, 228)*

"Food security," of course, also is a key concept of the SDGs, particularly of SDG 2, "End hunger, achieve food security and improve nutrition and promote sustainable agriculture." The intersectionality of SDG 2 with SDG 1 (End Poverty) and SDG 3 (Health and Wellbeing) is obvious, as are the conceptual limits. First, "achieve food security" is a somewhat lofty ideal, a message without addressee, as long as it does not oblige governments to actually *feed* people – merely "ensuring access" to food can, as experience from my ethnographic fieldwork demonstrates below, actually translate into the kind of food insecurity that is hard to observe but widely prevalent in Indian Country, a double burden of undernutrition and overweight. Second, Target 2.1 specifies the kind of diet that should be made available: "safe, nutritious and sufficient food all year round." This sounds good but it only equals level 2 of 3 increasing levels of diet quality defined by the FAO (FAO et al. 2020). This so-called "Nutrient Adequate Diet" is different from level 3, "Healthy Diet" in that it does not include "a more diverse intake of foods from several different food groups" and is not adapted to "a country's individual characteristics, cultural context, locally available foods and dietary customs" (FAO et al. 2020, 73). So, it has to be concluded that at a closer look, the promises of SDG 2 from the viewpoint of Indigenous people have serious limits in that they actually do not represent a real departure from the status quo.

However, since the mid-1990s, "food sovereignty" has emerged as a mobilizing frame for social movements, which directly counter the concept of "food security" (Edelman 2014). In particular, the global peasant movement La Vía Campesina claimed the term and disseminated its definition as "'the right of each nation to maintain and develop its own capacity to produce its basic foods, respecting cultural and productive diversity'"; this was motivated initially by the World Trade Organization's failure to "adequately address the issue of agricultural subsidies in the United States and Europe" (McKay et al. 2014, 1175). Ever since, the concepts have been the subject of what MacRae (2016) calls a "deeply polarized debate" between "two 'food-world-views'":

> On the other side [of the 'food security' coalition of capital and state, CB] is a vision, shared largely by local communities, organisations of small farmers and consumers, NGOs and academic researchers not affiliated to the international agri-food research system, of a global food system built from the bottom up – of multiple agricultural systems and food cultures built on the foundation of local ecologies and communities [...]. Food security is a core concept in the former view, while food sovereignty has become so in the latter [...].
>
> *(Macrae 2016, 228)*

How do native communities fit into this complicated picture? In the general literature on food and nutrition, Indigenous communities are usually counted among the most vulnerable U.S. populations, as I said before, in my view, a problematic ascription. For sure, however, most Indigenous communities are affected by food insecurity (Jernigan et al. 2017) and by interventions based on what Gadhoke and Brenton call "nutritionism": "a reductionist framework [...] that was more focused on nutricentric dietary guidelines [...] than on a more holistic view of food being something greater than the sum of its nutrient parts" (Gadhoke and Brenton 2017, 207). For many Indigenous communities, *food sovereignty* has become a new cultural and social revitalization project (Mihesuah and Hoover 2019; Lemke and Delormier 2017, 7; Kamal 2018; Vazquez 2011; Donlin 2015; Desmarais and Wittman 2014; McMullen 2004; Perry 2013, Coté 2016), which shares a lot of similarities with the Indigenous language regeneration and other cultural revitalization movements I have concerned myself with in my media-related research (Bender 2011). Coté suggests placing Indigenous food sovereignty within a context of self-determination as developed by Cherokee scholar Jeff Corntassel in his notion of "sustainable self-determination" (Coté 2016, 10; see also Corntassel 2012). Lemke and Delormier observed that parallel to this development of a local Indigenous interest in food sovereignty,

> several global initiatives were started and reports produced, in collaboration across sectors and disciplines, engaging in wide-ranging consultations with governments, academia, civil society and other actors [...]. Most of these reports highlight the importance of local and Indigenous knowledge, agroecology, and women's contributions for the necessary shift in direction of our agriculture and food systems, toward more environmentally sustainable and socially just modes of production and consumption.
>
> *(Lemke and Delormier 2017, 7)*

How this is all related remains unclear, especially the question of how Indigenous food sovereignty is, actually, connected to the adoption of the concept by the global peasant movement *La Vía Campesina* (Rosset and Martinez-Torres 2013; Edelman 2014), and the question of whether Indigenous food sovereignty is a discrete development and independent movement, to begin with. A second inconsistency in the literature, in my view, concerns the question of Indigenous modernity (Bender 2011). Many accounts on Indigenous food sovereignty emphasize Indigenous people's vulnerability as marginalized groups sitting on marginalized lands in arctic, arid, or high mountain areas. Yet, I argue, in terms of social and political relations, Indigenous people are far from isolated. In particular, tribal communities in the United States can be seen as agents in complicated political negotiations with the settler state and other outside institutions, an "ongoing accomplishment" (Garfinkel 1967) in the work of sovereignty on many scales, from the reservation level to national and international arenas. The "subtle changes in the scale and location of sovereignty" that McKay et al. found in the publications of La Vía Campesina – "from the national to the local and from the accrual of sovereignty in the hands of the nation-state to those of 'peoples'" (1176) – can be seen to have been maneuvered by tribal communities while they continuously exercised their sovereignty on many fields of which food is but one. Whyte even argues that "food sovereignty should be seen – in part – as a strategic process of Indigenous resurgence that negotiates structures of settler colonialism" (Whyte 2016). Therefore, in what follows, I mostly avoid the term "food sovereignty" and substitute it with "food-related sovereignty" which I will describe as landscapes or, to use a term coined by Cristina Grasseni, as Indigenous "ecologies of practice" (Grasseni 2007) in order to understand the Indigenous practice of ecology. In doing so, I will also pay special attention to the work of translation that is accomplished in tribal institutions and agencies, such as tribal administrations, schools, colleges, commissions, and departments. In these agencies, outside policies (usually of a neoliberal ilk, of course) are being translated into strategies of tribal sovereignty.

A NOTE ON METHODOLOGY

The data on which this chapter is based were collected in connection with my research into Indigenous sovereignty and health carried out in annual field trips of various lengths between 2012 and 2017. Initially, I focused on diabetes as an everyday experience in Indian Country, until I realized how crucial the field of health is as an arena for the constitution and defense of tribal sovereignty. Consequently, I started to pay much more attention to the people working in tribal and super-tribal health administrations, in health-related organizations and tribal health education, and to the strategies and practices of their specific work of attaining and securing what I call *Sovereign Health* (Bender, in preparation).

OJIBWE FOOD PRACTICES: HISTORIES OF TRANSFORMATION AND INNOVATION

The native people living in the woodland area of the Great Lakes traditionally hunted, fished, gathered wild rice, and cultivated gardens. They made skilled use of birch bark to construct lightweight containers, frame boats, and characteristic dome-shaped houses, today known as "wigwam" (Ritzenthaler 1978). In the seventeenth and early eighteenth centuries, the Algonquian-speaking Ojibwe located around Sault Ste. Marie acted as middlemen, traders, and brokers between the French colonists in the East and the Siouan-speaking Dakota in the West, acquiring for themselves a comfortable position in the trans-regional fur trade. The Dakota were at that time economically adapted to the Woodlands, hunting, fishing, and gathering wild rice just as their Eastern Ojibwe neighbors did in the area of Wisconsin and Minnesota. However, when the French bypassed the Ojibwe in the course of the mid-eighteenth century and started trading directly with the Dakota, the cooperation between the groups came to a screeching halt and the region west and south of the western tip of Lake Superior became a contested territory in a long-lasting guerilla war between Ojibwe and Dakota hunters (Warren 1885). As the Dakota were driven west, the Ojibwe established themselves permanently at the southern shore of *Gitchie Gami* (a.k.a. Lake Superior) and on Madeline Island, the largest of the Apostle Island, located approximately three miles off the southern coast of Lake Superior, a sacred place of origin. According to one of their most prominent legends, they were led to Madeline Island by a supernatural being in the form of a migis shell and shown to the ample rice beds of the adjacent Chequamegon Bay. In the course of the eighteenth century, the Ojibwe extended their hunting and trapping range from Chequamegon Bay into the interior of the woodland south of Lake Superior, which the Dakota had been driven out of. Around 1745, a group of Ojibwe hunters formed a permanent settlement which grew in size after a French trader, who had married into an influential Ojibwe family, established a trading post (Rasmussen 1998).

In 1825, the United States invited the Ojibwe, Dakota, and other Indian tribes to meet at Prairie du Chien to negotiate a treaty of "peace and friendship." In actuality, the federal government was interested in stabilizing the area for western expansion and acquiring land from the Ojibwe. However, before it could begin negotiations for resources and land cession treaties, it first had to establish tribal boundaries. Ojibwe-Dakota enmity was a convenient pretext (Loew 2001, 58). In ensuing treaties of 1837 and 1842, the Ojibwe were forced into surrendering a vast territory, "almost two-thirds of present-day northern Wisconsin, a portion of central Minnesota, and much of Michigan's Upper Peninsula" (Loew 2001, 60). Another treaty signed in 1854 established four Ojibwe reservations in Wisconsin, Red Cliff, Bad River, Lac Courte Oreilles, and Lac Du Flambeau.[3]

GREAT LAKES INDIGENOUS STAPLE FOOD: MANOOMIN

The Great Lakes area, particularly Minnesota and Northwestern Wisconsin, is known for its abundant beds of manoomin (English: wild rice, Latin: *Zizania aquatica*). In 1947, the German anthropologist Julius Lips and his wife Eva Lips spent a summer's worth of fieldwork with an Ojibwe community in the area of Nett Lake in Northern Minnesota, studying their economy as a case of what they called "harvesting cultures" (German: Erntevölker), a concept Julius Lips had come up with in order to transgress the conventional archaeological and culture-historical dichotomy between food gatherers and food producers. His aim was to describe in detail how the carefully planned communal harvesting of a year's supply of wild rice by Ojibwe people of Wisconsin and Minnesota during the two weeks of Indian Summer is different from the nomadic gathering of a large number of sparsely growing plants. Hunter-gatherers such as Indigenous Australians know up to 300 food plants. A "harvesting culture" such as the Ojibwe might know 50 to 100 food plants, including medical plants; however, about one plant, they know everything: *manoomin*. The concept of *Erntevolk* characterizes economies that actually "invented" food production. They combine the extractive practices of gathering food with the (mostly) sedentary lifestyle of food producers, such as different notions of property, a higher degree of social cohesion, and more elaborate storage techniques (Bender 2020; Lips 1928, 1953, 1956).

Present-day Ojibwe are well aware that they have a long history of protecting the plant and ensuring their access to it. Raster and Hill (2017) refer to the so-called White Pine Treaty of 1837 to point out that in the nineteenth century, Ojibwe reserved for themselves and all the generations to follow the right to hunt, fish, and harvest wild rice on the ceded territories. "[T]his acknowledgment by extension recognizes the Ojibwe's right to food sovereignty" (Raster and Hill 2017). Growing in shallow lakes with a steady water level, manoomin has to be harvested in the late summer or early fall by teams of two people, one of whom poles a canoe through a rice bed so that the other one can bend the rice stalks over the rim with two arm-long, lightweight sticks and knock the kernels into the boat. Traditionally, any two people can go ricing together: a husband and a wife, two brothers or sisters, cousins or friends, a parent and a child. At home, more people will be waiting to help in the hard work of scorching the rice (which has to be done on the same day as the harvest), and in the thrashing and winnowing, which can be done days later. Harvesting manoomin is an important activity in the annual cycle. It provides rice farmers with extra income and gives tribal families and tribally run schools an invaluable opportunity to introduce children to culturally and spiritually significant activities that connect land, food, body, and spirit. Manoomin plays a key role in Ojibwe origin stories and is the focal dish at the center of every ceremony, from harvesting feasts to life-cycle rituals to the elaborate performances of the Midewin, a.k.a. Grand Medicine Society.

Manoomin also plays an important role in Ojibwe concepts of health and the good life. In 2011, I conducted a series of interviews with a middle-aged tribal member from one of the Ojibwe reservations in Wisconsin who had weaned himself off of his diabetes and blood pressure medication by resorting to a diet of wild rice, venison, and berries:

Alan Rush: That was after I had a fire and my house burned in the summer of 2005. And we were out of home. So, what I did, I remodeled my garage and moved in there. [...] I was there alone, and basically cooked for myself and everything like that. My belief, I'm a Midewin, the old way that was given to the Ojibwe, the Anishinaabe people. So, sitting that winter, after taking my insulin, back then I was taking like 80 units, and all the pills. Seemed like I wasn't doing good, it wasn't getting any better. So I start thinking, OK if I'm a Midewin, I'm gonna start eating like one. Gonna live like one. So, I just thought about what the Anishinaabe people, how they ate, their meals or what food they consumed before Columbus era: Venison, wild rice, the berries, anything that I could think of that was here, then. There was no McDonalds, no grocery store. So, I had canned venison, frozen venison, and I like to fish, so I had plenty of fish, and wild rice, and I got away from drinking pop. It was just drinking water, and then when I was starting like that, it was hard to regulate the blood sugars. Cause I was taking the pills and the insulin. I lowered the amount of insulin I was taking, and still it was too much. My blood sugars dropped too low. With the medicines, they were counteracting the sugar levels, keeping 'em lower. That's what I was figuring. So, I took myself off insulin and quit all the pills.

As I have described in more detail elsewhere (Bender 2020), present-day Ojibwe ricing bundles an important traditional subsistence strategy with modern concepts of tribal territoriality and sovereignty and, thus, constitutes an Indigenous alternative to what Lauren Berlant described as the "rhizomatic" extensions of sovereign state power into bodies (Berlant 2007). However, the sacred resource of the Ojibwe has been in jeopardy for quite some time. Raster and Hill (2017) discuss how genetic research carried out at the University of Minnesota "effectively" cleared "the way for genetic modification" of manoomin in order to "increase productivity and profitability for Minnesota wild rice farmers and to boost Minnesota's competitiveness with the California wild rice industry" (Raster and Hill 2017, 268). This also raises serious questions as to how the naturally growing native manoomin is affected by such experiments.

Climate change, by impacting water temperature and availability, is jeopardizing "the ability of wild rice to grow and thrive in its traditional range" (Lynn et al. 2013, 550). In response to these threats, the Fond du Lac Ojibwe in Minnesota, for instance, have begun to control

> water levels on the lakes by operating water control structures (dams), ditch maintenance, and beaver dam management. Two technicians work full time on water level management and data collection. The Program Manager and the other technicians assist on these activities and also work on restoration planning and implementation.[4]

Since 2017, the Leech Lake Band of Ojibwe in Minnesota "is moving to expand its wild rice harvest from a sporadic enterprise involving mostly tribal members to a full-fledged business with international reach" (Rao 2017). In 2016, the tribe had sold wild rice to the U.S. Department of Agriculture for $270,000 to be redistributed to the recipients of the USDA Food Distribution program (see the next paragraph). In March 2017, the tribe showcased its manoomin at a large food expo in Japan with the aim to get access to Asian markets. A 2017 USDA grant under a program for smaller food producers paid for the tribe to hire a sales and marketing manager. His first public statement was, however, not commending the tribe's innovative wild rice operation, but publicly embarrassing it for the fact that it "never had a professional business plan": "'I'll be frank with you, it's been very unorganized and it's not sales-oriented [...]'" (Rao 2017) – a speech which, in my view, is all too reflective of the patronizing parlance of outside business development specialists condescending down to native communities to "help them."

FOOD STAMPS AND "COMMODS"

When I started my inquiry into food practices, I initially worked from the assumption that traditional subsistence strategies such as gathering manoomin, hunting, and fishing, provided tribal members with an autonomy that recipients of food stamps and food items from the USDA Food Distribution program did not have. In my mind, traditional subsistence strategies stood for tribal sovereignty, and reliance on food programs stood for dependence and vulnerability. It did not take me long, however, to find out that in reality, there was no such thing as a sharp distinction between people who went ricing and hunting and people who went to the Food Distribution. Rather, all tribal members, dependent on their actual economic situation, relied on a mix of strategies to make a living, combining wage work with social assistance and traditional subsistence. This provided them with a key independence: the independence from the job market. A male tribal member in his mid-1960s told me:

Art Miller: People stay. This is their home land, this is our homeland. And so, many people can augment their salaries, their seasonal work, get laid-off, they get unemployment, get commods, but they can always hunt, fish, in the summertime, or somebody will bring them fish. Or deer meat. They can go out and gather some of the wild foods. And people bring them things. There is still a social safety net in the tribe and the family. They look out for one another. They don't follow the work.

The "commods" that Art Miller mentions here are the food items handed out through the USDA Food Distribution, which is managed on the ground by tribal employees. Daniel Hawk, a tribal member in his late fifties and a seasoned director of a tribal Food Distribution program at one of the Ojibwe Tribes of Wisconsin, explained to me how tribal members actually use the program, and how they resist paternalistic tendencies in the way it is administered by the United States Department of Agriculture (USDA).

Daniel Hawk: [USDA] is trying to put additions to the food package all the time. It takes them a long time to get one item in the food package, you know. The process is quite long and takes months, […] a year, two years now. […] They gotta thoroughly check out these food products to make sure that they're gonna be healthy, low in sodium and all that. Before they make it available for us. They have strict guidelines on all that. […] Some of the products they have taken out of that food package, and they didn't give anybody any choice in the matter, they just took it. One of the items was butter. Everybody loved the butter. They just suddenly just took it away.

Cora Bender: Because it's unhealthy?

Daniel Hawk: Because there is so much cholesterol. Everybody really put up an uproar and hollered and complained, but it did no good. [smiles] Yeah, the government said, "You can't have it no more, it's too unhealthy." [Instead, they gave us] Blue Bonnet Light. To me, it ain't much good. I've tried it. […] If they had to use it, they wouldn't probably use it, either. […]

Cora Bender: How about other favorite items among the commodities?

Daniel Hawk: Well, the hamburger's always been a favorite, since they added it on in the program - I don't know how many years back. We issue a lot of that. So, things like the hamburger and the macaroni, you always hear about those. The mac soup that everybody loves to eat, the hamburger, mac and tomato soup, that's one of the favorites, you know.

Cora Bender: Isn't that what they call 'hangover soup'?

Daniel Hawk: Yeah, that's what they refer to as hangover soup. […] if there was always a favorite among tribes, you know, that's hangover soup. And you got flour and oil, basically you can make fry bread. You got canned milk or dry milk. Some people use that. So, that's two of the staples, hangover soup and fry bread.

Cora Bender: Which is both delicious!

Daniel Hawk: Yeah, they're both good. I eat them all the time myself.

Daniel Hawk also provided me with a key insight into the meaning of food security, or rather, *food insecurity* in the reservation setting:

Cora Bender: Looking forward into the future, what would you like to see change?

Daniel Hawk [long pause]: Well, I would say that they should give out a little bit more food to each household, especially the smaller households, the singles, even the two-households. [The food package] is supposed to supplement. But it lasts for half a month only. Have a little bit more so you can stretch it out to most of the month, let's say. That's what I'd like to see. [Not too long ago,] people from [the town of] Sumner came to the Tribal Office, and they asked me, 'Why are so many people from the reservation coming to the [Sumner] food shelf?' [I said] 'Basically a single household does not get enough food from us to last them through a month, that's why they're all coming over to you and asking for a hand-out also.' That's the big problem with single households. The ones that don't work and just stay with family, friends, to help supplement them and have something to eat all month. They got to live with friends or family."

Daniel Hawk: Some years back, this lady from [the town of] Spring Lake food shelf was actually trying [to enforce] a guideline where if they were getting commodities, they couldn't get stuff at the food shelf. And she was asking me if she could get a list of the food clients here. And I said, no, no, I don't give you that, that's confidential information. You know, people are trying to get enough food for the month! I see no problem, you know. I see nothing wrong with that! All the food they can get, these smaller households, the single households, especially.

While, unfortunately, tribal sovereignty does not reach far enough to change the size of the federal food package, at least it protects tribal members' identity and thus helps them to better navigate the forbidding landscape of county and town food shelves and church-run soup kitchens.

Native people statistically appear in the lowest income range of all ethnic groups in U.S. society. According to the 2017 Census, "[t]he percentage of American Indian and Alaska natives living in poverty in 2017 was estimated to be 26.8%. This compares to 14.6% for the nation as a whole" (National Congress of American Indians 2020). However, due to their rights of self-determination and tribal ownership of their land and natural resources, native people are in the unique situation to counter food insecurity with strategies of food-related sovereignty. By "food-related sovereignty," I mean not only the traditional culturally specific subsistence strategies such as rice that are the subject of food sovereignty activism. The term also covers strategies derived from the sovereign status of the tribe, such as protecting tribal members' data and identities from inquisitive outside food assistance bureaucracies. What is more, it also covers embodied practices of sovereignty that transcend the limits of a tribal locality and are shared all over Indian Country. New food traditions invented from "commods," such as fry bread (bannock) and hangover soup, are the staple foods of intertribal powwows all over North America, and provide a visceral cultural bond between tribal people of different nations.

REGENERATING FARMING PRACTICES FOR FOOD SOVEREIGNTY

When Lydia Seltzer, a Choctaw descendant working as the manager of the Sustainable Agricultural Research Station at a large tribal community college tries to involve members of the tribal community with the work at the College Farm, she frequently receives responses such as, "'We're hunter-gatherers. We don't farm!'"

Lydia Seltzer: This is somewhat disappointing, because the Ojibwe have thousands and thousands of years of experience, of stories and of things that history, anthropology and archaeology can attest to with discoveries of seed saving techniques, garden plots, tools, and things like that. So, they were indeed farmers!

Asked whether the tribal community's interest in Indigenous agricultural research is a specialty of her reservation, she says no.

Lydia Seltzer: This struggle to reclaim the agricultural heritage of the Indigenous peoples is occurring in many places. However, the excitement now is being renewed, and that is because of this new search for Indigenous seeds, and bringing back the crops that they have historically eaten in the past. People want to be involved. They want to know and learn more about the history and the means of growing, preparing, consuming, preserving and sharing the foods the way their grandparents and great grandparents did. Young people want to be involved and are eager to learn and participate in experiential agricultural activities. My hope is with the young people, because they really love it, even at the early childhood education level.

Working at the LCO Sustainable Agricultural Research Station for almost ten years, Lydia Seltzer remembers how in the beginning, in her early years there, successful production of vegetables and plants "became less and less successful, mostly due to poor soil conditions." Because of poor agricultural practices on the farm site for many decades, the soil was becoming more compacted "with properties not unlike concrete" and "topsoil would blow away with strong winds."

Over the past five years, there has begun to be a turnaround of fortunes regarding food production in harmony with soil health restoration. In the fall of 2019, the College Farm was able to give away almost 3,000 pounds of vegetables and fruit, not counting the seeds and plants that they handed out to community members so they could use them to grow at home or in the community gardens the College Farm provides. "Like many other Native American peoples, [our tribal communities] were pushed onto a reservation with less than desirable land," writes tribal member and community educator Sherrole Benton.

> Although the reservation is within their traditional homeland, the band suffered losses of prime wild rice beds, berry patches, sugar bushes, and hunting grounds. Their original village [...] was established in 1745 on the shores of the winding Chippewa River. After the federal government permitted a power company to build a dam in 1921, 15,300 acres of the river valley were flooded. The people were forced to relocate

> to higher ground and leave behind wild rice beds, fertile gardens, homes, schools, stores, cemeteries, and historical features left by the ancients. Today, [the Community College] is taking steps to address the reservation's soil quality.
>
> *(Benton 2019)*

Lydia Seltzer: Our land was covered by glaciers at one time, and then there was the forest, and then they cut the forest, and created cutover farms. So, we have over a hundred years of poor agricultural practices, and it gets to a point where the soil is unable to produce anything of substance. But we're trying to turn that around by employing different techniques, and we're starting to see results. Three years ago, I only had a crate full of potatoes. The next year I had three hundred pounds, this summer we had nine hundred pounds to give away to the community. It all has to do with the soil.

A key element of this work is intertribal networking:

Lydia Seltzer: Most tribes are trying to accomplish the same thing. We're all working together and of all the things we've done together, food sovereignty, growing food, sharing food knowledge, sharing seed knowledge is what is uniting all of the Indigenous people. All the initiatives going on throughout the world, all the initiatives by the Indigenous peoples and their allies, and most importantly sharing information and sharing seeds! Sharing the seed stories, these are all important elements of our traditions and histories. Growing good food, historically significant food, is a very uniting factor among the people.

The farm also cooperates with University of Wisconsin Department of Extension and other institutions and organizations such as the Spooner Agricultural Research Station, University of Wisconsin, Madison and the Intertribal Agricultural Council. Lydia Seltzer has observed that in the past few years, there has been a change in the dynamics of these partnerships.

Lydia Seltzer: Like the UW [University of Wisconsin] used to *teach* Indians how to grow! But in the last several years, this has changed. Now, they are wanting to learn from the tribes. Instead of telling us what we should be doing to grow crops, you know, now they are, 'here, we have science and we have people, we have resources, we'll do some training. But we want to assist you and learn from your knowledge and wisdom of traditional agriculture!

Versus "we're gonna show you how to dig a hole, put a seed in and water it!, that's what it seemed like to me" [laughs]. The universities are recognizing that the tribes are very aware of sustainability. When you talk about 'sustainable', they've been sustainable even through adverse times! Agricultural and plant knowledge has survived, and is well and becoming healthier all the time.

This is a matter of considerable satisfaction, given how modern agriculture was historically pushed onto native people as a means of forced pacification and colonial domination:

Lydia Seltzer: I did a presentation last year in Madison, and the topic was on 'getting Native people interested in their agricultural heritage again'. Because of historical trauma, they had turned their back on agriculture. Because at the boarding schools, it was farming, farming and more farming! [The Native students] would go to school in the morning, and then [the school administration] would send them out to different farms in the area - not to learn how to farm but to be indentured laborers.

Under these conditions, traditional knowledge about Indigenous gardening has to be gathered and reconstructed from a number of different sources.

Cora Bender: How do you gather knowledge about the traditional plants that were used by the tribes?

Lydia Seltzer: Mostly it's by sharing information with other people, the elders, other tribes of the Great Lakes Chippewa nations. I do a lot of research, too. People I know get a lot of useful historical information about the history of farming from the anthropologists who went to the tribes like Frances Densmore. She worked with the Chippewa Indians, writing and recording details of their lives. They write about the foods and they write about the practices way back there in the 1800s and more. I recently read a book about LaPointe, about Madeline Island around the time when the explorers and voyageurs came here, and they were talking that there were gardens there. That was in the late 1500s.

The farm is funded through research grants. In the past, grants were given by the First Nations Development Institute,[5] by the Kellogg Foundation and others. With these grants, the College Farm has done projects such as pollinator research and potato research. According to Amber Marlow, the college's dean of continuing education and customized training, a few years ago, the farm ran a beginner producer program, "'funded by the USDA Socially Disadvantaged Farmer Rancher Program that was for working with families and providing education and awareness about growing their food'" (Benton 2019). Presently, the farm applies mainly for USDA sustainable agricultural research grants.

Lydia Seltzer: Right now, we have a big soil health grant that we're working with because we're trying to turn our soil around, making it healthy and thus productive.

Another challenge the College Farm research addresses is the short growing season of the area.

Lydia Seltzer: We have about a 120-day growth period. And there are a lot of things that don't grow in it, so we try to find the plants that do. [...] This last summer [2018, C.B.], our last frost was on June 14. Then we got a frost early in October. And all our 90-day corn froze. So, if the tribe depended on that for food for the winter, they most likely would have starved. But we also grew a 60-day Indigenous corn. It all ripened, and is wonderful; and we got several gallons of seeds out of it, so. This year, we're going to plant that.

The College Farm is also an extension education department of the tribal college with a mission to involve tribal members in gardening and growing food.

Cora Bender: What are some of the reactions that you get from tribal members?

Lydia Seltzer: They love it! [] Last year, we had about twenty people coming to the farm per day all summer long. Lots of them are elders. They're excited about it. So, we rematriated Bear Island corn which is the corn of the Ojibwe people. – We call it 'rematriating', not 'repatriating', because agriculture is female! – I got this corn as a gift three years ago, and it grows really well. One elder came every couple of weeks to check on it, you know, and I just gave her some. And she'd hold the corn like a baby! She taught me how to listen to the corn-? It sounds crazy. When I first took her out to look at it, she had this beautiful look on her face, and she asks, "do you hear it?", I'm like, "hear what?" She goes, "they're singing to us!" And I listened, and when the wind blows, every leaf had a different tone, and as it quivers in the wind. And she called it singing, and she taught me to listen to the corn singing. And the next year, she came in and said, "they really like it here, they are so happy!" I felt like tears coming out of my eyes, you know! That was so moving. She held that corn so tight when I gave it to her!"

Global climate change makes itself felt locally. According to "local land management studies" quoted by Benton (2019), "[in] recent years, unusually bad storms damaged garden projects on the [LCO Ojibwe College] farm. Extreme swings in wet years and dry years are affecting the environment and water levels" (Benton 2019, online). LCO College president Russell Swagger has

> confidence that people will look to tribal communities and ask, 'What are tribal communities doing that's different than other communities? […] we're part of the solution and strengthening leadership, strengthening governance, and educating people so they know what they can do.'
>
> *(Benton 2019)*

THE MESSAGE OF INDIGENOUS FOOD-RELATED SOVEREIGNTY: THE OPPOSITE OF POVERTY IS SELF-DETERMINATION

Above, I discussed examples of strategies and practices of food-related Indigenous sovereignty in the Upper Midwest area of the United States on the background of recent literature concerning Indigenous food sovereignty and the impact of climate change. In particular, I looked at practices of traditional subsistence, i.e., harvesting manoomin, strategies to combine several forms of food assistance in a situation of structurally enforced food insecurity, and at the engagement of a modern tribal knowledge culture in the regeneration of Indigenous gardening. What do these examples contribute to a complex understanding of Indigenous food-related sovereignty?

First, in my view, it needs to be emphasized once more that "food security" is not so much "a view […] implemented by many national governments" (MacRae 2016, 228), but has become a kind of "corporate oxymoron" (Benson and Kirsch 2010) and branding gimmick masking international neoliberal and neocolonial agricultural strategies.[6] Some regional agricultural cooperation, such as the wild rice Project of the University of Minnesota discussed by Raster and Hill (2017), can be seen to emulate this; and in the social reality of reservation life, the promises of "food security" have been trickling down through so many layers of control and manipulation that they actually arrive at the bottom as their direct opposite: as the threats of a structurally enforced food *insecurity* in the context of punitive social policy (Nosrati and Marmot 2019).[7] By contrast, food sovereignty is picked up by many tribes as a promise toward the future of tribal communities, no matter what their current situation is. It serves as a constant reminder to an American public that tends to victimize native people that in the minds of native people, the opposite of poverty is not "enough" (i.e., "security") but *self-determination.*

However, just as "food security" can be seen to have been hijacked by forces that actually produce the reverse outcome of the promise, "food sovereignty" and the regenerative agriculture it promotes are also at risk of a "possible corporate take-over" (Rosset 2018) or of getting emulated by the proponents of an emergent economic model called "regenerative capitalism" that "purports to protect the biosphere while improving profits and competitiveness" (Falls 2019, 157). This vision of a "green Anthropocene" (or a green "capitalocene" [Moore 2017]), for that matter, might be a background to why the USDA, otherwise known as an integral part of the capitalist "American Food Enterprise" (Markowitz and Brett 2010), makes grants available to foster and assist the U.S. local food sector and, more specifically, Indigenous farming and food sovereignty.

Indeed, comparing sources of income and sources of funding relevant in the different cases described above shows that the ethnographic situation is slightly more complex than the dichotomies of the "food security vs. food sovereignty"-debate suggest. Beginning with the first case, traditional harvesting of manoomin is a key strategy to maintain and replenish Ojibwe people's cultural distinctness, spirituality, and notions of health and the good life. Intimately tied in with Ojibwe relations to land, manoomin practice constitutes an alternative sovereignty that permeates and bundles up bodies, homelands, and politico-cultural sovereignty. Yet, in the age of climate change, the deep undomesticated-ness of manoomin is more and more subject to attempts at manipulation by Western science (genetics), efforts at protection and care as well as strategies of expansion and international marketing by Indigenous communities and tribal governments in cooperation with USDA-funded specialists.

Nontraditional Indigenous food strategies in connection with food insecurity, such as the USDA Food Distribution program, are generally not discussed within the framework of Indigenous food sovereignty. For this reason, I decided to use the more loose-fitting term "food-related sovereignty" to cover all the efforts and the hard work of translation Indigenous people put into this type of food practice. The USDA is seen here to function as the key outside agency that, by not allowing sufficient food packages for a month, forces food insecurity onto native people while tribal agents try to alleviate its worst effects. They do their best to convert the meager provisions into some kind of food security, albeit a most precarious one, by protecting the identity of tribal members-recipients from the monitoring of outside food shelves. The strongest point of Indigenous sovereignty in this case is its cultural innovation: its capability to turn food handouts into (inter)tribal culture. Irrespective of what food purists and health educators have to say about the nontraditional provenance and unhealthiness of fry bread and hangover soup – the legendary status of these Indigenous staple dishes all over Indian Country and their enormous importance for an intertribal pow-wow culture is indisputable. Finally (and ironically so?), the USDA can be seen to sponsor the future of Indigenous food sovereignty as it funds many of the programs run at different tribal agricultural research stations. As the two previous examples have already demonstrated, it becomes especially obvious in the case of tribal farming that tribal sovereignty is not so much about the sources of the funding. Rather, it is about the work invested by tribal entities to translate and convert these monies into opportunities to advance and expand native self-determination, among them first and foremost the tribal ownership and use of land and the tribal right to the enforcement of treaties. In this respect, as has been mentioned before, Indigenous agricultural regeneration projects have many interesting similarities with Indigenous cultural revitalization movements, more specifically, media projects and language regeneration which are also, in many cases, sponsored through federal grants or non-Indian audience donations. One such media project, the FM radio station WOJB, licensed to the Lac Courte Oreilles tribe, has been successfully funded for many years through pledge drives that solicit money from a non-Indian audience in order to pay for native programming. Has this process been free of contradictions, free of conflict? No. Actually, the long history of WOJB can be subsumed in a definition of a native radio station as "a radio station that Native people have conflicts about" (Bender 2011, 182). I suggest we take a similar route when it comes to native food-related sovereignty. The "lack of specificity about the sovereign" deplored by Edelman in his critique of food sovereignty is, in my view, actually a lack of ethnographic attention to the situational assertion and exercise of sovereignty. We must have a better grasp on the meaning of the "contradictory notion of sovereignty" embedded in food sovereignty (McKay et al. 2014, 1175). We need to become more aware of the work of sovereignty carried out in tribal colleges, agricultural research stations, health centers, and tribal administrations, i.e., at the cutting edge where Indigenous actors take on state policies and convert them into tribal sovereignty.

RECOMMENDATIONS

Asked by the editors to develop a set of recommendations, I would like to emphasize that as a Cultural Anthropologist working in Indian Country, I never felt it was my place to recommend a certain course of action for tribal entities or individual actors to take. Much to the contrary, I have always seen it as my prime task to discuss Indigenous lifeways and strategies as examples from which to learn insights into culture, media, and globalization which would not be available any other way. This is also how I approach the task of making recommendations with respect to the SDGs. My main idea is that in engaging with the SDGs, Indigenous peoples will be able to give a unique feedback to the world on what the SDGs are "really" worth. Consequently, I avoid directing my recommendation at a specific address, neither that of tribal nor that of "outside" actors. Ultimately, it will be sovereign tribal actors that determine how tribes make use of the SDGs in the future:

1. First, abolish the language of "vulnerability" that victimizes poor and marginalized people. Instead, adopt a point of view of self-determination when discussing initiatives to improve the present situation, including the goals and targets of the Agenda 2030.
2. Consider a broader initiative bringing tribal colleges, tribal governments, national Indian and UN Major Group representatives together in order to engage with the SDGs and review their meaning and usefulness for Indian Country. Urban Indigenous communities, tribes, as well as Indigenous political representation on a national level can benefit from an awareness of the SDGs and of their own crucial role for attainment of the SDGs by the United States (see Fredericks 2019).
3. Take Tribal Sovereignty as the main compass to navigate UN program parlance. Tribal sovereignty is not everything, but without tribal sovereignty, all the resounding concepts, especially "sustainability" and "resilience," amount to a very little net gain for Indigenous people.
4. Consequently, focus on using the SDGs strictly to the advantage of Indigenous people. As an example, SDG 2 links "end hunger" and "achieve food security" with "promote sustainable agriculture." SDG 2.3 specifically targets doubling "agricultural productivity and small-scale food producers, including Indigenous peoples." How can this target benefit Upper Midwest tribal strategies to secure their rights to manoomin protection and limit or even stop the genetic experiments conducted with manoomin at the University of Minnesota?
5. Use the SDGs to push for a clarification of what "end hunger" and "the right to food" actually mean. As my research demonstrated, mere "access" to food does not equal the ability to feed oneself with dignity. Quite to the contrary, being forced to frequent different food assistance programs every month contributes to chronic stress, depression, and a general "unwellbeing," actually, the opposite of SDG 3.
6. On a more general level, use the SDGs to acquire support for post-Corona reconstruction. Reconstruction is not limited to economic ends. In Indian Country, specifically, Corona has hit traditional knowledge culture and the transmission of culture-specific knowledge and Indigenous languages by killing elders (Healy 2021). This jeopardizes basic Indigenous lifeways and concepts of wellbeing. How can SDG 3 (Health and Wellbeing), SDG 4 (Quality Education), SDG 11 (Sustainable Communities), and SDG 16 (Peace, Justice, Strong Institutions) be useful in promoting a new tribal revitalization?

As I said before, the answers to these questions can only be given by Indigenous peoples themselves.

ACKNOWLEDGMENTS

This chapter is based on ethnographic research into Indigenous health and sovereignty which I carried out in recurrent field trips of various lengths in the years 2007, 2009, and between 2012 and 2017, while I taught at the Special Research College "Locating Media," University of Siegen, Germany. It is my pleasure to extend my sincerest thanks to the college board of directors who made my frequent research trips possible, and to the great interdisciplinary team of colleagues and students for many fruitful discussions. Also, I would like to thank all tribal governments and tribal health entities who allowed me to participate in the everyday lives of patients and professionals, my Anishinaabe and other interlocutors for their valuable time and invaluable input, and last but not least, my husband gaiashkibos for his feedback and unwavering support through thick and thin.

NOTES

1. General Assembly Resolution adopted on September 25, 2015, "Transforming Our World: the 2030 Agenda for Sustainable Development, https://www.un.org/en/development/desa/population/migration/generalassembly/docs/globalcompact/A_RES_70_1_E.pdf, 27.02.202.
2. "It was then argued that all countries with difficulties in national food supply should 'potentially' have sufficient access to food imports." (Windfuhr and Jonsén 2005, 21).
3. At the time, two Ojibwe groups, the bands at Sokoagon (Mole Lake) and St. Croix, were left out because they did not sign the treaty of 1854. They remained landless until the mid-1930s when small reservations were parceled out for them under presidential executive order (Lurie 2002; Loew 2001, 78).
4. http://www.fdlrez.com/RM/wildrice.htm, 27.02.2020; see also Lynn et al (2013, 550).
5. https://www.firstnations.org/, 27.02.2020.
6. Such as the "New Alliance for Food Security and Nutrition" launched in 2012 under G8 auspices (Dalgleish 2015); see also Falls 2019 on "green capitalism".
7. Food insecurity is a key factor contributing to obesity and other metabolic and cardiovascular diseases (Indian Health Service Division of Diabetes Treatment and Prevention n.d.).

REFERENCES

Bender, Cora (2011) *Die Entdeckung der Indigenen Moderne. Indianische Medienwelten und Wissenskulturen in den USA*. Bielefeld: Transcript.

Bender, Cora (2020) Collageable Lives: Julius and Eva Lips and the Anthropology of Native North America. In *'The Savage Hits Back' Revisited: Art and Alterity in the Colonial Encounter*, ed. Anna Brus, 1–15. Berlin: Reimer.

Bender, Cora. In Preparation. Ojibwe Food and "Communities of Practice": A View from Medical Anthropology.

Benson, Peter and Stuart Kirsch (2010) Corporate Oxymorons. *Dialectical Anthropology* 34 (1): 45–48.

Benton, Sherrole (2019) LCO's Community Garden is Stepping Stone to Food Sovereignty. *Tribal College Journal* 30 (3): 12–13. https://tribalcollegejournal.org/lcos-community-garden-is-stepping-stone-to-food-sovereignty

Berlant, Lauren (2007) Slow Death (Sovereignty, Obesity, Lateral Agency). *Critical Inquiry* 33: 754–780.

Brett, John A. (2010) The Political-Economics of Developing Markets versus Satisfying Food Needs. *Food and Foodways* 18 (1–2): 28–42.

Centers for Disease Control and Prevention (2020) CDC Data Show Disproportionate COVID-19 Impact in American Indian/Alaska Native Populations. Press release, August 19, 2020. https://www.cdc.gov/media/releases/2020/p0819-covid-19-impact-american-indian-alaska-native.html.

Corntassel, Jeff (2012) Practicing Sustainable Self-Determination. *Brown Journal of World Affairs* 18: 151–162.

Coté, Charlotte (2016) "Indigenizing" Food Sovereignty. Revitalizing Indigenous Food Practices and Ecological Knowledges in Canada and the United States. *Humanities* 5 (3): 57. https://www.mdpi.com/2076-0787/5/3/57

Cozzetto, K. et al. (2013) Climate Change Impacts on the Water Resources of American Indians and Alaska Natives in the U.S. *Climatic Change* 120: 569–584.

Dalgleish, Mandela C. (2015) The New Alliance: Gaining Ground in Africa. In *Force Multipliers: The Instrumentalities of Imperialism*. (The New Imperialism, vol. 5), ed. Maximilian C. Forte, 107–124. Montreal: Alert Press.

Desmarais, Annette A. and Hannah Wittman (2014) Farmers, Foodies and First Nations: Getting to Food Sovereignty in Canada. *Journal of Peasant Studies* 41 (6): 1153–1173.

Dhir, Rishabh Kumar (2016) *Sustainable Development Goals: Indigenous Peoples in Focus*. Geneva: International Labor Organization. https://www.ilo.org/global/topics/Indigenous-tribal/publications/WCMS_503715/lang--en/index.htm.

Dhurandhar, Emily (2016) The Food-Insecurity Obesity Paradox: A Resource Scarcity Hypothesis. *Physiology and Behavior* 162: 88–92.

Dinour, L. M. et al. (2007) The Food Insecurity-Obesity Paradox: A Review of the Literature and the Role of Food Stamps May Play. *Journal of the American Dietetic Association* 107 (11): 1952–1961.

Dittmer, Kyle (2013) Changing Streamflow on Columbia Basin Tribal Lands – Climate Change and Salmon. *Climatic Change* 120: 627–641.

Donlin, Elizabeth P. (2015) The Power of Food: The Ojibwe Food Sovereignty Movement. A Movement toward Regaining and Restoring Indigenous Lifeways through Food in Minnesota. Master Thesis, Norway: University of Oslo.

Doyle, John T. et al. (2013) Exploring Effects of Climate Change on Northern Plains American Indian Health. *Climatic Change* 120: 643–655.

Edelman, Marc (2014) Food Sovereignty: Forgotten Genealogies and Future Regulatory Challenges. *Journal of Peasant Studies* 41 (6): 959–978.

Estes, Nick (2019) *Our History is the Future. Standing Rock versus the Dakota Access Pipeline, and the Long Tradition of Indigenous Resistance*. London: Verso.

Estes, Nick et al. (eds.) (2019) *Standing with Standing Rock. Voices from the #NoDAPL Movement*. St. Paul: University of Minnesota Press.

Falls, Susan (2019) The Anthropocene Goes Green? *Economic Anthropology* 6: 157–159.

FAO, IFAD, UNICEF, WFP and WHO (2020) *The State of Food Security and Nutrition in the World 2020: Transforming Food Systems for Affordable Healthy Diets*. Rome: FAO. https://doi.org/10.4060/ca9692en.

Finoh, Maya (2020) Five Ways the Trump Administration Has Attacked the U.N. and International Human Rights Bodies. New York: American Civil Liberties Union. https://www.aclu.org/print/node/70252.

Fredericks, Carla (2019) Mapping the Sustainable Development Goals onto Indian Nations. In *Creating Private Sector Economies in Native America: Sustainable Development through Entrepreneurship*, eds. Robert J. Miller et al., 185–194. Cambridge: Cambridge University Press.

Gadhoke, Preety and Barrett P. Brenton (2017) Erasure of Indigenous Food Memories and (Re-)Imaginations. In *Food Cults. How Fads, Dogma and Doctrine Influence Diet*, ed. Kima Cargill, 205–218. Lanham, MD: Rowman and Littlefield.

Garfinkel, Harold (1967) *Studies in Ethnomethodology*. Englewood Cliffs, NJ: Prentice-Hall.

Grah, Oliver and Jezra Beaulieu (2013) The Effect of Climate Change on Glacier Ablation and Baseflow Support in the Nooksack River Basin and Implications on Pacific Salmonid Species Protection and Recovery. *Climatic Change* 120: 657–670.

Grasseni, Cristina (2007) *Skilled Visions: Between Apprenticeship and Standards*. London: Berghahn.

Grossman, Zoltan (2021) The Resilience Doctrine: Indigenous Nations Understand Disaster Resilience. Part 3 of a 4-Part Primer on Disaster Collectivism in the Climate and Pandemic Crises. *Counterpunch*, February 3, 2021. https://www.counterpunch.org/2021/02/03/the-resilience-doctrine-Indigenous-nations-understand-disaster-resilience/.

Healy, Jack (2021) Tribal Elders are Dying from the Pandemic, Causing a Cultural Crisis for American Indians. *New York Times*, January 12, 2021. https://www.nytimes.com/2021/01/12/us/tribal-elders-native-americans-coronavirus.htm.

Himmelgreen, David A. and Nancy Romero-Daza (2010) Eliminating 'Hunger' in the U.S.: Changes in Policy Regarding the Measurement of Food Security. *Food and Foodways* 18 (1–2): 96–113.

Hostetter, Martha and Sarah Klein (2020) Learning from Pandemic Responses Across Indian Country. *Commonwealth Fund*, September 30, 2020. https://www.commonwealthfund.org/publications/2020/sep/learning-pandemic-responses-across-indian-country.

Indian Health Service Division of Diabetes Treatment and Prevention (n.d.) Food Insecurity and Diabetes: What's the Connection? https://www.ihs.gov/MedicalPrograms/Diabetes/HomeDocs/Training/WebBased/Seminars/Transcript_Food_Insecur_508c.pdf.

Indian Law Resource Center (n.d.) Implementing the United Nations Declaration on the Rights of Indigenous Peoples. https://indianlaw.org/implementing-undrip.

Indigenous Peoples Major Group for Sustainable Development (2020) Thematic Report for the High-Level Political Forum of Agenda 2030 for Sustainable Development 2020. https://Indigenouspeoples-sdg.org/index.php/english/.

Jernigan, Valarie Bluebird et al. (2017) Food Insecurity among American Indians and Alaska Natives: A National Profile Using the Current Population Survey–Food Security Supplement. *Journal of Hunger and Environmental Nutrition* 12 (1): 1–10.

Kamal, Asfia G. (2018) A Recipe for Change: Reclamation of Indigenous Sovereignty in O-Pipon-Na-Piwin Cree Nation. PhD Thesis, Winnipeg: Faculty of Graduate Studies, University of Manitoba.

Lakhani, Nina (2021) Exclusive: Indigenous Americans Dying from Covid at Twice the Rate of White Americans. *Guardian*, February 4, 2021. https://www.theguardian.com/us-news/2021/feb/04/native-americans-coronavirus-covid-death-rate.

Lemke, Stefanie and Treena Delormier (2017) Indigenous People's Food Systems, Nutrition, and Gender: Conceptual and Methodological Considerations. *Maternal and Child Nutrition* 13: 3.

Lieberman, Amy (2018) SDGs Gain Traction in the US, But with a Domestic Twist. *Devex*, April 11, 2018. https://www.devex.com/news/sdgs-gain-traction-in-the-us-but-with-a-domestic-twist-92459.

Lips, Eva (1956) *Die Reisernte der Ojibwa-Indianer. Wirtschaft und Recht eines Erntevolks*. Berlin: Akademie-Verlag.

Lips, Julius E. (1928) Die Anfänge des Rechts an Grund und Boden bei den Naturvölkern und der Begriff der Erntevölker. In *Festschrift für Pater Wilhelm Schmidt*, Wilhelm Koppers, ed. Pp. 485–494. Vienna: Mechitharisten-Congregations-Buchdruckerei.

Lips, Julius E. (1953) *Die Erntevölker, eine wichtige Phase in der Entwicklung der menschlichen Wirtschaft. Rektoratsrede, gehalten am 31. Oktober 1949 in der Kongreßhalle zu Leipzig*. Berlin: Akademie-Verlag.

Loew, Patricia (2001) *Indian Nations of Wisconsin*. Madison, WI: State Historical Society Press.

Lurie, Nancy O (2002) *Wisconsin Indians*. Madison, WI: State Historical Society Press.

Lynn, Kathy et al. (2013) The Impacts of Climate Change on Tribal Traditional Foods. *Climatic Change* 120: 545–556.

MacRae, Graeme (2016) Food Sovereignty and the Anthropology of Food: Ethnographic Approaches to Policy and Practice. *Anthropological Forum* 26 (3): 227–232.

Maldonado, Julie K. et al. (2013) The Impact of Climate Change on Tribal Communities in the U.S.: Displacement, Relocation, and Human Rights. *Climatic Change* 120: 601–614.

Markowitz, Lisa and John A. Brett (2010) Introduction: The Public Interest and the American Food Enterprise: Anthropological Policy Insights. *Food and Foodways* 18 (1–2): 1–6.

McKay, Ben et al. (2014) The 'State' of Food Sovereignty in Latin America. Political Projects and Alternative Pathways in Venezuela, Ecuador and Bolivia. *Journal of Peasant Studies* 41 (6): 1175–1200.

McMullen, Jennifer (2004) Regenerating Indigenous Health and Food Systems: Assessing Conflict Transformation Models and Sustainable Approaches to Indigenous Food Sovereignty. Master Thesis, Canada: University of Victoria.

Mihesuah, Devon and Elizabeth Hoover, eds. (2019) *Indigenous Food Sovereignty in the United States: Restoring Cultural Knowledge, Protecting Environments, and Regaining Health*. Norman: University of Oklahoma Press.

Moore, Henrietta (2015) The Sustainable Development Goals: We're All Developing Countries Now. *Guardian*, 9.25.2015.

Moore, Jason W. (2017) The Capitalocene, Part I: On the Nature and Origins of Our Ecological Crisis. *Journal of Peasant Studies* 44 (3): 594–630.

Nakashima, D. J. et al. (2012). *Weathering Uncertainty: Traditional Knowledge for Climate Change Assessment and Adaptation*. Paris, and Darwin: UNESCO, UNU.

National Congress of American Indians (2020) Indian Country Demographics. https://www.ncai.org/about-tribes/demographics.

Nord, Mark et al. (2007) Measuring Food Security in the United States: Household Food Security in the United States, 2006. United States Department of Agriculture Economic Research Report 49, November 2007. https://www.ers.usda.gov/webdocs/publications/45889/12224_err49_1_.pdf?v=0.

Nosrati, Elias and Michael Marmot (2019) Punitive Social Policy: An Upstream Determinant of Health. *Lancet* 394 (10196): 376–377.

Pan, Liping et al. (2012) Food Insecurity Is Associated with Obesity among US Adults in 12 States. *Journal of the Academy of Nutrition and Dietetics* 112 (9): 1403–1409.

Perry, William W. (2013) Indigenous Food Sovereignty: Growing and Surviving as Indians. Master Thesis, McGill University, Canada.

Pingeot, Lou (2014) Corporate Influence in the Post-2015 Process. Aachen: Bischöfliches Hilfswerk Misereor Working Paper. https://www.brot-fuer-die-welt.de/fileadmin/mediapool/2_Downloads/Fachinformationen/Sonstiges/Corporate_influence_in_the_post_2015_process.pdf.

Pingeot, Lou (2016) In Whose Interest? The UN's Strategic Rapprochement with Business in the Sustainable Development Agenda. *Globalizations* 13 (2): 188–202.

Pipa, Anthony F. et al. (2020) *American Leadership in Advancing the SDGs to Achieve Equity and Sustainability*. Washington, DC: Brookings Institute. https://www.brookings.edu/blog/up-front/2020/11/12/american-leadership-in-advancing-the-sdgs-to-achieve-equity-and-sustainability/.

Rao, Maya (2017) Selling Rice to Japan? Minnesota Tribes Marketing Wild Rice to the World. *Star Tribune*, March 20, 2017.

Rasmussen, Charlie Otto (1998) *Where the River Is Wide: Pahquahwong and the Chippewa Flowage*. Odanah: Great Lakes Indian Fish and Wildlife Commission Press.

Raster, Amanda and Christina G. Hill (2017) The Dispute over Wild Rice: An Investigation of Treaty Agreements and Ojibwe Food Sovereignty. *Agriculture and Human Values* 34: 267–281.

Reo, Nicholas J. and Angela K. Parker (2013) Re-Thinking Colonialism to Prepare for the Impacts of Rapid Environment Change. *Climatic Change* 120: 671–682.

Ritzenthaler, Robert E. (1978) Southwestern Chippewa. In *Northeast*, ed. Brice G. Trigger. *Handbook of North American Indians: Northeast Vol. 15*, ed. William C. Sturtevant, 743–759. Washington, DC: Smithsonian Institution.

Rosset, Peter M. (2018) Peter Rosset Calls for Support of Local Agroecology Processes, 03. April 2018, https://www.youtube.com/watch?v=h9c6FLtddU.

Rosset, Peter M. and Maria E. Martinez-Torres (2013) La Vía Campesina: The Birth and Evolution of a Transnational Social Movement. *Journal of Peasant Studies* 37 (1): 149–175.

Scheyvens, Regina et al. (2016) The Private Sector and the SDGs: The Need to Move Beyond 'Business as Usual'. *Sustainable Development* 24: 371–382.

TallBear, Kim (2020) A Sharpening of the Already Present: Settler Apocalypse 2020. Youtube Video, https://www.youtube.com/watch?v=eO14od9mlTA.

United Nations Permanent Forum on Indigenous Issues (2019) Indigenous Peoples Have a Crucial Role in Implementing SDG 16, Concludes Permanent Forum. International Institute for Sustainable Development, May 9, 2019. https://sdg.iisd.org/news/Indigenous-peoples-have-a-crucial-role-in-implementing-sdg-16-concludes-permanent-forum/.

Vazquez, Jennifer M. (2018) The Role of Indigenous Knowledge and Innovation in Creating Food Sovereignty in the Oneida Nation of Wisconsin. Master Thesis, Iowa State University Graduate Theses and Dissertations 10137.

Voggesser, Garrit et al. (2013) Cultural Impact to Tribes from Climate Change Influences on Forests. *Climatic Change* 120: 615–626.

Warren, William W. 1885. (1970) History of the Ojibway Nation. Minneapolis, MN: Ross and Haines. [Originally published as "History of the Ojibways: Based upon Traditions and Oral Statements." In *Collections of the Minnesota Historical Society* 5: 29–394].

Whyte, Kyle P. (2013) Justice Forward. Tribes, Climate Adaptation and Responsibility. *Climatic Change* 120: 517–530.

Whyte, Kyle P. (2016) Indigenous Food Sovereignty and Settler Colonialism. In *Routledge Handbook of Food Ethics*, eds. Mary Rawlinson and Caleb Ward, 354–365. London: Routledge.

Williams, Terry and Preston Hardison (2013) Culture, Law, Risk, and Governance: Contexts of Traditional Knowledge in Climate Change Adaptation. *Climatic Change* 120: 531–544.

Windfuhr, Michael and Jennie Jonsén (2005) *Food Sovereignty: Towards Democracy in Localized Food Systems*. Bourton-on-Dunsmore: ITDG Publishing.

4 "How Decolonized Are We?" The Colonial Legacy of Commodity Foods and Food Insecurity Expressed by the Voices of Southwestern Native American Chefs

Jacquelyn N. Heuer

CONTENTS

INTRODUCTION

Traditional food systems represent a body of knowledge that has significance for any cultural group, contributing not only to their culture but also to their overall health and well-being (Companion 2008; Gadhoke and Brenton 2017; Gurney et al. 2015; Satterfield et al. 2016). Though the definition of traditional food systems is often discussed and contested, within this chapter, traditional foods and systems

DOI: 10.1201/9781003014942-4

refer to the foods of Indigenous peoples that were historically collected from the surrounding environment and were culturally significant (Kuhnlein and Receveur 1996). Among the Southwestern (SW) Pueblos, such as the Acoma, Hopi, San Felipe, Santo Domingo, Tewa, and Zuni communities, agricultural practices were common (Cleveland et al. 1995; Robison 1992; Waldman 2006; Wall and Masayesva 2019). The Apache, Arapaho, and Navajo (Diné) were nomadic hunter–gatherers who regularly raided the Pueblos (Waldman 2006). Over time, the Navajo learned horticultural methods from their Pueblo neighbors (Sasaki and Adair 1952). SW tribes cultivated various crops, including squash, beans, sunflowers, cotton, tobacco, and numerous corn varieties. In addition, many SW tribes raised turkeys and chickens and later acquired sheep and goats from the Spanish. These tribes also hunted local wild game and gathered edible plants from their surrounding environment (Sasaki and Adair 1952; Waldman 2006; White 1973).

While SW tribes were not forcibly relocated like many other Native American tribes, they were confined to reservations. Oral stories from the Zuni indicate that the United States federal government played a role in the disruption of traditional food systems through the imposition of new agricultural policies (Cleveland 1998). Agricultural policies, like many other policies surrounding the forced acculturation and assimilation of Indigenous populations, were rooted in racism, meaning that they established a racial bias and prejudice that determined sources of institutional power that systematically worked against Native Americans (Washington and Williams 2019). This strategy strove to bring Native Americans, including the SW tribes, into "modern," "Western," or "American" cultural and lifestyles by controlling aspects of Native American culture, including education, religion, and language. Changes to agricultural policy worked to appropriate valuable natural resources (e.g., water) and strove to replace traditional practices with "modern" practices including canal irrigation, ranching, and agribusiness. Given the large scale of these practices, the consolidation of small farms was encouraged. To help facilitate this, the government began substituting individual land rights for communal rights (Cleveland 1998; Vlasich 2005). SW tribes were also encouraged to replace their ancestral crops with commercial and hybrid crops, which the federal government argued would encourage the growth of the cash economy (Cleveland et al. 1995; Cleveland 1998; Vlasich 2005).

The ramifications of these agricultural shifts are palpable today, as federal policies have shaped Indigenous land use, traditional agricultural practices, and dietary consumption patterns, thereby limiting access to traditional foods, contributing to a loss of food sovereignty, and exacerbating food insecurity among tribes (Gurney et al. 2015; Osterkamp and Longstaff 2004; Wall and Masayesva 2004). The same forces that shaped agricultural practices in the SW also increased the dependence on the introduced "white man" foods, such as coffee, sugar, flour, cereal, rice, beans, salt pork, and beef (Conti 2006). The provision of government rations led to the formation of the Food Distribution Program on Indian Reservations (FDPIR) in 1973 (Byker Shanks et al. 2015). Since its inception, the nutritional quality of foods provided by FDPIR has been critiqued, as early provisions consisted of highly processed foods such as canned meats, juices, pasta, and processed cheese (Mucioki et al. 2018). While changes to FDPIR have sought to improve the nutritional content of the foods consumed, dietary quality remains a concern for many Native American communities (Byker Shanks et al. 2015; Mucioki et al. 2018). Today, many Native Americans continue to lack access to healthy, high-quality, and culturally appropriate foods due to the limited availability of grocery stores, the increased prevalence of fast food chains, and a lack of healthy foods available at convenience stores (Jernigan et al. 2012; Loh et al. 2020). As a result, many of these "white man" or "Western" foods continue to be consumed by Indigenous populations, with some scholars arguing that this continued acceptance of Western foods contributes to the ongoing colonization and cultural genocide of Native Americans (Mihesuah 2016; Milburn 2004; Wiedman 2012).

As a result of the forced acculturation and assimilation of Native Americans, Indigenous foodways were disrupted, destroyed, and sometimes, lost altogether; these disruptions have not only contributed to the health disparities among Native American populations today, but have also resulted in a lasting historical trauma that has been carried down through the generations (Gadhoke and Brenton 2017). While some SW groups, such as the Hopi, were able to retain their Indigenous agricultural knowledge, dietary changes still occurred, especially as more individuals have had to abandon agriculture in favor of more economically stable work (Soleri and Cleveland 1993). Among SW Native Americans, health disparities are a major concern. As Lombard et al. (2014) note, SW Native Americans have higher rates of stomach, gallbladder, liver, myeloma, and kidney cancers when compared to non-Hispanic Whites. Moreover, the Navajo Nation faces rates of type 2 diabetes that are two to four times higher than those of non-White Hispanics (Lombard et al. 2014). While the causes of these health disparities are multifaceted, research has indicated that they are linked to a low consumption of healthy foods, including fresh fruits and vegetables (Lombard et al. 2014; Sarkar et al. 2019; Wiedman 2012).

Access to healthy foods and food security are key concerns among Native Americans (Jernigan et al. 2020; Pindus and Hafford 2019). Between 2000 and 2010, 25% of Indigenous populations in the United States were food insecure, a rate more than twice that of White/Caucasian Americans (Jernigan et al. 2017). Moreover, a 2016 study of FDPIR found that households enrolled in the program consisted of very low-income populations with high rates of food insecurity – 34% experienced low food security and 22% experienced very low food security (Pindus and Hafford 2019). Research has estimated that 85% of reservation residents receive food from FDPIR (Gurney et al. 2015). In 2019, it was estimated that the United States Department of Agriculture supplied food to an average of 83,800 individuals from 276 tribes through FDPIR (USDA 2020).

While tribe-specific studies on food insecurity are lacking, recent research indicates that food insecurity rates may be even higher. Among a sample from the Navajo Nation, 76.7% of individuals experienced some level of food insecurity (Pardilla et al. 2013). Similarly, a recent study among Indigenous populations in the Klamath River basin of Oregon and California found that approximately 92% of individuals within these tribes are food insecure (Sowerwine et al. 2019). The COVID-19 pandemic has only worsened food insecurity rates among Native Americans. Disruptions to food supply chains have exposed many issues within the American food system, including the presence of food deserts on reservations. Reservations tend to be geographically isolated; as a result, residents often must drive to their nearest grocery store that may be an hour or more away only to find empty shelves during the pandemic (Eschner 2020; Heuer et al. 2020; UN 2020).

Food security on reservations has long been a concern, with commodity food programs being introduced in the 1950s to address the high levels of food insecurity and malnutrition on reservations. These programs have had lasting implications, primarily due to the low-quality foods provided and the failure to incorporate traditional foods (Gadhoke and Brenton 2017; Gurney et al. 2015). Moreover, the processed foods that are typically included in these programs have been associated with the endemic of diet-related chronic diseases (e.g., obesity and type 2 diabetes) among Native Americans (Gurney et al. 2015). Obesity has become a major concern within the last two generations, with the rising rates of obesity being linked to the increase of high-fat foods and highly processed carbohydrates available through these food assistance programs and the decrease in daily activity; meanwhile, diabetes has increased exponentially, at a rate 234% higher than all other ethnic groups in the United States (Companion 2008).

Today, the lack of access to traditional foodways is intrinsically linked to cultural loss and revitalization programs, food security and sovereignty initiatives, environmental changes and degradation, and negligent laws and policies that may make accessing traditional foods and foodways difficult (Gurney et al. 2015). The loss of lands and dependence on government rations, coupled with ever-increasing concerns of contaminants (e.g., metals and organochlorines) in traditionally harvested resources such as fish and wild game, have led to an increased dependence on commercial foods and a decreased use of traditional foods (McAuley and Knopper 2011).

As Hoover and Mihesuah (2019) note, one cannot address Indigenous food security without addressing Indigenous food sovereignty, as the two issues are intertwined and continue to shape the health not only of SW Native Americans, but for Indigenous populations across the globe. As a result, there are several clear connections between the issues of Indigenous food security, food sovereignty, and the Sustainable Development Goals (SDGs) outlined by the United Nations (UN). Moreover, as the UN Food and Agriculture Organization (FAO) annual reports on food security and nutrition have noted, food security, nutrition, economic opportunity, and climate change are intrinsically intertwined. As research has demonstrated, food insecurity among Native Americans has been linked to poverty and has negatively influenced health disparities among these populations (Bauer et al. 2012; Jernigan et al. 2020; Lombard et al. 2014; Pardilla et al. 2013; Sowerwine et al. 2019; Wiedman 2012). These issues clearly connect to SDGs 1, 2, 3, and 10, which advocate for ending poverty in all its forms, ending hunger and ensuring food security, promoting well-being, and reducing inequality, respectively. Given these factors, food sovereignty presents a sustainable solution to these issues by allowing Native American communities to address concerns.

Dietary transitions are not unique to Native Americans. Indigenous populations have actively addressed their food sovereignty while undergoing dietary transitions on a global scale, from Canada's First Nations (Batal et al. 2018; Kuhnlein et al. 2004; Young and Harris 1994) to Australia's Aborigines (Ferguson et al. 2017; O'Dea 1992; Sherriff et al. 2019), among others (Chee et al. 2019; O'Meara et al. 2019; Piya and Joshi 2018; Soares et al. 2019). Many of these food movements serve as counter-hegemonic movements, challenging the hegemony, or dominance, of globalized and neoliberal food policies that have bolstered an increased dependence on industrialized agriculture (Coté 2016; Rose and Lourival 2019). As such, these movements deemphasize the focus on food as a commodity and strive to address the social and racial injustices that have led to inequality within the food system (Fairbairn 2012).

Given the dietary shifts that have occurred among Indigenous populations across the globe, this research sought to examine the perceptions that individuals enrolled in the culinary program at the Southwestern Indian Polytechnic Institute (SIPI) in Albuquerque, New Mexico had of their traditional, or ancestral, foodways. While the overarching goal of the research was to explore perceptions of traditional foods among the SIPI culinary students, the objective of the research was to understand the numerous components of traditional food systems, including how they are maintained, how they are reproduced, and how the knowledge is passed down through the generations. Throughout this research, the participating Native American culinary students and professional chefs were able to consider the lasting impacts of colonization, especially as it pertained to how the food security and food sovereignty of their communities has been shaped (and continues to be shaped by) dietary acculturation and subsequent transitions.

METHODS

The data for this research were collected for my master's thesis at New Mexico State University (NMSU) in Las Cruces, New Mexico. During my time there, I partnered with SIPI and collected data over two years, from May 2015 until February 2017, utilizing a multimethod design. I began with an extensive review of the literature, including a review of past ethnographic work on Native Americans of the SW (Bakker 1999; Cleveland et al. 1995; Cleveland 1998; Cushing 1920; Robison 1992; Sasaki and Adair 1952; Soleri and Cleveland 1993; Vlasich 2005; White 1973), as well as a review of published Native American cookbooks (Frank 2002; Niethammer 1974; Swentzell and Perea 2016). Using these ethnographic works, I formulated a semi-structured interview guide that examined key themes of defining traditional foodways, colonization and acculturation, dietary transitions, loss of knowledge of culture, and the conservation and modification of traditional foods, among others. Next, I conducted interviews with SIPI students who were enrolled in the culinary program, as well as the director of the culinary program, Chef Bailey. The students who participated in this research came from tribes across the country and ranged in age from 19 to 53 years. Of the ten students interviewed, four students were Navajo, one student was Acoma, and one student was Inupiat Nome. Additionally, four students held multiple tribal memberships: White Mountain Apache/San Carlos Apache, Northern Arapaho/Navajo, San Felipe/Santo Domingo, and White Mountain Apache/San Carlos Apache/Hopi/Tewa. Meanwhile, Chef Bailey, while not a Native American himself, has dedicated his career to understanding traditional foodways and as a result, has gained the respect of his students.

In addition to these interviews, I also interviewed three professional Indigenous chefs – Walter, Lois, and Claudia – whose insights helped me to better understand the challenges faced by professional chefs who seek to raise public awareness of traditional foodways. Claudia is of Purépecha descent, holds a PhD in sociocultural anthropology, and is the cofounder and coowner of a Native-based food catering company in the Los Angeles area. Meanwhile, Lois is Kiowa/Shepardic, holds a PhD in culinary anthropology, and owns her own catering company in the Santa Fe area, where she works with the third chef, Walter, who is from the Navajo Nation. The purpose of interviewing these chefs was twofold: first, the interviews made it possible for the research to assess multigenerational perceptions of traditional foods and second, the interviews helped to establish the ideological differences between Native American culinary students and seasoned Indigenous chefs.

Finally, to complete my research, I conducted participant observation with the culinary students during their final semester in the culinary program. During this observation, I asked the students to prepare several recipes that I had preselected from *Foods of the Southwest Indian Nations* (Frank 2002), asking the students to explain their choices in the kitchen, especially if they elected to deviate from the recipes.

It should also be noted that throughout the research process for my thesis, I was consistently considering my positionality by being reflexive of my research and the trends that I was seeing, not only in the literature but also in the interviews and observations with the culinary students and chefs (Palaganas et al. 2017; Watt 2007). As a Caucasian woman of European descent working on a graduate thesis in anthropology, I was fully aware of past research transgressions that have contributed to an overall wariness within Indigenous communities of Western research (Cochran et al. 2008). I was painfully aware of my privilege, especially as I was actively engaging in the troupe of studying a marginalized group (McCorkel and Myers 2003). I had no desire to come across as a "White savior" and was concerned that my discussions with Indigenous culinary students and chefs would be construed as such, especially since my research would be published as a thesis. I was also concerned that individuals would feel as though this research was appropriating Indigenous foods, culture, and voices. While this research was designed and framed using Western theories, I wanted this research to reflect the voices of the individuals that I interviewed and therefore I have elected to focus primarily on the direct quotes from the research participants.

Given this, it was determined to shape my data collection and analysis through the use of decolonizing methodologies and Indigenous Ways of Knowing (IWOK). Within Indigenous studies, there is a movement toward decolonizing methodologies; this movement primarily seeks to transition who is responsible for the dominant discourses surrounding Indigenous research (Tuhiwai Smith 2012). As a result, decolonizing methodologies offer an opportunity for researchers and community members alike to critique the roles of power and dominant culture in establishing narratives. Similarly, IWOK acknowledges the importance of Indigenous knowledge, especially when addressing issues such as colonization, structural racism, and health disparities. IWOK encourages the active participation of Indigenous communities within Western research and in doing so, recognizes the merit of epistemologies that may differ from Western scientific thinking (Cochran et al. 2008; Simonds and Christopher 2013).

COMMODITY FOODS AND THE CONTINUING COLONIZATION OF NATIVE AMERICANS

Today, Native American communities are facing a food crisis, brought about by colonization and the dietary changes which followed, namely the increased consumption of processed foods and the decreased consumption of healthy, land-based foods (Rudolph and McLachlan 2013). According to Mirsky (1981), numerous factors contribute to this change in food habits. These factors are defined by Mirsky (1981, 130) as "impersonal forces," and can include life-altering changes, such as cultural contact, urbanization of an area, and technological change. Other forces of dietary change are nondirected forces – neither planned nor directed; these forces include the delocalization of food and economic forces, such as industrialization, which have shaped agricultural practices and food consumption in the SW (Kuhnlein and Receveur 1996).

Many of the culinary students that I spoke to were familiar with their traditional foodways, having grown up on the dishes that their parents and grandparents cooked. Yet despite the attempts of Native Americans to maintain traditional foods throughout the generations, there are still purveying issues of continued acculturation and colonization of Native American populations. Pedro described this continuing acculturation and colonization not as a blatant force, but rather inconspicuous oppression:

> I always feel like maybe there was some type of cuisine that we did eat, like a lot that was traditional and stuff, but it's just like, maybe we have it a little bit, but it's more just the way we've been colonized. And maybe we've lost our traditional foods, our, what we used to eat and how we used to prepare it. Everything was just so different.

By using commodity foods and Western ingredients, the diets that Native Americans are consuming have been evolving, moving more toward a Western diet. As George lamented, "When you look at traditional food then to now, everything's so Westernized, with Westernized ingredients!" The Westernization of the diet has affected the culinary teachings of the students, making it so that in some cases, they did not grow up learning how to prepare traditional foods. For other students, the move toward a Western diet was ironic, given that many of the foods consumed by early settlers in America were provided to them by Native Americans. Loujuana explained,

> I think traditional foods are really important due to the fact that when the settlers first came here, they didn't know what to do with the land, they didn't know how to grow their food, and that's what our people had, what they did for them. We gave them that knowledge and we still have that knowledge to this day and we're still here. I mean, we helped a whole different race have a sustainable life here on our land. That's quite amazing. We helped them grow their food and everything, and here we are, still, a hundred years later, still growing the same foods and making the same traditional foods. We're still strong. There's some things that have been modified in time, but that's just time, working its way.

While Native Americans want to consume healthier foods, the continued presence of Western and American foods, including "fast" and "junk" foods, pose challenges to Indigenous health and well-being (Kuhnlein et al. 2006; Lombard et al. 2014; Milburn 2004; Whiting and Mackenzie 1998). These impacts include smoking, alcohol abuse, decreased physical activity, increased stress, and an increase in health issues, such as obesity, diabetes, and cardiovascular disease (Jernigan et al. 2020; Kuhnlein and Receveur 1996; Redwood et al. 2009). These health issues, as well as others, relate to the "three chronicities of modernity:" inactivity, overconsumption of calories, and chronic psychological stress (Wiedman 2012, 603). The overconsumption of calories often directly relates to a poor diet, especially when the diet consists of processed foods, fatty meats, and poor access to fresh fruits and vegetables (Conti 2006).

FOOD SYSTEMS AND HEALTH DISPARITIES IN SW NATIVE AMERICANS

Given the health issues faced by Native Americans, locally initiated programs seek to combat the issues at hand. Some key programs include the Tohono O'odham Community Action (TOCA) program and the Hawaii Diet™ program, both of which focus on the consumption of Indigenous foods as a method for managing diabetes (Fazzino 2008; Hoover and Mihesuah 2019; Nabhan 2004). Meanwhile, another program, the Inter-Tribal Bison Cooperative, seeks to reintroduce bison on reservation lands, thereby encouraging the consumption of traditional foods while also striving for food sovereignty (Lulka 2006). More recently, the Navajo Nation formed the Diné Community Advocacy Alliance (DCAA), which utilizes grassroots-level community health advocacy to address obesity, diabetes, and other chronic health conditions within the community (Livingston 2019). Through programming and activism, the DCAA was able to pass the Healthy Diné Nation Act of 2014, which implemented the Unhealthy Foods 2% Sales Tax. The revenue from the additional sales tax placed on preidentified processed and unhealthy foods has helped to fund community health programs for exercise and recreation, health education, and community food and water initiatives, among others (Livingston 2019).

Historically, many of these community food programs did not address the historical and racist causes of food insecurity and hunger among Native American populations (Rudolph and McLachlan 2013). The racially based policies that systematically deprived Native Americans of their land, forced tribes to relocate, and led to the extermination of tribal culture through forced acculturation all shaped disparities in food access (Loh et al. 2020; Odoms-Young 2018; Washington and Williams 2019). Many of these policies continue to shape food access, determining where supermarkets are located and influencing which foods are stocked by local grocery stores (Jernigan et al. 2012; Reese 2018). These inequities in food access are indicative of the burden of disease among Native Americans; as such, while they are identifiable, they are difficult to combat. As Adelson (2005, S58) notes, those who are the poorest, the most disempowered, and the sickest are oftentimes engaged in a constant struggle to change or remove themselves from their circumstances. Unfortunately, this is not always possible because of the internalization of hegemonic influences; in the case of Native American populations, health disparities reflect generations of historical trauma and persistent inequality shaped by structural racism (Adelson 2005; Reese 2018).

Public health interventions recommended for the majority of diet-related health issues were typically based on Western or allopathic biomedicine and were often imposed upon populations, with very little regard or attention to the needs of the population in question (Adelson 2005). For instance, the foods provided by food assistance programs (e.g., FDPIR) have historically consisted of unhealthy, processed foods that lack cultural relevance (Dwyer 2010; Lulka 2006; Vantrease 2013). As a result, these programs reproduced colonial power structures, making it difficult to address the root cause of the health disparities (Rudolph and McLachlan 2013). However, as public health practitioners have learned, incorporating IWOK and other decolonizing epistemologies within such public health education programs is imperative, as Indigenous communities deserve to have culturally relevant and appropriate interventions (Cochran et al. 2008; Simonds and Christopher 2013).

These solutions are imperative to addressing health disparities within Native American communities, especially when considered within the context of the UN SDGs to promote well-being (SDG 3) and reduce inequality within countries (SDG 10). Until the policies and structures that promote these health inequities within Native American communities are addressed, poverty (SDG 1) and food insecurity (SDG 2) will continue to persist, contributing to the continuing colonization and oppression of Indigenous populations.

The lasting implications of historical trauma and structural racism are reflected in Native American cuisine today. Frybread, which is recognized by many to be a traditional food, despite its link to colonization, serves as a prime example of the hegemonic relationship between food and culture. As Pedro exclaimed, "You know everybody thinks that like, traditional foods, that they just say right away, 'Frybread.' Boom! That's traditional food. But it's more like, that's all people had to eat." For a majority of the culinary students, frybread is a complex food because it has cultural significance and is also a symbol of the colonization of their people. While seen as a universal food today, fry bread was introduced into the Native American diet after the introduction of wheat flour as a commodity (Smith and Wiedman 2001). As a result, fry bread is often viewed in relation to commodity foods, which causes disruptions to traditional diets. Loujuana explained,

> I was thinking about, [...] how frybread helped us go throughout long journeys, but another thing that brought up to my mind was commodity food. Like some of our traditional foods have been replaced with things that I see as commodity food because I grew up with that food. But we also learned how to manage with that, make things that we used to make with that. And some recipes would just change consistently.

Often served at gatherings and festivals, frybread is recognized by many as a traditional food consumed by many Native Americans (Smith and Wiedman 2001). However, in reality, the conceptualization of fry bread as a traditional food is a complex cultural issue. According to Vantrease (2013, 55), "The flat discs of fried dough were created roughly 150 years ago, with ingredients and implements – wheat flour, lard, and steel pots – introduced by Europeans and provided by the U.S. government."

As a result, frybread reflects government dietary assimilation efforts in the United States, making it a complex, conflicted food symbol, one that still, to this day reflects the continuing, but hidden, power of colonization. However, fry bread also continues to be an important cultural food, born out of political consciousness.

While "fry bread came about as a necessity to keep Indian people alive in times of starvation," (Vantrease 2013, 58) fry bread also operates as a counter-hegemonic symbol, empowering Native Americans, as it stimulates an ethnic pride within communities because it represents a cultural tradition that emerged at a time when Native Americans lost so much. According to Wendland (2010, 201–202), counter-hegemonic movements arise out of a "contradictory consciousness," which often seek to make possible meaningful political change. In this sense, the continuing practice of cooking fry bread is one of embodiment and practice, in which Native Americans still struggle to appropriate the "white man's" food and make it their own. Fry Bread may have not been created with the express intent to counter the colonization efforts of the time, but the continued perseverance and popularity of the dish today certainly seems to indicate a more conscious understanding of the complex hegemony at play.

However, as scholars have argued, the continuing consumption of frybread and subsequent use of flour is a contentious discussion within Native American communities. On one hand, the use of flour indicates a continuing legacy of colonization, reflecting the days when government-issued foods were the only foods available to Indigenous populations (Vantrease 2013). As Anjalene pointed out, the adaptation of frybread was necessary for survival and as such, continues to play an important role in her tribe's culture and traditions:

> Everybody eats fry bread, although it's made with flour that was given to us, it's considered sacred food because it helped along a lot of tribes during their long walks. So, it's considered to have a lot of cultural significance now, because it played an important role. So, I think it has to do a lot with what sustained us during the hard times, because a lot of the times, that's what sort of gave us our defining moments.

On the other hand, as Mihesuah (2016) argues, the fried flour continues to colonize Indigenous bodies and populations today, contributing to the rising rates of chronic diet-related diseases, such as obesity and type II diabetes, while simultaneously threatening food sovereignty and making it difficult for populations to "decolonize" their diets.

RECLAIMING HEALTH AND WELL-BEING

In the instance of food sovereignty, decolonizing methodologies work as a counter to the hegemonic influence of colonialism and more recently, neoliberalism. In the past decades, neoliberalism has been utilized to explain the shifts within the economy. Alkon and Mares (2012, 348) define neoliberalism as "the political economic philosophy that asserts the primacy of the market in attending to human needs and well-being and reorients the state towards the facilitation of market mechanisms." This places the responsibility for well-being on the individual, regardless of the other influences that may have affected the ability for the individual to remain healthy.

For Native Americans, neoliberalism has only served to continue the perpetuation of colonization, as the current policies shaping the food system have largely restructured the ways in which Indigenous populations are able to select culturally relevant foods, thereby shaping their daily dietary choices (Alkon and Mares 2012; Caraher and Coveney 2004).

As a countermovement, food sovereignty shifts beyond the provisioning of food to inequalities of land distribution, resource management, and the commodification of food crops (Mares and Alkon 2011). As such, the counter frame to the corporate food regime occurs on two levels: first, Native Americans must be actively and consciously aware of their role, and second, Native Americans must also be able to make use of their role within the realm of food sovereignty (Fairbairn 2012). Today, many Native Americans understand the counter-hegemonic potential of food sovereignty. The movements deployed often move beyond agriculture, focusing on a resurrection of traditional foods while also emphasizing locally sourced and culturally appropriate foods (Grey and Patel 2014).

The chefs that I interviewed focused on the incorporation of traditional foods in the cuisine as a primary element of their culinary styles, utilizing their positions as chefs to improve food sovereignty for Native populations. For Claudia, Walter, and Lois, this incorporation allowed them to highlight traditional foods in their dishes while simultaneously raising awareness about these ingredients and Native dishes for their clients who may be unfamiliar with these foods. Lois and Walter, who run a catering company, incorporate Indigenous techniques into their catering menu, as Lois explained,

> And so, here's process – an ancient technique, right? Archaeologists found all these pottery shards and they're like, 'Wow! Native cooks were really sloppy.' No… They didn't break their pots. This is what they did. Took food, wrapped it in corn husk, wrapped it in clay, sealed the clay, put the clay in ash or the oven, broke it open, there's the shards, and ate it. So, all I'm doing is this ancestral technique and serving it new. There are the ingredients. Wild rice, greens, river trout. There it is. So old, that's new. Alright? So, my culinary training allows me to say okay, I know how it was done thousands of years ago. Could we cook it in a fire? Sure! Is that practical in a situation where I'm serving hundreds of people? Not necessarily. So, let's use modern, we can turn the oven up to 500, put all these things in there, crack it open, serve it. And we do it. We have classes at the cooking school, we do it for events, we do it here, we do it everywhere! And so, you can take this old, and you can… I'm a chef, I'm trained, I know what I'm doing, and I can implement that. And then, here it is. Old, look, it's new. Amazing! Right?

For Lois, a large part of her culinary style relies on making people aware of Native American cuisine, highlighting its richness and diversity. Lois' cuisine emphasizes the "magic eight," which are corn, beans, squash, chile, tomatoes, potatoes, chocolate, and vanilla. Each of these ingredients was brought from the New World to the Old World, and as a result, became prominent elements of European and Asian culinary styles. As Lois explained,

> So, think about these plants for a minute and what… Italian, tomato. Asian, chile. Corn, beans, and squash didn't exist. None of these, none of these. No French chocolate. No…

> And these two sisters always go together. Look at every dessert recipe. What do you add? Vanilla and chocolate. They work together. Irish potato. English fish and chips. Russian potato, Russian vodka. Look at how these changed Old World.

However, Lois' culinary style is not just influenced by the traditional foods that she uses. She also considers how Native cuisine can be used to help others. As she explained,

> And it's helping Native people find their own voice. It's battling obesity, its battling type 2 diabetes, and it's also serving delicious, amazing, beautiful Native food to corporate clients. And taking that and working with a lot less in Native communities, and so being a chef is about serving food, about feeding people, about nurturing, about life, about serving Native foods.

Each chef's culinary style also serves to increase awareness of traditional foods within the general public. As Claudia explained,

> We are not in the dark and many of us have podcasts, blogs, use social media platforms, create decolonizing curriculum, participate in community events and talks to spread the word and share the ancestral wisdom. What I do mostly see and have witnessed time and time again, is being able to raise and increase awareness through the production of food, which is really the production of ancestral knowledge that becomes plated to tell a story. One that embodies resilience, culture, tradition, and teaches lessons of health, food, and flavor.

For Walter, it's the ancestral knowledge that is especially important, because the knowledge of traditional foods is not always passed down through the generations, which leads to a loss of knowledge. This loss of knowledge can lead many to feel lost in life, which can then lead to social issues. Walter described the situation,

> You know it's always good with kids, they teach us, we become their students and they teach us. You know, you pass down to them. If you don't pass anything down, your grandma and grandpa didn't pass anything down to me, where would I have been? That's the question I was asking this morning when I was laying and I was like, huh… How did I get here? And the time you ask yourself questions, where did I came from, before? What am I here for? What is it? Which direction am I going? […] Because we've got problems on our reservation, alcohol, at the time. Now it's drugs, now it's both, today. So, it's, you know, and we try to encourage the little ones, and the older ones, and the unfortunate ones, my heart goes out to them, you know.

Lois and Walter both enjoy using their positions to give back to the community, from feeding the homeless to working on diabetes prevention within communities. Lois is certified with the CDC as a diabetes educator and is currently writing a curriculum for Native American communities to teach cooks, community health workers, and community members how to cook simple, healthy meals. In many instances, Lois explained, such action is needed because people have lost sense of who they are as a culture, and as such, have lost the foods as well:

> I think Native communities, in some instances the cord was broken. How do you do this? Well, let's re-fix that cord, let's repair it. Sort of like a violin string. You can still play the violin with only, what are there four? Four or five… Maybe six. Alright, let's say there's six strings, and one is broken. You can still play it, but it doesn't quite work. But we can repair it.

Chef Bailey voiced a similar concern, reflecting on his role as an educator for the younger generation of Native Americans. Though the culinary program at SIPI was meant to be a stepping stone to a fruitful career, Chef Bailey explained how he thought the program could be so much more:

> This generation, they feel broken, they feel lost, they feel no pride. They don't communicate with anyone, not even themselves. And one of the things that I work very hard and very diligently on is getting them to realize that they are somebody, and they are somebody that has something to offer. And if they can walk out of here with their head held high, and believe in themselves, and believe that they have every ability and every tool that they can use to find whatever the answer may be, that's all that matters. It doesn't matter what they do for a living. It matters that they believe in themselves. That's what my program is about. It's not about food, it's about a person.

In addition to placing an emphasis on the person and helping his students develop a better understanding about themselves, Chef Bailey spends a great deal of time honing skills that will be useful in multiple facets of daily life for the students:

> I could care less if they stay in food or if they're doing something else. What I want them to take away from the program, is that they learned how to think critically, they learned how to do for themselves, they've learned how to work as a team, but rely on their own knowledge, that they have the ability to find the answer. I want them to realize and take away that they're an adult and they're capable and they're proud. I think that's the most important thing, that they walk away knowing they are whole, you know.

RECLAIMING FOOD SOVEREIGNTY IN A CHANGING CLIMATE

Despite the growing support for food sovereignty within Native American communities, there are still major challenges that need to be overcome, especially in today's political and economic climate. While this research did not directly address the concerns of managing food security and population health amidst climate change, the implications of climate change were implicitly discussed by all. Claudia and Walter both discussed the importance of adhering to a plant-based diet, which they argued was a healthier option for Native American communities and the environment. Walter credits the interest in traditional foods to the growing health issues, among both Native and non-Native Americans. As he explained, many of today's health concerns among Native Americans were caused by the commodity foods on the reservations but going back to a plant-based diet has its benefits, both culturally and physically.

This emphasis on a plant-based and organic diet also ties the future of traditional foods to the future of sustainable foods, as many Native American chefs work to incorporate organic and sustainably raised foods. For Lois, one of the most important components of this relationship is supporting Native American farmers who are practicing sustainable agriculture. In addition to knowing where her ingredients come from, Lois is proud to support Native-owned and Native-operated farms. She explained her reasoning,

> I buy hand-harvested wild rice from tribes in Minnesota and Wisconsin and are Native owned and Native operated and I'm paying wholesale, $10.80 a pound. And most other chefs in restaurants go, "How can you do that?" Because I am playing a role. I buy something that's Native, I perpetuate them going out on the canoes, in the boat, to harvest the rice, to keep the environment safe, to keep the tribe economically viable. Yeah. I've no problem paying that. That's what it costs.

The cost, as Lois pointed out, is one of the key determinants for many chefs. Whereas some chefs may choose to purchase conventionally produced ingredients, Lois believes that the consumer pays for these items in more ways than one, explaining,

> We always have the metaphor [that] food is our medicine. That's Native. And what happened? When you drive up to a window and you order a number six, is that food is our medicine? No. What happened? The commodification, greed, corporations… And I'm not anti-science, I'm pro-science. Genetically modifying things to make money, not for the well-being of the planet, of the world? That's not Native!

Lois continued, emphasizing the importance of using higher-quality ingredients, even if it means having smaller portions. She purchases sustainably raised meat, including elk and bison. While these ingredients are more expensive, Lois feels that they make a difference, both for consumers and producers. While the portions may be smaller, they are of higher quality, and more importantly, they adhere to Lois's philosophy of "buying Native, supporting Native."

In the future, buying Native foods and supporting Native communities may prove to be more difficult due to climate change. Researchers have cautioned for years that warming temperatures threaten the wild rice harvests for Native American communities in the Midwest (Hersher 2018; Lynn et al. 2013). Given the relatively short growing season for rice, rising temperatures threaten to cut the growing season even shorter while also creating new competition for rice as other plants begin to flourish in the warmer waters (Hersher 2018). These factors all lead to troubling trends for wild rice harvests and consumption, as the decreases in the availability of wild rice threaten the traditional food systems that rely on these foods (Lynn et al. 2013). Given this, the agricultural practices within traditional food systems present a solution to meeting the UN SDGs, providing avenues for the sustainable production and consumption of foods (SDG 12), while simultaneously protecting the diversity of local ecosystems (SDG 14 and 15).

As the climate continues to change, food systems and food sovereignty are consistently at risk of deterioration on a global scale (Powys Whyte 2019). This is due to the way that climate change affects growing seasons; there may come a time where a majority of foods are no longer able to be grown because the climate is no longer conducive to the practice (Lynn et al. 2013). This would affect access to food for several populations; however, numerous Indigenous and scientific reports identify Indigenous populations as one of the populations that will suffer the most from climate change (Powys Whyte 2019). This access would be especially hindered if it were a crop that was exported on a global scale, such as the quinoa is from Bolivia (Walsh-Dilley 2013). Such a restriction to access could affect diet, potentially rendering work done with traditional food systems as useless.

IMPACTS OF COVID-19 ON NATIVE AMERICAN FOOD SECURITY

In light of the COVID-19 pandemic, it is important to consider the lasting impacts that this global crisis will have on Native Americans, not only in terms of epidemiology but also in relation to food security. As Lakhani (2020) notes, when Native Americans first heard of the pandemic, they wasted no time in preparing for the novel virus. As history has taught us, diseases have been used by European colonizers as a way to colonize and purposely kill more than 70% of the populations who were Indigenous to North America. Data from Native American tribes demonstrate that their initial concerns about COVID-19 were well-founded, with the Navajo Nation having an infection rate of 2,680 cases per 100,000 people, the Pueblo of Zia having an infection rate of 3,319 per 100,000 people, and the Pueblo of San Felipe having an infection rate of 3,301 per 100,000 people (Akee 2020; Lakhani 2020). It should also be noted that the latter two tribes have small populations: 934 people in the Pueblo of Zia and 3,544 people in the Pueblo of San Felipe (Lakhani 2020).

Unfortunately, these disproportionately high rates of COVID-19 are likely linked to historical inequities and health disparities. For instance, Native American households are 3.7 times more likely to lack complete indoor plumbing than other households in the United States. In addition, many of the tribal businesses that support communities have been closed in hopes of reducing COVID-19 infection rates. Unfortunately, these businesses are the very same sources of income that help fund tribal health clinics and community programs (Mineo 2020). Moreover, diabetes has been identified as a potential COVID-19 risk factor and Native Americans are three times more likely to be diagnosed with diabetes than their white counterparts (Akee 2020).

The effects of COVID-19 will undoubtedly continue to compound, especially when considered within the context of Native American food security. COVID-19 has had a multi-directional ripple effect throughout the food system, shaping the ways in which food is supplied and consumed (Heuer et al. 2020; UN 2020). Ultimately, these ripple effects are also impacting food security, especially with the rising rates of unemployment and other associated economic constraints (UN 2020). Prior to the pandemic, an estimated 14.3 million American households were food insecure; however, after the pandemic, it is estimated that an additional 17.1 million individuals experienced food insecurity (Feeding America 2020; Siddiqi et al. 2020).

The effect of food insecurity within Indigenous communities during the pandemic is even more profound, given that many Native Americans reside in food deserts and grocery stores have frequently been bare during the pandemic (Simms Hipp 2020). Fortunately, Native Americans, like many others, were able to turn toward cultivating their own foods in their communities. Programs such as the Seeds and Sheep program in the Navajo Nation were launched to not only address concerns about food insecurity, but to also continue to strive toward food sovereignty (Ortiz 2020). While it is difficult to say what the future holds for Native Americans in the wake of the COVID-19 pandemic, one thing is certain. The continued historical legacy of colonization and racism is still shaping the health of Native Americans today and will likely compound the ways in which COVID-19 shapes food security for Native Americans.

THE FUTURE OF TRADITIONAL FOOD SYSTEMS

Fortunately, despite the challenges to food security and food sovereignty in Native American communities, traditional foods have a very bright future, thanks in large part to the growing number of Native American chefs. While these aforementioned disruptions to Native American cultural and culinary practices have impacted how traditional foodways are shaped and maintained, these Indigenous food practices are experiencing a resurgence. Thanks to community efforts surrounding food sovereignty, Indigenous populations have been reconnecting with their traditional foodways in response to rising rates of obesity and type II diabetes, as well as growing concerns over a general lack of access to food, poverty, environmental degradation, pollution, and depletion of resources (FAO 2018, 2019; Hoover and Mihesuah 2019). This coupled with the growing food scene and interest in Indigenous foods has placed a greater spotlight on Native American cuisine in recent years. As a result, the future of Native American cuisine can continue to build on the momentum of current programs. Unfortunately, this momentum is not without its risks, as Claudia pointed out:

> I say that the future of Indigenous foods is stronger than ever before in the colonial history of food. It is strong and resilient and has finally felt safe to speak truth to power within the culinary world. My worry is that it will be appropriated by nonIndigenous chefs as a way to continue to erase the Native from the culinary scene, making it a hipster trend. I would not want to see this for all the lessons, teachings, and stories will be lost in translation. However, witnessing the rise of Native chefs, I feel that Indigenous cuisine will be more respected and that community members may begin to re-center these foods in their household kitchens.

For students who are just embarking on their culinary journey, working within the realm of Native American cuisine can be daunting, but both Claudia and Lois believe that the students can learn how to do so by working with more seasoned Native American chefs. Lois recommended that Native American culinary students do their research, learning about who is working in the industry and to stay abreast about what is currently happening in the realm of Native American cuisine. She also stressed the importance of finding balance, stating,

> And realize you're trying to do, you're in two worlds. So, the non-Native world is fast and maybe they don't want to recycle, maybe they want to throw everything away and as you're starting out it's hard because you're scared, and you want to just do because you don't want to lose your job. But always try and keep what feels appropriate to you, your ethics, your values.

Claudia suggested working as a stagiaire with Native chefs, stressing the importance of learning the different tastes and techniques. She said, "There are many of us doing this work and can pass down culinary knowledge that has been granted to us through our culinary endeavors to re-indigenize and decolonize."

Lois also stressed the importance of not getting caught up on the idea of decolonizing, explaining,

> You know, everybody's like, "I'm going to decolonize!" Really? What does that mean? I'm speaking to you in English. How decolonized are we? You're in a Western setting, doing a Western graduate thesis. I'm in a Western kitchen. We're not going to completely decolonize. I'm not going to play that game and fool... Can I do a, so rather than say decolonize, I'm now of the genre, or of the movement where I'm just saying indigenize. We're not undoing, we're moving into indigenizing. So, it moves past the trauma, I think. It moves past the historical trauma; it moves into a positive realm. Indigenize. Cool. That's great.

While decolonizing the food systems is not entirely possible, re-indigenizing the food system certainly is, especially with Native American chefs bringing traditional foods to the forefront in the culinary world. By re-indigenizing cuisine, Native American chefs are not only bringing well-deserved and long overdue recognition to Native cuisine, but they are also revitalizing the culture and health of Native communities and people.

RECOMMENDATIONS

Moving forward, several approaches may be taken to address the intersections of Native American food security, food sovereignty, and health within the context of climate change. Using the 2030 Agenda for Sustainable Development, these recommendations may be linked to specific SDGs. First and foremost, food insecurity among Native Americans is intrinsically linked to SDG 1: end poverty in all its forms everywhere. As Bauer et al. (2012) noted, food insecurity among their study population on a rural reservation was correlated with high rates of poverty. Poverty not only decreases the ability of an individual or family to purchase food but also influences countless other barriers to food security, including the access that individuals have to healthy, affordable foods (Bauer et al. 2012; FAO 2019; Jernigan et al. 2020; Lombard et al. 2014; Pardilla et al. 2013; Sowerwine et al. 2019; Wiedman 2012).

Food security and food sovereignty are also linked to SDG 2: end hunger, achieve food security and improved nutrition, and promote sustainable agriculture. Given this, programs and policies aimed at addressing food security among Native Americans must begin incorporating healthier foods, especially within the commodity food assistance programs. In doing so, these programs would not only address the nutritional inferiority of commodity foods when compared to traditional foods (Companion 2008) but could also work within the community to provide cultural programs that reconnect communities to their ancestral foods and practices (Fazzino 2008; Hoover and Mihesuah 2019; Lombard et al. 2014; Lulka 2006).

Native American food insecurity has also been linked to diet-related chronic diseases (Bauer et al. 2012; Jernigan et al. 2017; Wiedman 2012), thereby connecting the issue to SDG 3: ensure healthy lives and promote well-being for all at all ages. Providing affordable, nutritious foods as part of food assistance programs would be beneficial to ensure the achievement of this goal. While FDPIR has made improvements to the program, more change is still needed to ensure that Native Americans have access to healthy, culturally relevant foods (Byker Shanks et al. 2015; Mucioki et al. 2018). Moreover, by addressing the connections between poverty, food insecurity, and health, strides would also be made to address SDG 10: reduce inequality within and among countries. As Gadhoke and Brenton (2017) note, United States' Indigenous populations tend to have proportionally higher health disparities than when compared to other ethnic groups in the United States; these health disparities are linked to the lasting historical trauma and inequalities that continue to be perpetuated by structural racism in the United States.

As the COVID-19 pandemic has clearly demonstrated, there are many vulnerable populations who have struggled because of the pandemic. As a result, social programs are needed that will extend protections for those individuals who are struggling with poverty, food insecurity, and chronic health disparities. As Cohen et al. (2020) have noted, food insecurity and poor health outcomes are often entwined in a cyclic outcome. Moreover, as Himmelgreen et al. (2020) have posited, food insecurity and diet-related chronic diseases often exacerbate one another, thereby contributing to poor health outcomes.

As the 2019 UN FAO report on food security and nutrition suggests, increasing economic opportunities for Indigenous populations is imperative to dietary diversity within communities. Moreover, Indigenous communities, along with other marginalized populations, are more likely to struggle financially during economic downturns and crises. Given these factors, the UN (2020) recommends expanding existing food security monitoring systems, ensuring that COVID relief packages reach populations that are the most vulnerable, and strengthening social protection systems. Within Native American communities, such recommendations would ensure that accurate data on food insecurity rates among individual tribes are recorded and would also help to address the structural inequalities that contribute to food insecurity on reservations.

Lastly, addressing Native American food insecurity links to SDG 12: ensure sustainable consumption and production patterns. Given how Indigenous populations in the United States have managed responsible environmental stewardship for generations, it stands to reason that the interweaving of food security and food sovereignty could allow for the resurgence of responsible food production and consumption patterns. Just as the Inter-Tribal Bison Cooperative succeeded in restoring ecological balance and food sovereignty to the participating tribes (Lulka 2006), similar initiatives could succeed with other core food sources. Such initiatives would also link to additional SDGs, as they would not only make it possible for populations to practice less intensive agricultural methods, thereby taking steps to address climate change (SDG 13) but would also make it possible to protect the ecological diversity below water and on land (SDGs 14 and 15, respectively) through the practice of responsible hunting, fishing, and harvesting practices. Moreover, re-investing in sustainable solutions would also help to ensure the stability of Indigenous food systems, thereby reducing risk for food insecurity, increasing food sovereignty, and also increasing resilience against fluctuations in the food supply chain.

While climate change poses a challenge to ensuring Indigenous food security and food sovereignty, Indigenous populations have repeatedly demonstrated their resilience through their efforts to revitalize and re-indigenize their traditional, ancestral foodways (Coté 2016; FAO 2018). However, as the 2018 UN FAO report on food security and nutrition notes, Indigenous populations have adapted to a variety of climates and as a result, have generations of knowledge that may be utilized to adapt to the changing climate. For instance, many of the traditional agricultural practices from the SW Pueblos may provide assistance for growing food in dry climates (Soleri and Cleveland 1993; Wall and Masayesva 2019). In doing so, Indigenous communities, including the SW Native American tribes, would be able to help ensure food security within their communities while also continuing their pursuit of food sovereignty in the midst of turbulent economic and climate changes.

REFERENCES

Adelson, N. (2005) The Embodiment of Inequity: Health Disparities in Aboriginal Canada. *Canadian Journal of Public Health* 96 (2): S45–S61.

Akee, R. (2020) How COVID-19 is Impacting Indigenous Peoples in the U.S. *PBS News Hour*, May 13, 2020. https://www.pbs.org/newshour/nation/how-covid-19-is-impacting-indigenous-peoples-in-the-u-s

Alkon, A. H. and T. M. Mares (2012) Food Sovereignty in US Food Movements: Radical Visions and Neoliberal Constraints. *Agriculture and Human Values* 29 (3): 347–359.

Bakker, B. M. (1999) Nourishing Gifts: Native and Traditional Foods of the Southwestern Pueblos. In *A People's Ecology: Explorations in Sustainable Living*, ed. G. Cajete, 21–52. Santa Fe: Clear Light Publishers.

Batal, M., L. Johnson-Down, J. C. Moubarac, A. Ing, K. Fediuk, T. Sadik, C. Tikhonov, L. Chan and N. Willows (2018) Quantifying Associations of the Dietary Share of Ultra-Processed Foods with Overall Diet Quality in First Nations Peoples in the Canadian Provinces of British Columbia, Alberta, Manitoba and Ontario. *Public Health Nutrition* 21 (1): 103–113.

Bauer, K. W., R. Widome, J. H. Himes, M. Smyth, B. Holy Rock, P. J. Hannan and M. Story (2012) High Food Insecurity and Its Correlates among Families Living on a Rural American Indian Reservation. *American Journal of Public Health* 102 (7): 1346–1352.

Byker Shanks, C., T. Smith, S. Ahmed and H. Hunts (2015) Assessing Foods Offered in the Food Distribution Program on Indian Reservations (FDPIR) Using the Healthy Eating Index 2010. *Public Health Nutrition* 19 (7): 1315–1326.

Caraher, M. and J. Coveney (2004) Public Health Nutrition and Food Policy. *Public Health Nutrition* 7 (5): 591–598.

Chee, V. A., E. Teran, I. Hernandez, L. Wright, R. Izurieta, M. Reina-Ortiz, M. Flores, S. Bejarano, L. U. Dào, J. Baldwin and D. Martinez-Tyson (2019) 'Desculturización,' Urbanization, and Nutrition Transition among Urban Kichwas Indigenous Communities Residing in the Andes Highlands of Ecuador. *Public Health* 176: 21–28.

Cleveland, D. A. (1998) Indian Agriculture, United States Agriculture, and Sustainable Agriculture: Science and Advocacy. *American Indian Culture and Research Journal* 22 (3): 13–29.

Cleveland, D. A., F. Bowannie, Jr., D. F. Eriacho, A. Laahty and E. Perramond (1995) Zuni Farming and United States Government Policy: The Politics of Biological and Cultural Diversity in Agriculture. *Agriculture and Human Values* 12 (2): 2–18.

Cochran, P. A. L., C. A. Marshall, C. Garcia-Downing, E. Kendall, D. Cook, L. McCubbin and R. M. S. Gover (2008) Indigenous Ways of Knowing: Implications for Participatory Research and Community. *American Journal of Public Health* 98 (1): 22–27.

Cohen, A. J., J. L. Rudolph, K. S. Thomas, E. Archambault, M. M. Bowman, C. Going, M. Heisler, T. P. O'Toole and D. M. Dosa (2020) Food Insecurity among Veterans: Resources to Screen and Intervene. *Federal Practitioner* 37 (1): 16–23.

Companion, M. (2008) *An Overview of the State of Native American Health Challenges and Opportunities*. Washington, DC: International Relief and Development.

Conti, K. M (2006). Diabetes Prevention in Indian Country: Developing Nutrition Models to Tell the Story of Food-System Change. *Journal of Transcultural Nursing* 17 (3): 234–245.

Coté, C. (2016) "Indigenizing" Food Sovereignty: Revitalizing Indigenous Food Practices and Ecological Knowledge in Canada and the United States. *Humanities* 5 (3): 57.

Cushing, F. H. (1920) *Zuni Breadstuff*. New York: Museum of the American Indian.

Dwyer, E. (2010) Farm to Cafeteria Initiatives: Connections with the Tribal Food Sovereignty Movement. National Farm to School Network, Urban & Environmental Policy Institute. http://www.farmtocafeteriacanada.ca/wp-content/uploads/2014/06/F2S-and-Tribal-Communities.pdf

Eschner, K. (2020) COVID-19 is Exposing Food Deserts around Native American Reservations. *Popular Science*. https://www.popsci.com/story/health/native-american-nations-coronavirus-food-security/

Fairbairn, M. (2012) Framing Transformation: The Counter-Hegemonic Potential of Food Sovereignty in the US Context. *Agriculture and Human Values* 29 (2): 217–230.

Fazzino, D. (2008) Continuity and Change in Tohono O'odham Food Systems: Implications for Dietary Interventions. *Culture & Agriculture* 30 (1–2): 38–46.

Feeding America (2020) The Impact of the Coronavirus on Food Insecurity. https://www.feedingamerica.org/sites/default/files/2020-04/Brief_Impact%20of%20Covid%20on%20Food%20Insecurity%204.22%20%28002%29.pdf

Ferguson, M., C. Brown, C. Georga, E. Miles, A. Wilson and J. Brimblecombe (2017) Traditional Food Availability and Consumption in Remote Aboriginal Communities in the Northern Territory, Australia. *Australian and New Zealand Journal of Public Health* 41 (3): 294–298.

Food and Agriculture Organization of the United Nations (2018) The State of Food Security and Nutrition in the World: Building Climate Resilience for Food Security and Nutrition. http://www.fao.org/3/i9553en/i9553en.pdf

Food and Agriculture Organization of the United Nations (2019) The State of Food Security and Nutrition in the World: Safeguarding against Economic Slowdowns and Downturns. http://www.fao.org/3/ca5162en/ca5162en.pdf

Frank, L. E. (2002) *Foods of the Southwest Indian Nations*. Berkley: Ten Speed Press.

Gadhoke, P. and B. P. Brenton (2017) Erasure of Indigenous Food Memories and (Re-)Imaginations. In *Food Cults: How Fads, Dogma, and Doctrine Influence Diet*, ed. K. Cargill, 205–218. Lanham: Rowman & Littlefield.

Grey, S. and R. Patel (2014) Food Sovereignty as Decolonization: Some Contributions from Indigenous Movements to Food System and Development Politics. *Agriculture and Human Values* 32 (3): 431–444.

Gurney, R. M., B. Schaefer Caniglia, T. L. Mix and K. A. Baum (2015) Native American Food Security and Traditional Foods: A Review of the Literature. *Sociology Compass* 9 (8): 681–693.

Hersher, R. (2018) Climate Change Threatens Midwest's Wild Rice, a Staple for Native Americans. *NPR*, August 7, 2018. https://www.npr.org/sections/thesalt/2018/08/07/632840187/climate-change-threatens-midwests-wild-rice-a-staple-for-native-americans

Heuer, J. N., G. R. Lehigh, K. Díaz Serrano, N. Romero-Daza and D. Himmelgreen (2020) Food Access in the Time of COVID-19: Reflections on the U.S. Food System During a Pandemic. *Practicing Anthropology* 42 (4): 13–17.

Himmelgreen, D., N. Romero-Daza, J. Heuer, W. Lucas, A. A. Salinas-Miranda and T. Stoddard (2020) Using Syndemic Theory to Understand Food Insecurity and Diet-Related Chronic Diseases. *Social Science & Medicine* 295: 113124. https://doi.org/10.1016/j.socscimed.2020.113124

Hoover, E. and D. A. Mihesuah (2019) Introduction. In *Indigenous Food Sovereignty in the United States: Restoring Cultural Knowledge, Protecting Environments, and Regaining Health*, ed. D. A. Mihesuah and E. Hoover, 3–25. Norman: University of Oklahoma Press.

Jernigan, V. B. B., E. J. D'Amico, B. Duran and D. Buchwald (2020) Multilevel and Community-Level Interventions with Native Americans: Challenges and Opportunities. *Prevention Science* 21 (1): 65–73.

Jernigan, V. B. B., K. R. Huyser, J. Valdes and V. Watts Simonds (2017) Food Insecurity among American Indians and Alaska Natives: A National Profile Using the Current Population Survey–Food Security Supplement. *Journal of Hunger & Environmental Nutrition* 12 (1): 1–10.

Jernigan, V. B. B., A. L. Salvatore, D. M. Styne and M. Winkleby (2012) Addressing Food Insecurity in a Native American Reservation Using Community-Based Participatory Research. *Health Education Research* 27 (4): 645–655.

Kuhnlein, H., B. Erasmus, H. Creed-Kanashiro, L. Englberger, C. Okeke, N. Turner, L. Allen and L. Bhattacharjee (2006) Indigenous People's Food Systems for Health: Finding Interventions that Work. *Public Health Nutrition* 9 (8): 1013–1019.

Kuhnlein, H. V. and O. Receveur (1996) Dietary Change and Traditional Food Systems of Indigenous Peoples. *Annual Review of Nutrition* 16: 417–442.

Kuhnlein, H. V., O. Receveur, R. Soueida and G. M. Egeland (2004) Arctic Indigenous Peoples Experience the Nutrition Transition with Changing Dietary Patterns and Obesity. *The Journal of Nutrition* 134 (6): 1447–1453.

Lakhani, N. (2020) Why Native Americans Took COVID-19 Seriously: 'It's Our Reality.' *The Guardian*, May 26, 2020. https://www.theguardian.com/us-news/2020/may/26/native-americans-coronavirus-impact

Livingston, D. (2019) Healthy Diné Nation Initiatives: Empowering Our Communities. In *Indigenous Food Sovereignty in the United States: Restoring Cultural Knowledge, Protecting Environments, and Regaining Health*, ed. D. A. Mihesuah and E. Hoover, 173–185. Norman: University of Oklahoma Press.

Loh, I. H., Angela C. B. Trude, F. Setiono, L. Redmond, B. Jock and J. Gittelsohn (2020) Dietary Intake of Upper Midwest and Southwest Native American Adults. *Ecology of Food and Nutrition* 5: 1–20.

Lombard, K. A., S. A. A. Beresford, I. J. Ornelas, C. Topaha, T. Becenti, D. Thomas and J. G. Vela. (2014) Healthy Gardens/Healthy Lives: Navajo Perceptions of Growing Food Locally to Prevent Diabetes and Cancer. *Health Promotion Practice* 15 (2): 223–231.

Lulka, D. (2006) Bison and the Food Distribution Program on Indian Reservations. *Great Plains Research* 16: 73–84.

Lynn, K., J. Daigle, J. Hoffman, F. Lake, N. Michelle, D. Ranco, C. Viles, G. Voggesser and P. Williams (2013) The Impacts of Climate Change on Tribal Traditional Foods. *Climatic Change* 120 (3): 545–556.

Mares, T. M. and A. H. Alkon (2011) Mapping the Food Movement: Addressing Inequality and Neoliberalism. *Environment and Society: Advances in Research* 2: 68–86.

McAuley, C. and L. D. Knopper (2011) Impacts of Traditional Food Consumption Advisories: Compliance, Changes in Diet and Loss of Confidence in Traditional Foods. *Environmental Health: A Global Access Science Source* 1 (10): 55–60.

McCorkel, J. A. and K. Myers (2003) What Difference Does Difference Make? Position and Privilege in the Field. *Qualitative Sociology* 26 (2): 199–231.

Mihesuah, D. (2016) Indigenous Health Initiatives, Frybread, and the Marketing of Nontraditional "Traditional" American Indian Foods. *Native American and Indigenous Studies* 3 (2): 45–69.

Milburn, M. P. (2004) Indigenous Nutrition: Using Traditional Food Knowledge to Solve Contemporary Health Problems. *American Indian Quarterly* 28 (3/4): 411–434.

Mineo, L. (2020) For Native Americans, COVID-19 Is 'the Worst of Both Worlds at the Same Time.' *The Harvard Gazette*, May 8, 2020. https://news.harvard.edu/gazette/story/2020/05/the-impact-of-covid-19-on-native-american-ccommunities/

Mirsky, R. M. (1981) Perspectives in the Study of Food Habits. *Western Folklore* 40 (1): 125–133.

Mucioki, M., J. Sowerwine and D. Sarna-Wojcicki (2018) Thinking Inside and Outside the Box: Local and National Considerations of the Food Distribution Program on Indian Reservations (FDPIR). *Journal of Rural Studies* 57: 88–98.

Nabhan, G. P. (2004) *Why Some Like It Hot: Foods, Genes, and Cultural Diversity*. Washington, DC: Island Press.

Niethammer, C. (1974) *American Indian Cooking: Recipes from the Southwest*. Lincoln: University of Nebraska Press.

O'Dea, K. (1992) Diabetes in Australian Aborigines: Impact of the Western Diet and Life Style. *Journal of Internal Medicine* 232 (2): 103–117.

Odoms-Young, A. M. (2018) Examining the Impact of Structural Racism on Food Insecurity: Implications for Addressing Racial/Ethnic Disparities. *Family & Community Health* 41 (S2): S3–S6.

O'Meara, L., S. L. Williams, D. Hickes and P. Brown (2019) Predictors of Dietary Diversity of Indigenous Food-Producing Households in Rural Fiji. *Nutrients* 11 (7): 1629.

Ortiz, E. (2020) As the Coronavirus Pandemic Strains Supplies, Native Americans Fight Food Insecurity. *NBC News,* May 24, 2020. https://www.nbcnews.com/news/us-news/coronavirus-pandemic-strains-supplies-native-americans-fight-food-insecurity-n1213116

Osterkamp, L. K. and L. Longstaff (2004) Development of a Dietary Teaching Tool for American Indians and Alaskan Natives in Southern Arizona. *Journal of Nutrition Education & Behavior* 36 (5): 272–274.

Palaganas, E. C., M. C. Sanchez, V. P. Molintas and R. D. Caricativo (2017) Reflexivity in Qualitative Research: A Journey of Learning. *Qualitative Report* 22 (2): 426–438.

Pardilla, M., D. Prasad, S. Suratkar and J. Gittelsohn (2013) High Levels of Household Food Insecurity on the Navajo Nation. *Public Health Nutrition* 17 (1): 58–65.

Pindus, N. and C. Hafford (2019) Food Security and Access to Healthy Foods in Indian Country: Learning from the Food Distribution Program on Indian Reservations. *Journal of Public Affairs* 19 (3): e1876. https://doi.org/10.1002/pa.1876

Piya, L. and N. P. Joshi (2018) Food Basket of a Highly Marginalized Indigenous Community in the Mid-Hills of Nepal: Transition and Responsible Factors. Paper from the 30th International Conference of Agricultural Economists, Vancouver, B.C. https://ideas.repec.org/p/ags/iaae18/277071.html

Powys Whyte, K. (2019) Indigenous Climate Justice and Food Sovereignty: Food, Climate, Continuance. In *Indigenous Food Sovereignty in the United States: Restoring Cultural Knowledge, Protecting Environments, and Regaining Health*, ed. D. A. Mihesuah and E. Hoover, 320–334. Norman: University of Oklahoma Press.

Redwood, D., M. C. Schumacher, A. P. Lanier, E. D. Ferucci, E. Asay, L. J. Heizer, L. Tom-Orme, S. L. Edwards, M. A. Murtaugh and M. L. Slattery (2009) Physical Activity Patterns of American Indian and Alaskan Native People Living in Alaska and the Southwestern United States. *American Journal of Health Promotion* 23 (6): 388–395.

Reese, A. M. (2018) "We Will Not Perish; We're Going to Keep Flourishing": Race, Food Access, and Geographies of Self-Reliance. *Antipode* 50 (2): 407–424.
Robison, J. K. (1992) Agriculture and Economy at Acoma Pueblo, 1598–1821. Master's thesis, Department of History, University of Montana.
Rose, N. and I. Lourival (2019) Hegemony, Counter-Hegemony and Food Systems Literacy: Transforming the Global Industrial Food System. *Australian Journal of Environmental Education* 35 (2): 110–122.
Rudolph, K. R. and S. M. McLachlan (2013) Seeking Indigenous Food Sovereignty: Origins of and Responses to the Food Crisis in Northern Manitoba, Canada. *Local Environment* 18 (9): 1079–1098.
Sarkar, D., J. Walker-Swaney and K. Shetty (2019) Food Diversity and Indigenous Food Systems to Combat Diet-Linked Chronic Diseases. *Current Developments in Nutrition* 4 (S1): 3–11.
Sasaki, T. and J. Adair (1952) New Land to Farm: Agricultural Practices among the Navajo Indians of New Mexico. In *Human Problems in Technological Change*, ed. E. H. Spicer, 97–111. New York: Russell Sage Foundation.
Satterfield, D., L. DeBruyn, M. Santos, L. Alonso and M. Frank (2016) Health Promotion and Diabetes Prevention in American Indian and Alaska Native Communities—Traditional Foods Project, 2008–2014. *MMWR Supplements* 65 (1): 4–10.
Sherriff, S. L., L. Baur, M. G. Lambert, M. Dickson, S. J. Eades and S. Muthayya (2019) Aboriginal Childhood Overweight and Obesity: The Need for Aboriginal Designed and Led Initiatives. *Public Health Research & Practice* 29 (4): e2941925. http://dx.doi.org/10.17061/phrp2941925
Siddiqi, S. M., J. Cantor, T. Dubowitz, A. Richardson, P. A. Stapleton and Y. Katz (2020) Food Access: Challenges and Solutions Brought on by COVID-19. *RAND Blog*, March 31, 2020. https://www.rand.org/blog/2020/03/food-access-challenges-and-solutions-brought-on-by.html
Simms Hipp, J. (2020) Hunger in Native America and Our Resilient Response. *Food Research & Action Center*, June 1, 2020. https://frac.org/blog/hunger-in-native-america-and-our-resilient-response
Simonds, V. W. and S. Christopher (2013) Adapting Western Research Methods to Indigenous Ways of Knowing. *American Journal of Public Health* 103 (12): 2185–2192.
Smith, J. and D. Wiedman (2001) Fat Content of South Florida Indian Fry Bread: Health Implications for a Pervasive Native-American Food. *Journal of the Academy of Nutrition and Dietetics* 101 (5): 582–585.
Soares, G. H., F. C. de Almeida Carrer, M. G. Haye Biazevic and E. Michel-Crosato (2019) Food Transition and Oral Health in Two Brazilian Indigenous Peoples: A Grounded Theory Model. *Journal of Health Care for the Poor and Underserved* 30 (3): 1037–1052.
Soleri, D. and D. A. Cleveland (1993) Hopi Crop Diversity and Change. *Journal of Ethnobiology* 13 (2): 203–231.
Sowerwine, J., M. Mucioki, D. Sarna-Wojcicki and L. Hillman (2019) Reframing Food Security by and for Native American Communities: A Case Study among Tribes in the Klamath River Basin of Oregon and California. *Food Security* 11: 579–607.
Swentzell, R. and P. M. Perea (2016) *The Pueblo Food Experience Cookbook: Whole Food of Our Ancestors*. Santa Fe: Museum of New Mexico Press.
Tuhiwai Smith, L. (2012) *Decolonizing Methodologies: Research and Indigenous Peoples*. London: Zed Books.
United Nations (2020) Policy Brief: The Impact of COVID-19 on Food Security and Nutrition. https://www.un.org/sites/un2.un.org/files/sg_policy_brief_on_covid_impact_on_food_security.pdf
United States Department of Agriculture (2020) Food Distribution Program on Indian Reservations. https://fns-prod.azureedge.net/sites/default/files/resource-files/fdpir-program-fact-sheet-2020-for%20website.pdf

Vantrease, D. (2013) Commod Bods and Frybread Power: Government Food Aid in American Indian Culture. *Journal of American Folklore* 126 (499): 55–69.
Vlasich, J. A. (2005) *Pueblo Indian Agriculture*. Albuquerque, NM: University of New Mexico Press.
Waldman, C. (2006) *Encyclopedia of Native American Tribes*, 3rd Edition. New York: Checkmark Books.
Wall, D. and V. Masayesva (2019) People of the Corn: Teachings in Hopi Traditional Agriculture, Spirituality, and Sustainability. In *Indigenous Food Sovereignty in the United States: Restoring Cultural Knowledge, Protecting Environments, and Regaining Health*, ed. D. A. Mihesuah and E. Hoover, 209–222. Norman: University of Oklahoma Press.
Walsh-Dilley, M. (2013) Negotiating Hybridity in Highland Bolivia: Indigenous Moral Economy and the Expanding Market for Quinoa. *Journal of Peasant Studies* 40 (4): 659–682.
Washington, K. N. and D. E. Williams Jr. (2019) Using a Role-Driven Race Equity Reform Approach to Mitigate the Effects of America's History of Racism on Food Insecurity. *Professional Agricultural Workers Journal* 7 (1): 11–21.
Watt, D. (2007) On Becoming a Qualitative Researcher: The Value of Reflexivity. *Qualitative Report* 12 (1): 82–101.
Wendland, C. L. (2010). *A Heart for the Work: Journeys through an African Medical School*. Chicago, IL: University of Chicago Press.
White, L. (1973) *The Acoma Indians: People of the Sky City*. Glorieta: Rio Grande Press.
Whiting, S. J. and M. L. Mackenzie (1998) Assessing the Changing Diet of Indigenous Peoples. *Nutrition Reviews* 56 (8): 248–250.
Wiedman, D. (2012) Native American Embodiment of the Chronicities of Modernity: Reservation Food, Diabetes, and the Metabolic Syndrome among the Kiowa, Comanche, and Apaches. *Medical Anthropology Quarterly* 26 (4): 595–612.
Young, T. K. and S. B. Harris (1994). Risk of Clinical Diabetes in a Northern Native Canadian Cohort. *Arctic Medical Research* 53 (2): 64–70.

5 Food Insecurity and Resilience in a Rapidly Warming Arctic

Don Callaway

CONTENTS

DOI: 10.1201/9781003014942-5

INTRODUCTION

During the last decade, the North Slope Borough (NSB) has conducted three survey research efforts. Using an extensive 22-page questionnaire, information on a wide variety of topics is collected from a statistically significant number of households in the eight communities that constitute the NSB. These surveys have two major intents, one is to provide an accurate enumeration of the population, a key dimension of the NSB budget and the second is to provide accurate information for needs assessments as NSB departments seek support through grants and other proposals. This chapter selects a limited number of variables and topics from a much larger data set to understand the social, cultural, and economic context of Inupiaq households and how these factors plus the impacts of climate change on subsistence contribute to extremely high proportions of food insecurity (Callaway and Smith 2008).

BACKGROUND

Demography

Slightly over 8,000 individuals reside in eight communities on the NSB. Seven of these communities are small villages ranging in size from 261 to 749 individuals. These seven communities are, on average, over 85% of Inupiaq individuals. An eighth community Utqiagvik has slightly over 5,000 individuals about two-thirds of which are Inupiat. Utqiagvik is the central administrative, economic, and logistical hub of the North Slope Borough. In addition to these 8,000 residents, there are about 2,000 workers who commute and work at Prudhoe Bay (an enclave) and surrounding oil fields, mostly working a schedule of two or three weeks "on" (seven days per week) and two or three weeks "off" (usually commuting home to urban areas in Alaska, Texas, and all points south).

Food Insecurity

In general, 7.4% of households in the United States face "low food security" with an additional 4.9% facing more serious circumstances of hunger regarded as "very low food security." Thus, within the United States, 12.3% of households face some form of food insecurity. In contrast, 36%, or triple the proportion, of the Inupiaq households on the North Slope face some form of food insecurity.

This average proportion of 36% actually masks considerable variation between the communities. Communities One through Four, in the tables below, have about twice the food insecurity (41% to 22%) when compared to the other four communities. Communities "One" through "Four" will be briefly highlighted in the discussion and tables below and will be known as "highly" food insecure. In addition, community "One" and community "Three" will be singled out for a more detailed "case study" discussion. Community "One" is an interior community and highly dependent on land mammals, primarily caribou, while community "Three" is coastal and very dependent on marine mammals.

Subsistence Harvests

Subsistence is the harvest and sharing of natural resources and is practiced extensively among Inupiaq households within the NSB. In 2012, NSB Inupiaq households harvested an average of 155 kg usable weight of wildlife resources per person per year. The harvest broken down by resource category is – [16 kg fish, 35 kg land mammals, 81 kg marine mammals, and 5 kg birds/plants] (Fall 2016). The five coastal communities harvest and consume more marine mammals (seals, walrus, and whales) while the two interior communities harvest more land mammals (primarily caribou). In the four highly food insecure communities, these wildlife harvests comprised more than half the total diet of 70% of the Inupiaq households.

Poverty

About 10% of the households within the state of Alaska are below the poverty threshold. In contrast, 27% or nearly triple that proportion of Inupiaq households on the North Slope in 2018 were below the poverty limit. The four highly food insecure communities average 40% of their Inupiaq households below the poverty threshold, twice the average proportion of the remaining four communities. Inupiaq per capita income in the highly food insecure communities was about $12,500, three-fourths that of the remaining communities, and one-fourth of the U.S. average in 2018.

Employment

Adult male and female Inupiat that are in the labor force find it very difficult to obtain full-time employment. Communities One through Four range in size from 261 to 555 individuals of which about 87% are Inupiat. These extremely small communities have very limited opportunities for employment. Nearly all the available jobs are in the service sector and are provided by the North Slope Borough, the school district, and village corporations. Most of these jobs are filled by local Inupiat, supplemented in a few cases by nonlocals, mostly Anglo, who bring highly technical (and well-paying) skills such as engineering. In these small communities, everyone knows what few jobs are available and who occupies them. Lack of infrastructure, technical skills, raw materials, and distance from markets all generate against expanding the opportunity for local jobs. In fact, in a number of communities, young adults (and older individuals) often emigrate in the search for employment. This emigration often skews local population pyramids.

Full-time employment for Inupiaq adults in the workforce, for the highly food insecure communities, varies between 35%–54%, while the effective unemployment rate varies between 33% and 44%. Alaska in 2018 had the highest unemployment rate within the nation at 6.5%, this was mostly due to high rates of seasonal extraction work (e.g., commercial fishing) and the high rural unemployment documented above. Since most of the population in Alaska is concentrated in three urban areas, the rural unemployment is extraordinarily high. For the North Slope, unemployment is seven times the urban areas of Alaska and ten times the national average.

The two major reasons cited by Inupiaq respondents as to the reason for their unemployment are "couldn't find a job" (44%) and "family responsibilities (e.g., taking care of an elderly parent)" at about 20%. Interestingly conflicts between employment and the ability to engage in subsistence activities were only mentioned by 2% of respondents. This is probably because less than 2% of Inupiaq adults work for the oil industry. The oil industry's schedule of work would interfere with subsistence pursuits and this impediment plus a variety of other reasons leave this as an unlikely source of employment in the future.

Income

Despite the low employment figures the oil fields in Prudhoe Bay and its environs are an important source of income for Inupiaq households. Income to Inupiat flows from three main sources, including capital gains "taxes" on the oil field infrastructure to the local North Slope Borough in amounts of around $300 million per year. These monies are then used by the NSB to provide services (electricity, water, housing) and hire local Inupiat to deliver these services. Another source of income flows through the Arctic Slope Regional Corporation (ASRC), a regional corporation in which NSB Inupiat own shares. ASRC has revenues of over $2 billion per year money that comes through a wide variety of investments and services including providing a multitude of services to the oil fields. Each household of Inupiaq shareholders received an average of $22,000 in ASRC dividends for 2018. Finally, oil field revenues help to fuel the Alaska Permanent Fund Dividends (PFD), which are given each year to all Alaska residents and provide about $6,400 in 2018 to an average Inupiaq household of four persons.

In the four highly food insecure NSB communities, about 60% of Inupiaq household income is derived from dividends (Regional and Village Corporations and the PFD), while about 37% comes from wage income.

CLIMATE CHANGE THREATS TO MARINE AND TERRESTRIAL MAMMAL HARVESTS

In the last 60 years, the mean winter surface temperature in Alaska and Western Canada has increased by 3°–4° C. This is more than triple the change in average temperature at the equator. In addition, between 1968 and 1990, precipitation has increased by about 30%.

Status of the Arctic Sea Ice

The reduction of Arctic sea ice provides the most profound, iconic, and readily observable outcome of global warming. Measured in September, at the nadir of its extent, the Arctic ice cap has been reduced from nearly 12 million km^2 at the turn of the twentieth century to 4.15 million km^2 in 2019. This represents a reduction of 65% during the last 100 years with the majority of this reduction coming during the last decade.

Impacts of Sea Ice Reduction

Sea ice provides habitat for sea mammals and birds, and is the basis for the existing food chain in the Bering Sea. Walrus, especially females and pups, depend upon the retreating perimeter of the sea ice as a conveyor belt whose edge they ride northward as the margins of the sea ice melt throughout the summer months. The sea ice edge provides a special environment for the upwelling of nutrients within the water column. The ice edge also provides a platform for walrus as they dive to the sea bottom in search of crustaceans (clams and crabs) and other food. Walrus pup mortality has increased as Bering Sea researchers aboard boats report the crying of abandoned pups in open sea locations.

Walrus, seals, and bowhead whales are the major sources of food for marine mammal hunters. The retreating ice is causing difficulties in the harvesting of these species. All marine mammal hunters now assert that hunting in current ice conditions is far more dangerous. In addition, they must venture much further out from shore into deeper and rougher open waters. More boats are needed for safety reasons and those boats must be larger, with bigger engines that burn increasing amounts of fuel, which is itself experiencing rising prices. In short, marine mammal hunters now face decreasing levels of prey populations, which must be harvested in increasingly dangerous conditions, where the cost of these activities is sharply rising while the hunters are experiencing depressed economic conditions.

The impacts of climate change on terrestrial mammals such as caribou are detailed in the case study discussion of Community One. In general, tundra fires, an almost unheard of event, destroy enormous amounts of caribou graze. In addition, the northward expansion of less nutritious shrubby ecosystems diminishes caribou health. Finally, a changing climate has increased the impact of parasites and winter icing on calf survival (Winfree et al. 2014).

ARCTIC INDIGENOUS COMMUNITIES AND CLIMATE CHANGE

The traditional way of life in much of rural Alaska is at risk. Alaska Native villagers are undergoing a series of challenges related both to climate change and to deteriorating economic circumstances. Rapid climate change brings a multitude of physical impacts to villages from erosion, subsidence, floods, and storm surges that in some cases require significant emergency response efforts, massive investments in infrastructure, and full-scale community relocation. Other climate changes include shifts and dislocations of subsistence species, which has the potential to negatively impact traditional practices and diet. This, and is leading, in several prominent cases, to increased food insecurity and negative social, emotional, and physical health impacts. In addition, we are now entering a new age where fluctuations exist not in the components of an ecosystem but in the demise of entire ecosystems. Current marine mammals and tundra species may totally be gone in the next 50 years.

Current economic conditions include increasing unemployment, and decreasing flows of money and services to rural areas all coupled with spiraling increases in cost of living as rising energy prices preclude many households from heating their houses and/or purchasing the gas and technology needed for hunting and fishing. In addition, relocation of extended families and in some cases whole communities to urban areas may destroy traditional support networks.

Traditional Resilience Strategies

Two of the traditional adaptations to deal with environmental and subsistence uncertainty have been to

1. Have flexible harvest strategies and compensate for short falls in one resource type by harvesting more from other available resource categories.
2. Utilize social networks, which spread the risk from uncertainty, by sharing available subsistence harvests, technology, labor, and income widely within and between extended families.

One traditional strategy employed by Inupiat and others is to maintain a consistent amount of harvest in terms of pounds over time by varying the composition and proportion of those harvests on a year-to-year basis. In general, when one resource such as marine mammals becomes unavailable or inaccessible, harvesting more of another resource, e.g., caribou or white fish, tends to make up the shortfall (Magdanz, Utermohle, and Wolfe 2002). Climate change is already impacting marine mammals such as walrus and seal populations, which are already in sharp decline with the retreating Arctic ice cap, and caribou, as mentioned earlier, have already suffered a 50% decline. Thus, climate change presents a new, more encompassing threat, in that multiple subsistence resource categories may be at risk at the same time, although from different climate drivers. These impacts limit the opportunity within a community to ramp up the harvest of alternative species.

Resilience – Sharing through Extensive Social Networks

In general, the most substantial traditional practice to limit the risk of starvation involves a complex strategy of sharing harvests within and between extended families. This strategy has historically evolved into social networks that dynamically share and reciprocate subsistence resources, cash, and domestic labor (e.g., babysitting) relationships that exist within and between extended families. These transactions and relationships buffer Indigenous communities to change and scarcity, scarcity in the availability of subsistence species, scarcity in employment and wage work, and the vicissitudes of services delivered by state and federal entities. This strategy continues to be a mainstay, however, increased immigration, demographic dependencies, storm surges, flooding, melting permafrost, community relocation, and shrinking incomes may stretch these networks to the breaking point.

This chapter will primarily discuss the impacts of climate change on issues of food security for small, frontier, and remote (FAR), not connected by any road, communities in the NSB with additional material drawn from the Northwest Arctic Native Association (NANA) region. With two exceptions, the "hub" communities of Utqiagvik (Barrow) with about 5,000 residents and Kotzebue with about 3,500 residents. The small communities, on average, are more than 85% Alaskan Native (Inupiat) and range in size from 250 to 700 residents. Inupiaq households are composed of, on average, about four persons per household.

METHODS

During the last decade, the NSB has funded and conducted three extensive survey research projects (2010, 2015, and 2019) on the eight communities within the NSB – Anaktuvuk Pass, Atqasuk, Utqiagvik (formerly Barrow), Kaktovik, Nuiqsut, Point Lay, Point Hope, and Wainwright. Three reports from these survey efforts, "The 2010 [2015 & 2019] Economic Profile and Census" are derived from an extensive 22-page survey questionnaire. This questionnaire covers a variety of topics including – demography, housing, subsistence activities, health, employment, and income from a variety of sources and 22 questions on food security.

In 2019, the sample size was 1,083 households of which 870 (80%) were Inupiaq households, 143 were Caucasian (13%) with the remaining 7% of households being from a variety of other ethnicities. Sampling in the seven villages attempted to contact all households although effective response averaged about 85%. A 40% random sample was conducted in the largest community Utqiagvik (pop. 5,256). From this sample, the Standard Error of the Proportion was calculated to be +/–2.2%. (NSB 2015, 2019)

Interviews were conducted during a 3-month period from January to March 2019 and recall responses were requested for the 12-month period preceding the interview. Trained NSB residents conducted all survey interviews with translation into Inupiaq where appropriate. All responses were coded and the codes were entered in Excel spreadsheets, these spreadsheets then served as the basic input to two SPSS programs. One SPSS program consisting of approximately 340 variables contained all household information with each row of the data matrix representing one household. A second SPSS program contained demographic data where the data matrix consisted of one row per person.

FOOD SECURITY QUESTIONS

The 22 questions on food security used in this research were derived from extensive research on food security issues among small Alaska Native communities (ICCA 2015). This initial research compared actual amounts of food eaten by people with food insecurity measures. The report that summarized the Alaska research contains a detailed statistical analysis, based on Cronbach's alpha that reduced several variables on food insecurity into two major items. We used the Alaska analysis as the basis for these questions rather than the USDA series of questions.

Using the Alaska findings, we asked questions on two general topics – (a) levels of concern or worry about having enough food and (b) whether respondents in our research had actually experienced episodes where their family or family members, during the last 12 months had not eaten because they did not have any food. These two topics provided results very comparable to USDA categories of "low food security" and "very low food security." In addition, we used a number of follow-up questions to determine whether these insecurities arose from availability of subsistence resources or store-bought foods. Subsequent follow-up questions explored the potential reasons for lack of access to either resource. For example, for traditional resources questions were asked about availability of hunters, illness, lack of technology (boats, ATVs), lack of income for gasoline and ammunition, and most importantly, for the topic of this chapter, the abundance of local resources and the impacts of climate change. With respect to store-bought foods, questions were asked about income, employment, cost of living, availability of access to stores and market basket inventories for community stores, and so forth.

PRELIMINARY RESULTS AND COMPARISON TO U.S. NATIONAL PARAMETERS

Although concerns about healthy meals and the actual lack of any food are two separate questions, Table 5.1 is a crosstab of those two questions. Out of the 703 Inupiaq households for which we have comprehensive data on both measures, 209 (30%) Inupiaq households indicated that in the last 12 months, they had found it difficult to get food for healthy meals. Out of the same sample of 703 Inupiaq households, 153

TABLE 5.1
NSB 2019 – Cross-Tabulation "Last Year Were There Times Your Household Found It Difficult to Get Food for Healthy Meals?" By "Last Year Were There Times When Members of Your Household Did Not Have Enough to Eat?"

Inupiaq Households in Eight Communities of the North Slope Borough		HH Head – Health – Last Year Were There Times When Members of Your Household Did Not Have Enough to Eat?		Total
		Yes	No	
HH Head – Health – Last year were there times your household found it difficult to get food for healthy meals?	Yes	107	102	209
	No	46	448	494
Total		153	550	703

(22%) said that there were times during the last year when household members did not have enough to eat. One hundred and seven Inupiaq households responded "yes" to both questions.

As mentioned earlier, the "difficulty getting healthy meals" corresponds very closely with the USDA category of "low food security," while the "did not have enough to eat" corresponds with the more serious USDA classification of "very low food security." Within the United States, in general, the USDA categorizes 7.4% of American households as having "low food security."

As mentioned above, 30% of Inupiaq households within the NSB are similarly classified in the 2019 survey project, that is, Inupiaq families on the North Slope have four times the proportion of households facing "low food security." An additional 4.9% of U.S. households are classified as having "very low food security," this compares to 22% of Inupiaq households. In general, 12.3% of U.S. households face some form of food insecurity, whereas 36% (omitting overlaps, i.e., the 107 "yes/yes" responses) of Inupiaq households (triple the U.S. proportion) experience some form of food insecurity.

Table 5.2 has been organized so that the first four columns represent the four communities with the highest scores on the food insecurity measures (found on rows one and two). The first column in Table 5.2 contains the variable descriptions, e.g., "difficulty in obtaining food for healthy meals." The first two variable rows contain the two measures of food insecurity. It also has a number of variables asked of respondents as to the reasons why they have difficulty in obtaining healthy meals or why they have gone without meals. In addition, a number of measures of subsistence use, and economic indicators are provided. Each of the entries in the eight communities is limited to their "Yes" responses as reported as a percentage, although one variable, "have you been able to obtain all the traditional food you need" contains the percentage of "No" responses. Finally, two variables contain the average household and per capita income for Inupiaq households in U.S. dollars.

Table 5.3 takes all the responses and rank orders the response among the eight communities. So for the first question, has the respondent "found it difficult to get food for healthy meals?" Community Two with 47% of the respondents saying, "Yes" is ranked number "1." Community Three with 46% "Yes" responses has a proportional response that is within the Standard Error of the Proportion (2.2%) and thus is also given a rank of "1." Community One and Four at 36% and 35% respectively are given a rank of "2," while the remaining four communities (five through eight) have percentages close enough that they are all given the rank of "3." Similar (rough) rankings are then given on each variable for each community. Communities One and Three are the focus of the analysis since they represent the highest scores ("1" and "2") for the food insecurity measures.

The rank ordering for each variable is used to help to identify those attributes that are most highly explanative of the "food insecurity" measures. For example, Community Two (blue highlights), which is tied for the highest rank on the food insecurity measure "found it difficult to get food for healthy meals" ranks the highest (1) on the major reason for this being that respondents couldn't get "enough store-bought food" but has a very low rank (4) for lack of subsistence food as being a major impediment to obtaining healthy meals.

TABLE 5.2
Inupiat Households – Attributes of Food Insecurity

Inupiat Households Attributes of Food Insecurity		Community One	Community Two	Community Three	Community Four	Community Five	Community Six	Community Seven	Community Eight
		%	%	%	%	%	%	%	%
Found it difficult to get food ot healthy meals?	Yes	36%	47%	46%	35%	21%	24%	23%	21%
Members of your household did not have enough to eat?	Yes	36%	16%	26%	33%	19%	18%	20%	17%
Found it difficult to get food for healthy meals?	Yes	36%	47%	46%	35%	21%	24%	23%	21%
Healthy Meals – Because you couldn't get enough subsistence food?	Yes	47%	32%	41%	45%	60%	64%	56%	35%
Health Meals – Couldn't get enough store-bought food?	Yes	70%	88%	75%	59%	74%	83%	72%	47%
Members of your household did not have enough to eat?	Yes	36%	16%	26%	33%	19%	18%	20%	17%
Have you been able to obtain as much traditional food as needed?	No	27%	21%	37%	33%	12%	39%	10%	18%

(Continued)

TABLE 5.2 (*Continued*)
Inupiat Households – Attributes of Food Insecurity

Inupiat Households Attributes of Food Insecurity		Community One	Community Two	Community Three	Community Four	Community Five	Community Six	Community Seven	Community Eight
		%	%	%	%	%	%	%	%
Not get enough subsistence foods because – no active hunter?	Yes	20%	42%	46%	39%	54%	47%	33%	30.0%
Not get enough subsistence foods resources are not abundant?	Yes	45%	36%	55%	32%	40%	56%	50%	57%
Not get enough subsistence foods because climate change has affected harvesting?	Yes	65%	20%	65%	51%	45%	33%	71%	64%
Not get enough subsistence foods because – no snow machine or ATV?	Yes	25%	63%	55%	41%	52%	24%	33%	47%
% HH's depend on subsistence for half or more of their diet	%	78%	58%	68%	73%	57%	58%	80%	77%
Could not afford to purchase food?	Yes	43%	31%	45%	47%	30%	14%	31%	22%
Could not afford – had to pay bills	Yes	67%	93%	89%	92%	90%	86%	59%	80%

(*Continued*)

TABLE 5.2 (*Continued*)
Inupiat Households – Attributes of Food Insecurity

Inupiat Households Attributes of Food Insecurity		Community One	Community Two	Community Three	Community Four	Community Five	Community Six	Community Seven	Community Eight
		%	%	%	%	%	%	%	%
Could not afford to purchase food – food cost to much	Yes	71%	100%	88%	89%	88%	67%	50%	74%
Could not afford to purchase food – not enough income	Yes	70%	92%	76%	53%	81%	75%	55%	64%
Could not afford to purchase food – not working	Yes	48%	55%	56%	47%	69%	29%	59%	68%
% Wage income of total HH income	%	42%	34%	36%	35%	59%	56%	27%	47%
% Dividend income of total HH income	%	52%	60%	61%	62%	36%	41%	60%	46%
Ave. HH income	$	68,057	51,489	43,503	46,064	81,395	65,995	46,109	75,814
Per capita income	$	17,977	10,815	9,574	12,257	21,267	17,432	11,047	17,636
Household with income below the poverty guidelines	Yes	16%	50%	51%	39%	22%	24%	39%	16%

TABLE 5.3
Inupiaq Households in Eight North Slope Borough Communities: Levels of Food Insecurity Associated in Rank Order of Social and Economic Attributes

Inupiat Households – Attributes of Food Insecurity	Community One Rank	Community Two Rank	Community Three Rank	Community Four Rank	Community Five Rank	Community Six Rank	Community Seven Rank	Community Eight Rank
Found it difficult to get food for healthy meals? (% yes response)	2	1	1	2	3	3	3	3
Members of your household did not enough to eat? (% yes response)	1	5	2	1	4	4	3	4
Found it difficult to get food for healthy meals? (% yes response)	2	1	1	2	3	3	3	3
Healthy meals – because you couldn't get enough subsistence food? (% yes response)	3	4	3	3	1	1	2	4
Health meals – couldn't get enough store-bought food? (% yes response)	2	1	2	3	2	1	2	4
Members of your household did not have enough to eat? (% yes response)	1	5	2	1	4	4	3	4
Have you been able to obtain as much traditional food as needed? (% "no" 1 = highest)	2	3	1	1	5	1	5	4
Not enough subsistence foods because – no active hunter? (% yes response)	5	2	2	3	1	2	3	3

(Continued)

TABLE 5.3 (*Continued*)
Inupiaq Households in Eight North Slope Borough Communities: Levels of Food Insecurity Associated in Rank Order of Social and Economic Attributes

Inupiat Households – Attributes of Food Insecurity	Community One Rank	Community Two Rank	Community Three Rank	Community Four Rank	Community Five Rank	Community Six Rank	Community Seven Rank	Community Eight Rank
Not enough subsistence food resources are abundant? (% yes response)	2	3	1	3	2	1	1	1
Not enough subsistence foods – climate change has affected harvesting? (% yes response)	2	5	2	3	4	5	1	2
Not get enough subsistence foods because – no snow machine or ATV? (% yes response)	5	1	2	3	2	5	4	3
% HHs depend on subsistence for half or more of their diet (% yes response)	1	4	3	2	4	4	1	1
Could not afford to purchase food? (1 = highest)	1	3	1	1	3	5	3	4
Could not afford – had to pay bills (1 = highest)	4	1	2	1	1	3	5	3

(*Continued*)

TABLE 5.3 (*Continued*)
Inupiaq Households in Eight North Slope Borough Communities: Levels of Food Insecurity Associated in Rank Order of Social and Economic Attributes

Inupiat Households – Attributes of Food Insecurity	Community One Rank	Community Two Rank	Community Three Rank	Community Four Rank	Community Five Rank	Community Six Rank	Community Seven Rank	Community Eight Rank
Could not afford to purchase food – food cost too much (1 = highest)	4	1	2	2	2	4	5	3
Could ot afford to purchase food – not enough income (1 = highest)	3	1	3	5	2	3	5	4
Could not afford to purchase food – not working	3	2	2	3	1	5	2	1
% Wage income of total HH income (1 = highest)	2	3	3	3	1	1	5	2
% Dividend income/total HH income (1 = highest)	2	1	1	1	4	3	1	3
Ave. HH income (1 = highest)	3	4	5	5	1	3	5	2
Per capita income (1 = highest)	2	5	5	4	1	2	4	2
Household with income below the poverty guidelines (1 = highest)	4	1	1	2	3	3	2	4

OTHER PROCESSES AND VARIABLES THAT MAY CONTRIBUTE TO FOOD INSECURITY

There are a number of reasons or independent variables that lead to high indices of food insecurity. Many are elucidated in the variables contained in these tables, some are not and are contingent on special circumstances both historical and contemporary that lead to the extremely high proportions of food insecurity in Inupiaq populations of the North Slope.

Some of these contingent events include historical events such as the initiation and collapse of the "Alaska Bypass." Initiated in 1972 the "Alaska Bypass" allowed pallets containing 1,000 pounds of shrink wrapped goods (including food) to be shipped by air from Alaskan urban areas, such as Anchorage and Fairbanks, to remote rural (mostly Alaska Native) villages under extremely cheap rates subsidized by the U.S. Postal Service. This allowed these extremely remote Native villages to import significant amounts of food and goods that if shipped under normal air postage rates would cost two or three times the subsidized rates. In 2010, the Postal Service ran a $73-million-dollar deficit supporting this program. The program was closed around 2011. This had several dramatic effects, the already high cost of living in these rural communities (2.5× urban Alaska) to increase substantially. Secondly, the "Alaska Bypass" subsidized at least five airlines that flew between urban areas and remote villages and between remote villages. Now one airline, perhaps two, depending on the locale, service these villages making travel and freight much more sporadic and expensive.

Some commodities, such as fuel oil, are shipped by single barge trips during the summer months. However, this mode of transportation is not appropriate for some goods such as perishable foods. In addition, on more than one occasion barges bringing bulk food items, e.g., canned goods and foods with a long shelf life, have failed in their delivery to some communities because of ice conditions or if dropped off at alternative sites, have failed to be recovered. Other attempts to resupply (e.g., through the attenuated local flight services) have proved inadequate.

Other more sporadic and unpredictable events may make nonsubsistence (store-bought foods) unavailable. Extremely small communities of 200 to 400 people are extended beyond the breaking point in administering the many demands and responsibilities of federal and state services (e.g., the school lunch program or dealing with the fiscal, purchasing, and other paperwork associated with stocking a store). An illness to one individual, a family crisis, or any number of small but desperate events may cause a school lunch program to miss a deadline and fail for part of the school year. Similar events impact the administration of small stores. For example, one community only has one store, open sporadically with almost no inventory.

SUBSISTENCE FOODS

Nearly every Inupiaq household (>95%) on the North Slope uses subsistence foods, and nearly two-thirds depend on subsistence foods for more than half their diet. So changes in accessibility or availability of subsistence foods can have major impacts on food security. In addition, there can be any number of events or processes that can influence access and availability to the harvest of subsistence foods. Processes outside the natural environment can also affect subsistence harvests. For example, low or unpredictable income influences the purchase of subsistence technology, including the purchase of boats, motors, ATVs, and snow machines. In addition, gasoline (@ $10 gallon), ammunition, and maintenance of the equipment all require considerable amounts of cash.

Detailed Community Analysis

Two communities (One and Three) will be analyzed in some detail. Space allotted to this chapter does not allow an in-depth analysis of the four communities (One to Four) with the highest food insecurity scores, let alone a consideration of all eight communities on the North Slope. In addition, Community One and Community Three provide a high contrast with Community One an interior community heavily dependent on the harvest of caribou while Community Three is a coastal community with a heavy dependence on the harvest of marine mammals; however, both communities suffer from the substantial impacts of climate change representing very different ecosystems. Finally, both communities, out of all eight, have the highest response to the two key food insecurity measures. Note, however, that the first four communities, with different greyscale highlights, represent a significant gap between their food insecurity proportions when compared to the last four.

COMMUNITY ONE: "NOT ENOUGH TO EAT" – VERY LOW FOOD SECURITY

Community One is an interior tundra oriented village and has the highest proportion of Inupiaq households (36% – Rank 1) who reported there were times during the previous 12 months that they did not have enough to eat. Food security values also vary across time (Fall and Kostick 2018). There are numerous reasons why more than a third of households report these high levels of "very low food security." For this community, we begin with the fact that 78% of the households report that they rely on subsistence foods (foods hunted, gathered, and collected from the environment) for more than half of their diet.

A significant segment of households note a combination of factors that contribute to their not having enough to eat. The chief reason they cite is that they have not been able to obtain as much traditional food as they need. They credit this lack of subsistence to the lack of abundance and/or accessibility to their key wild food resource – caribou.

CLIMATE CHANGE IMPACTS ON CARIBOU HERDS

In 2014, the average caribou harvest was 1,255 edible weight per household or about 391 pounds per capita. Note that caribou, by weight, account for about 90% of the wildlife harvest they consume. Per capita harvest of caribou for Community One fluctuates considerably over time. The per capita harvest in 1998 was 103 pounds, in 2002 it was 158 pounds and the harvest of 391 pounds in 2014, as mentioned above, was the highest in two decades (Brown et al. 2016). Note, the harvest numbers for

2018, the year the questions on food security were asked, were down considerably although we don't have the exact numbers.

Ten of the thirteen communities in northwest Alaska (75%), for which we have good empirical data, depend on caribou for a substantial part of their diet. Of the two communities for which we have decent time series data (Kivalina, Noatak) both report substantial decreases, by nearly half, in their harvest and consumption of caribou.

Climate change was linked by about two-thirds (65% – Rank 2) of the Inupiaq households as a major reason why caribou are not abundant. Cody Sullivan (2018) reports that worldwide overall abundance of reindeer and caribou has declined 56% from a total estimated population of 4.7 million individuals to about 2.1 million individuals over the past two decades. Five herds in particular, in the Alaska–Canada region, experienced such drastic declines that recovery isn't in sight.

In the United States, out of the four tracked herds, three peaked sometime between 2003 and 2010 only to decline 57% by 2017 (Sullivan 2018).

The hypotheses linking climate change and caribou decline are as follows (Mallory 2017):

- Increasing temperatures in some areas bring an expansion of less nutritious shrubs
- Increase of parasitic infections
- Increased frequency of winter icing (making access to lichen much more difficult)
- Increased tundra fires create vast areas that caribou tend to avoid

In addition to "natural" fluctuations and the complex impacts of climate change there are contingent social and economic factors. For example, caribou herds accessed by Community One sometimes come under substantial pressures from nonlocal hunters, who ignore hunting regulations and access the herd through "outfitters" that fly them in, drop them off, and return to pick them up (Dau 2005). In addition, coastal communities are having considerable difficulty harvesting marine mammals; the reasons for this will be analyzed in the consideration of Community Three. In response to decreased marine mammal harvests (also impacted by climate change factors), some coastal communities substantially increase their hunting of caribou (a traditional "resilience" practice), which puts increased pressure on the herd and has implications for caribou-dependent communities.

"UNABLE TO OBTAIN HEALTHY FOODS" – LOW FOOD SECURITY

Community One also ranks second in having difficulty in obtaining healthy meals (low food security). Thirty-six percent of the households in the community cited this as a problem. Of those Inupiaq households that have "low" food security, a full 70% name the inability to obtain store-bought food as the major problem. Not being able to afford the purchase of food was the major reason mentioned by nearly half (Rank 1) of the "low" security households. This is somewhat surprising given that average Inupiaq household income for Community One is nearly $68,000 and per capita income is nearly $18,000 per person. Despite the extremely high cost of living mentioned before, this level of income is above average for Inupiaq households on the North Slope. The important factor for all the communities on the North Slope is not necessarily the amount of income but its source.

Wage income provides a steady and consistent stream of income for a household. However, dividend income, that is, dividends, is given to shareholders of regional and village corporations (plus the Alaska Permanent Fund dividend) amount to half or more of the total household income from all sources. Dividend income is not paid out consistently but may occur quarterly or annually (or even ad hoc each year). Thus many Inupiaq households, especially in the winter months, run out of money and often have to choose between paying for heating oil or food. For Community One, these income difficulties are exacerbated by extreme difficulty in the transportation logistics of getting food to the community and/or sporadic management practices in the timely purchasing of food to restock the local store.

COMMUNITY THREE: "UNABLE TO OBTAIN HEALTHY FOODS" – LOW FOOD SECURITY

Community Three had the highest score for "low food security" with nearly half the Inupiaq households in the community reporting that they had difficulty in obtaining food for healthy meals. The major reason stated for this inability to obtain healthy food was "we could not afford to purchase food." This reason was stated by almost half of the respondents (46% – Rank 1). A major reason for not being able to purchase food was lack of employment; most of the low food security households had no working members.

In addition, for a number of reasons that cannot be addressed here, Community Three had more than 40% of its Inupiaq population under the age of 15, certainly an exacerbating influence on lack of wage income, although it needs to be repeated that small communities like this have only a small number of available wage jobs, mostly linked to a Borough or Village government. All these income problems are indicated in Tables 5.2 and 5.3.

Community Three has the lowest per capita income on the North Slope ($9,500 – Rank 5), and one the highest proportion of Inupiaq households below the poverty threshold, with half of all Inupiaq households below the poverty threshold (Rank 5). Needless to say, Community Three has five times the number of households below the poverty threshold when compared to the state of Alaska proportions. Community Three also has the double burden of extremely low income compounded by nearly two-thirds of total Inupiaq household income coming from dividend sources. Not only is there very little income, but also much of what income is available is sporadic and unpredictable.

These income shortfalls also need to be understood in the local context. Community Three is one of the most difficult to access in terms of transportation and in terms of bringing freight (including food) to the community. Using a market basket from 2015 (where all prices have increased since then) – the cost of living is exorbitant, with fresh fruit, only sporadically available, is several dollars per pound. Wheat bread is $6.15 a loaf, a 13-oz box of cereal (Special K) is 6.95 a box, a 5-lb sack of rice is $11.35, a 32-oz carton of milk is $4.15, a one pound box of margarine is $15.15, and a pound of chicken thighs are $16.79 (NSB 2015). Finally, the local store is often closed because of lack of inventory, lack of staff, and a complete lack of profit.

"NOT ENOUGH TO EAT" – VERY LOW FOOD SECURITY

In 2019, the community reports a very high proportion (26%) of households saying they did not have enough to eat (very low food security). Of these households with very low food security, two-thirds mentioned their inability to obtain traditional foods as the major reason for them not having enough to eat and nearly all these households attribute the shortfall in harvesting marine mammals to climate change (see below).

The 2018 survey reveals slightly over two-thirds (68%) of Inupiaq households in Community Three rely on the harvest of wildlife resources for half or more of their diet. A community harvest survey was done in 2012 in which the average household harvested 2,896 pounds of wildlife resources, while the average per capita harvest was 594 pounds. On a per capita basis marine mammals constituted 317 (54%) pounds per person and 188 (32%) pounds per person came from large land mammals, primarily caribou. It is important to point out a survey done two decades previously found that marine mammal harvests constituted 72% of the communities diet, a drop of 25% in the intervening years leading to 2012.

FOOD AND AGRICULTURE ORGANIZATION (FAO) 2019 REPORT

This extensive background section contained in the beginning not only provides a needed context to understand this chapter's analysis it also provides a critical and necessary backdrop for the editor's request to integrate the analysis contained in this chapter with the Food and Agriculture Organization (FAO) 2019 report – "Food Security Information Network (FSIN) 2019 Global Report on Food Crises" and to consider how the circumstances of the U.S. Norther Arctic described in this chapter are relevant to the United Nations Sustainable Development Goals (SDGs).

The FAO 2019 report is a devastating description and analysis of acute food insecurity in 53 countries, regions, subregions,and populations of special significance (e.g., migrants) from Afghanistan to Zimbabwe. The food insecurity experienced in Northern Alaska and the United States in general is classified as "low food security" and "very low food security."

> Households classified as having *low food security* have reported … food acquisition problems and reduced diet quality, but typically have reported few, if any, indications of reduced food intake. Those classified as having *very low food security* … reported that he or she was hungry at some time during year but did not eat
>
> *(Coleman-Jensen et al. 2017)*

Thus, under the worst case in the United States, parents may forgo eating so that their children can eat, often with older children having minimal or no meals so that the youngest children can eat. This is not to minimize these impacts, especially for certain sections of the U.S. population. Very low food insecure elders have increased risk of chronic health conditions:

- 60% more likely to experience depression
- 53% more likely to report a heart attack
- 52% more likely to develop asthma
- 40% more likely to report an experience of congestive heart failure (Ziliak and Gundersen 2013)

In contrast, *acute food insecurity* as described in the FAO 2019 report is defined as any manifestation of food insecurity that threatens lives or livelihoods. In essence, acute food insecurity in the final IPC "famine" phase carries with it the palpable specter of immediate starvation and death. For the people of the Democratic Republic of the Congo or Yemen, food insecurity in the United States is a problem "we can only dream of having."

The FAO 2019 reports four major drivers of food insecurity:

1. Conflict
2. Climate-related shock
3. Economic-related shock
4. Population displacement

As has been developed throughout this chapter, climate and economic impacts have been delineated, as a major driver, not considered, because of space limitations, is the possibility of community displacement and relocation as a driver. This driver has not yet occurred on the North Slope but is an increasing phenomenon for small Alaska Native communities in coastal and riverine Alaska. Thankfully, the kinds of conflicts described in the FAO 2019 report have not occurred in the United States.

One caveat must be placed on these generalizations. Historically, Alaska Native communities that have been relocated have been associated with increased levels of alcoholism, drug use, domestic violence, and a variety of other social and psychological pathologies. Climate change impacts in Alaska seem inexorable and it's quite possible a perfect storm of community relocation due to flooding and erosion, combined with substantial changes in the ecosystems that hinder or prevent traditional subsistence harvests and all these impacts exacerbated by a national economic depression (not to speak of a pandemic) that decreases or eliminates transfers to small rural communities, could lead to the dreadful circumstances experienced by the communities, regions, and nations described in the FAO report.

UNITED NATIONS SUSTAINABLE DEVELOPMENT GOALS (SDGs)

The United Nations 2030 agenda for sustainable development had at its core 17 Sustainable Development Goals (SDGs) to end poverty and its deprivations integrally linked with strategies that improve health and education, reduce inequality, and spur economic growth all the while addressing climate change and preservation of the environment. Although there are 17 major SDGs, each major SDG has up to 12 subgoals. Once again, given space limitations will only address a small subset of SDGs and provide a brief recommendation to implement the goal.

SDG 1.2 Reduce Poverty by at Least 50% by 2030

In fact, three survey research projects 2010, 2015, and 2019 reveal an increase during the last decade in the proportion (22%–27%) of Inupiaq households living below the poverty threshold (which is three times the state average). Only one of the four highly food insecure communities had a decrease in the proportion of Inupiaq households below the poverty threshold (29% to 16%) between 2010 and 2019 while in the other three communities the proportion has more than doubled in the last decade and now stands at half the population.

Given the paucity of available jobs detailed in the background to this chapter, one can have little optimism that this trend will stabilize let alone reverse. One recommendation might be to train young Inupiat in highly specialized occupations (e.g., engineer, teacher, or GIS computer) now held by nonlocals. Unfortunately, as the surveys reveal there is little enthusiasm to leave the village. Young men whose status in the community is linked to providing subsistence foods find little incentive in leaving their tight knit community and those that do, either at an early age or after high school, seldom return being employed by Native and other corporations in their urban offices. Young women with skills often emigrate for employment to hub communities or urban centers and settle in these locations.

Decreases in transfers from state and federal entities also give little optimism for improvement in economic conditions. The budget for the state of Alaska, once flush has been in substantial decline during the last decade. There are no income taxes within the state and the budget is almost entirely derived from taxes on oil production. Oil production is in substantial decline and in addition the deteriorating price of a barrel of oil all contribute to bare bones budgets. The federal government is a major employer in the state; however, shrinking program budgets bring decreases in employment and in transfers from federal programs.

SDG 2.1 – Universal Access to Safe and Nutritious Food by 2030

SDG 2A – Invest in Rural Infrastructure.

The analysis in this chapter, especially the detailed consideration of Community One and Three, indicates that food insecurity is the product of multiple drivers – historic bureaucratic decisions, high costs of transportation, ad hoc management failures, low incomes, and climate change impacts on subsistence harvests (see next SDG 13B).

"Low food security" has been linked to lack of access to nonsubsistence foods (i.e., Western store-bought foods). This access may be curtailed by multiple causes:

- Lack of income to purchase foods
    - Lack of employment
    - Unpredictable nature of transfers, especially dividend income
    - Difficult choices between paying for heat or eating

- Infrastructure and management deficits
  - Lack of stores or lack of stock within stores
  - High cost of store-bought foods due to transportation costs
  - Lack of management and fiscal skills

RECOMMENDATIONS

The major impediment, a lack of income, has been discussed in SDG 1 above and does not seem solvable under existing conditions or likely to be remedied by 2030. However, the logistical and infrastructural deficits can be remediated by the reinstatement of the "Alaska Bypass" process whereby air shipments of food and other domestic stuff are flown into remote communities on shrink wrapped pallets. The "Alaska Bypass" was possible because of a subsidy to the U.S. Postal Service (a government agency) at about $75 million in 2010 dollars (for all of rural Alaska). A reinstatement of this program would require an act of congress, an unlikely prospect. If it were possible it would solve multiple problems by allowing households (or multiple households) in communities without stores or with stores containing very limited inventory to directly purchase food at urban prices (e.g., Costco had a very efficient bush service) and have them shipped directly to the community for pickup. In addition, it would help minimize problems many small communities have in utilizing highly bureaucratic purchasing systems and paperwork, e.g., such as school lunch programs.

Another recommendation involves switching purchasing responsibility for food programs such as school lunch or meals on wheels for the elderly from the community to the service agency, usually located in urban areas. Under this scenario, the government service agent would need to directly (and perhaps repeatedly) contact the village to obtain the information about the number of eligible individuals and then arrange for the shipment to the community. Urban service agencies also have better communication with the air transportation services that deliver the food to the community and could arrange for reshipments when weather prevents delivery.

SDG 3.8 Achieve Universal Health Coverage

Most Alaskan Natives on the North Slope have access to free health care provided by the Indian Health Service. Longstanding treaties with the federal government guarantee all Native Americans and Alaska Natives free health care.

SDG 13B Promote Mechanisms to Raise Capacity for Planning and Management

A significant segment of this chapter deals with the impact of climate change on the harvest of subsistence (wildlife) resources. A variety of changes directly affect Inupiaq hunters. As ice retreats and open water expands, hunters are forced to harvest in much less safe conditions. More and bigger boats with larger engines are required to provide a safety backup and to traverse greater distances. All this added technology and its concomitant fuel requirements place considerable strain on already limited incomes. Decreasing ice coverage and greater areas of unstable first year ice are not only a safety issue for Inupiaq hunters, and the changing environment has very deleterious effects on marine mammals, especially ice edge seal specialists who now lack insulating snow and cover from protection for their pups. Many marine mammals are now not only less accessible, but also they are fewer in number. Similar problems and processes are discussed within the chapter with regard to land mammals and interior Inupiaq caribou hunters.

How does one make reasonable recommendations about the crushing inexorable total reconfiguration that climate change is bringing, especially for a group of 8,000 individuals on the lance point of these changes but with almost no leverage to affect the outcome? Given the current political climate, the vested interests involved, and the lack of commitment even from environmentalists in terms of sacrificing their current lifestyle, one can only be pessimistic about mitigating the problem.

However, some modest changes in bureaucratic structures, some expanded perspective on what natural resource management can be and some modest generosity in those that now make decisions and hold power can lead to substantial advances for Alaskan natives in adapting to climate change.

Currently, within the state of Alaska there are two entities, the Alaska Board of Fish and Game and the Federal Subsistence Board who use Western wildlife management techniques to regulate hunting and fishing within the state. For sake of brevity, we are going to ignore other powerful regulatory boards within the state, e.g., commercial fishing. The state board regulates state lands (23% of Alaska's total acreage) and the Federal Subsistence Board manages a whopping 72% of all the acreage in Alaska whereas Native entities own and manage about 10% of the total acreage with 1% of lands in Alaska in private ownership.

The State Game Board, under the former Governor Sarah Palin, had no Alaska Native Representation on the board and the board has long been influenced by sports hunting interests. The Federal Subsistence Board that has representatives from the U.S. Forest Service, National Park Service, BLM, and the U.S. Fish and Wildlife Service does have mandated Alaska Native Representation, although their influence is modest, especially when compared to the influence of environmental groups.

Both the state and federal entities use similar Western management techniques to arrive at their regulatory regimes. In this process, they rely on biologists, ecologists, and other specialists to provide data, information and evaluation of the number, condition and health of a variety of wildlife species. Oversimplifying, these entities use two tools to try and manage for "natural and healthy," or the "sustainable yield" of wildlife populations, depending on an agency's mandate. These two tools are establishing regulations for "seasons" and "bag limits." A season defines the period of time that a species, e.g., caribou, can be hunted. For example, a season may start in August and end in September or October for caribou. Harvesting caribou outside this period of time is illegal. But seasonal regulations are usually intrinsically linked to "bag limits," the total a single hunter may harvest during one hunt or the maximum number of animals that may be harvested from a specific herd. Managers monitor harvest and once the maximum has been harvested shut down the season.

In this idealized example, I am ignoring any number of complexities including restrictions that may be imposed on the technology used. In addition, most management agencies act as if they didn't manage these resources then there would be an absence of any management leading an open season on species and their possible eradication. Of course, this perspective ignores traditional management techniques that are applied by Native cultures to their harvest of animals. For example, traditionally there are substantial sanctions against hunters that harvest more than can be consumed. And, by consumption, the explicit implication is consumption of the whole animal.

Now substantial difficulties arise as climate change influences access to and the availability of a subsistence species. For example, lack of snow or frozen ground may make it difficult if not impossible for a hunter to access game over wet tundra. In this case, a modification of the "season" may increase access. In addition, subsistence hunters are interested in taking enough game to support their household and community and in terms of efficiency (their time, expense, and fuel) find it frustrating to harvest only two caribou per day when they could harvest all they need in a single hunt.

The problem arises with the lack of flexibility and response of the bureaucracies that set the regulations. Inertia, conflicting data, and influence of vested interests (e.g., err on the side of conservative limits) all militate against a quick response and effective adaptation to changing conditions.

A strong recommendation would be to empower local/Native actors to have the largest (or final) say in the construction of regulations, a kind of cooperative management regime on steroids. In addition, to streamline the process and to avoid competing interests (sports hunters vs. conservationists, local vs. out of state hunters), a merger of the state and federal boards is recommended.

As to the possibility of the enactment of these recommendations once again one has to be pessimistic. Historically land managers seldom cede their regulatory authority to others. With respect to the state/federal merger, the state resents (a polite word) federal control of so much of Alaska lands; many urban sports hunters and others are ideologically opposed to special treatment afforded to rural residents in federal law. A merging of these two entities would provide optimism for the potential of a solution to the Israeli/Palestinian conflict.

It is interesting to note the absence of an explicit sub-SDG on "environmental justice" in the United Nations discussion of SDG 16. In the recommendation suggested above for SDG 13B a clear case can be made for the initiation of participatory justice.

A brief consideration of environmental justice indicates two (of several) forms of justice. For example, distributive justice deals with the fair distribution of burdens and benefits of environmental actions. Several studies initiated in the 1980s disclosed the greater likelihood of poor and minority communities suffering siting of toxic landfill and other facilities compared to their white counterparts (Figueroa and Mills 2001).

In contrast, participatory justice asks the questions "How are these distributive decisions made?" and "Who makes them?" In general, the poor and minorities have little participation or influence in how environmental benefits and burdens are assigned.

Although discussions of both dimensions of environmental justice appear together in the literature, there has been a tendency (among academics) to favor the distributive dimension (Figueroa and Mills 2001). However, minorities and others that bear the brunt of environmental degradation favor participatory justice. For example, the Principles of Environmental Justice, adopted by the First National People of Color Environmental Leadership Summit in 1991:

> Include only 2 references to distributive justice in the 17 principles. The remaining principles emphasize participatory justice concerns of rights against discrimination, individual and group self-determination, and respect for diverse cultural perspectives
>
> *(Hofrichter and Gelobter 2002)*

For the Inupiat of northern Alaska, the possibility that the urban United States or the United States in general will share equally in the burdens of climate change, at this point, seems far-fetched. On the other hand, the attainment of some level of participatory justice, that is, their influence in making decisions to adapt and to help ameliorate the impacts of climate change they are currently experiencing seems more achievable.

CONCLUSIONS/SUMMARY

There are three main drivers of food insecurity for North Slope Inupiaq families and these drivers act in structural and ad hoc ways that provide complex pathways to food insecurity.

1. Poor access to store-bought (Western) foods.
2. Climate change impacts on the access to and harvest of wildlife resources (subsistence).
3. Decisions made historically by federal and state entities that have long-term consequences and contemporary social and economic circumstances that impede access to healthy foods.

1. Poor access to Western foods has four major sources.
   - A. Lack of stores or limited stock in existing stores.
   - B. Extremely high cost of food two to five times that of urban areas in the state.
   - C. Lack of income to purchase store-bought food.
     1. High unemployment and lack of full-time job opportunities.
     2. Inupiaq total household income is heavily dependent (>50%) on sporadic dividend income; unpredictable in amount and delivery time.
   - D. Bureaucratic and management difficulties in the consistent provision of programs such as school lunch programs and meals on wheels to elderly and in the stocking and availability of food in village stores.
2. Climate change has multiple direct and indirect impacts along with unanticipated feedback.
   - A. The dramatic decrease in multiyear ice has multiple implications.

1. Marine mammal hunters must travel much greater distances over dangerous open waters. This requires bigger boats, larger engines, more boats, and more fuel – huge increased cost burdens on low-income communities.
2. Changing ice conditions impact the survival rate of marine mammals such as ringed seals. With fewer seals more widely dispersed requires hunters to travel further distances, conduct more trips and face higher costs and increased hazards to their safety.

B. Large changes in terrestrial ecosystems.

1. Melting permafrost makes travel more difficult.
2. Novel and extensive tundra fires eliminate food for caribou.
3. Changing plant communities, e.g., the northern expansion of less nutritious shrubs directly affect caribou health, as do increased parasitic infections and winter icing conditions.

3. Historic bureaucratic decisions and contemporary management inadequacies.

A. State requirements for Inupiaq children to attend school have long-term consequences as Inupiat families alter seasonal camps and reside in permanent settlements.

B. Elimination of "Alaska Bypass" a program that subsidized the U.S. Postal Service in provision of low-cost freight of food stuffs to remote rural communities.

C. In small Native communities, management skills and capacities are razor thin and an illness in one management position can prevent timely purchase orders to restock local stores or to miss paperwork deadlines on food service programs.

These broad generalizations summarize the major drivers of food insecurity for North Slope Inupiaq households. However, it is important to recognize that any one of these factors by itself can necessarily cause food insecurity. However, as the case study analyses of Communities One and Three indicate, it is usually a combination of factors that lead to food insecurity.

Summary: Community One

In Community One, an interior community that is heavily dependent on one species, caribou, to provide 90% of their wildlife subsistence diet. They also had the highest proportion (36%) of Inupiaq households that actually went hungry during periods of the preceding year. Eight out of ten Inupiaq households in this community rely on the harvest of wildlife to provide the majority of food in their diet.

Heavily dependent on one species the community suffers when the herd decreases, which it has, and both biologists and hunters attribute the decrease to impacts from climate change described in the chapter. In addition, the herd is under hunting pressures from outside sports hunters and from Inupiaq hunters in nearby coastal communities. As coastal marine mammal hunters face increased difficulties they increase their harvest of other species, a resilience strategy described earlier.

Household income is a problem for purchasing store-bought goods, although this community has the second highest per capita income of the eight communities, and consistent with the three other highly food insecure communities, Community One derives a majority of household income from dividend sources with their attendant problems. Finally, management difficulties, weather delays, and transportation issues have on occasion interfered with sufficient food stocks in the local store.

Summary: Community Three

Community Three, a small coastal marine mammal-dependent community, had the highest score for "low food security" with nearly half the Inupiaq households reporting they had difficulty in obtaining store-bought food because they could not afford to purchase it. Most of the food insecure households had no working members. A contributing factor to this is high dependency ratios occasioned by skewed population pyramids with large bulges in the under 15 age groups. In addition, Inupiaq households in this community had the lowest per capita income within the NSB and more than half of the households were below the poverty threshold. Having no full-time store in the community, the nearest being about 100 miles away exacerbated all these problems.

Finally, two-thirds of Inupiaq households depended upon subsistence foods for a majority of their diet with marine mammals forming the majority of their harvests. Forty-one percent of the households said they could not obtain enough subsistence foods for their needs, either by harvesting or sharing with other households. A majority of hunters say that the abundance and access to marine mammals have decreased considerably with two-thirds attributing climate change as the major contributing factor.

COVID-19 IMPACT ON NORTHERN ALASKAN INUPIAQ COMMUNITIES

Historic Epidemics and Alaska Natives

In the early 1990s, as I was initiating my fieldwork in the Russian Far East, I took a long walk in Provideniya and ended up on top of a small peninsula with a beautiful view overlooking the bay. This area is devoted to a cemetery containing a number of graves and headstones. One grave had a headstone with the picture of a young girl etched into the granite. Surrounding the grave was a small fence and within that fence were a small concrete table and benches. It was the tradition in this community to celebrate absent loved ones not only with flowers but also to gather around the grave with a small repast and discuss and celebrate the memory of the departed family member. This experience caused me to reflect on the various cemeteries and abandoned communities I had visited in Arctic and Subarctic areas of Alaska.

For example, in an interview discussing the 1918–1919 pandemic, Alan Boraas, an anthropology professor at Kenai Peninsula College, said about half of the aboriginal population (of the Kenai Peninsula) died from the epidemic. In addition, from 1880 to 1920, at least eight Dena'ina villages were abandoned due to various epidemics and the few survivors moved and concentrated in larger communities. Boraas in Clarion (2018) states:

> Today, there are few reminders of influenza's effect on the peninsula. South of Kenai near Kasilof lies the old village site of Kalifornsky. Abandoned after the outbreak, a small graveyard inside a delicate white fence holds 16 unmarked graves, and one outside the fence, Dena'ina elder and writer Peter Kalifornsky's resting place. The graves inside the fence belong to village members who perished from disease (Clarion 2018).

Aboriginally, the Arctic was a tough place to make a living and survival was a spinning wheel of contingency. Of course, nothing prepared these peoples for the wave after wave of suffering brought by measles, smallpox, diphtheria, and tuberculosis – culminating with the influenza epidemic of 1918–1919. The flu epidemic crested late in Alaska, arriving in force during the fall of 1918 and culminating in the spring of 1919. In 1917, there were about 58,000 people living in Alaska of which about 48% were Alaskan Natives. In one detailed study of death certificates from 1918 to 1919, the authors estimate that Alaska Natives accounted for approximately 82% of the mortality. In addition, if one aggregates the mortality by 14-year age intervals (0–14,15–29, 30–44, and 45+), the deaths were fairly equally distributed among each age group, e.g., those 0–14 accounted for about 25% of the deaths (Health Analytics Unit 2018).

Moreover, mortality was geographically concentrated with what is now the Nome census area accounting for two-thirds of the mortality; the current North Slope Borough, the focus of this chapter, was responsible for less than 1% of the mortality. Of course, strict reliance on death certificates has its shortcomings and the authors cite other reasonable estimates that are double the number discussed in their analysis. The proportion of people who died from influenza among those diagnosed (case fatality rate) was >2.5%, which is at least 25 times greater than contemporary seasonal flu (i.e., not COVID-19), have a case fatality rate of <.1. Per capita, more people died in Alaska than anywhere else in the world except Samoa. Historians estimate 8% of the total Alaska Native population died during the 1918–1919 epidemic.

Contemporary COVID-19 Impacts

In early July 2020, I wrote the following analysis: The previous discussion acts as an introduction to the Coronavirus epidemic currently impacting the United States and the world. As detailed in the previous discussion, Indigenous people accounted for the vast majority of deaths in the 1918/1919 epidemic. Entire villages were decimated, leaving behind only small graveyards. If we count a generation as 20 years then five generations have occurred since this pandemic. However, the memory of the destruction that the 1918–1919 epidemic caused has been carried down by elders and is structuring the current village response.

Alaskan villages were some of the first communities to institute lockdown measures. The vast majority of the 200 small rural villages are inaccessible other than by air, although some intervillage river travel is accomplished by boat. Most villages are trying to eliminate passenger travel either into or from the village. So, with respect to controlling access to the community, their relative isolation proves useful (Campbell 2020).

For example, travel to Kotzebue, a northwest Arctic hub, requires that:

All travelers entering the Borough through Kotzebue must complete travel questionnaires and submit to COVID-19 testing administered by public health nurses from Maniilaq Health Center or provide satisfactory proof of negative test results, and await results of that testing before traveling within Kotzebue or to another village (Northwest Arctic Borough 2020).

However, there are also drawbacks to small Alaska Native communities as most lack any medical infrastructure. Until recently, serious illness or injury usually required the patient to fly out either to a hub community, such as Kotzebue or Utqiagvik or to Anchorage or Fairbanks. Unfortunately, shortly after the villages started to limit passenger travel the state also issued a prohibition of intrastate travel with the intention of slowing the spread of COVID-19. This had the consequence of some of the small bush airlines going out of business. In most places, emergency evacuation is still possible but transportation of goods is limited.

The structure of village life provides some benefits in that the vast majority of communities, over a period of a few months, are self-sufficient since the majority of their diet still comes from the subsistence harvest of wildlife resources. However, there are also significant costs associated with traditional village life. For example, houses are crowded, often with multigenerational families. In addition, due to insulation against the cold most houses have poor air circulation. There are also water and sewer issues that have to be dealt with, making many households more vulnerable in preventing the spread of a virus should it enter the community. In addition, many of the marine mammal dependent communities face increased difficulties, as their harvest techniques require close multi-household cooperation.

In 2020, Alaska had a population of about 710,000 individuals of which about 15% are Alaska Native. Of the approximately 107,000 Alaska Native, about half live in urban areas. As of late June 2020, there have been 12 deaths attributed to COVID-19 in Alaska. Two of these are Alaska Native (17%), two are Asian and seven are Caucasian (47%) and one is Pacific Islander. The 17% mortality for Alaska Natives is commensurate with their proportion within the total population and is in stark contrast to the mortality associated with the 1918–1919 epidemic. The North Slope Borough, the focus of this chapter, has four individuals who have tested positive for COVID-19 but have no mortality cases (APM 2022).

COVID-19 has proven lethal to older individuals and/or to individuals with underlying health conditions. Table 5.4 provides the percentage of NSB Inupiaq individuals with underlying health conditions and compares it to U.S. national proportions. With respect to diabetes and heart disease, NSB populations are at a lower risk than the U.S. population. Both populations are fairly similar with respect to asthma or breathing problems. And for a variety of reasons, NSB Inupiaq population has half the heart disease when compared to the general U.S. population. The real risk for the Inupiaq population, especially given the respiratory nature of COVID-19, is the huge proportion of NSB Inupiaq adults who smoke. In fact, a majority of them smoke and this poses a serious health vulnerability should COVID-19 enter the NSB at any significant level.

So as of the time of this writing (early July of 2020), Alaskan Native villages, relying on the experience of elders and respecting the sacrifice of earlier generations,

TABLE 5.4
NSB Inupiaq Underlying Health Conditions vs. U.S. Percent

Morbidity Adults 16+	NSB Inupiat %	U.S. Population %
Diabetes	6.2%	9.1%
Asthma/Breathing	9.9%	7.7%
High blood pressure	21%	~50%
Heart disease	5.5%	12.1%
Smoking	~50%	21%
~N	1,650	-

have accomplished a remarkable flattening of the COVID-19 curves and are self-isolating and protecting themselves hopefully until a vaccine is readily available. Nevertheless, given the attributes of these communities, small crowded housing, limited access to sanitation/clean water, and little medical infrastructure, should a case be discovered immediate action is required.

February 19, 2021

Considerable time, nearly seven months, has elapsed since the submission of my addendum concerning the COVID-19 impact on the inhabitants of the North Slope Borough (NSB). During July 2020, on a five-point scale [low, medium, high, very high, and extremely high], the NSB was considered to be at a "low" risk level. This risk assessment is based on cases per capita and test positivity. Other risk assessments use the same ordinal attributes but may focus singularly on per capita cases and not include test positivity – so evaluations, on seemingly the same scale, are not comparable.

By August 2020, the NSB risk assessment for COVID-19 had increased to "moderate" and by the end of the month was rated as "high" – [11 per 100,000 population (11:100,000)]. The situation worsened month by month and by November through January 2021, the risk assessment was "extremely high" (147:100,000) for 72 of the 90 days contained in those three months. The last few days of January and for the majority of February the risk assessment has been "high," although for the last week, it has increased to "very high" (45:100,000) (*Times* 2021).

During this pandemic, the United States has experienced about an 11.8% tested infection rate for the COVID-19. During this same period, the NSB tested infection rate has been about 10% (998/9,832). During this period, the mortality from COVID-19 in the United States has been about 1.8%. During the same period, the NSB mortality rate has been about half a percent. However, these mortality appraisals are incomparable for several reasons. Many of the severely ill NSB residents are transported to Anchorage and their deaths will be reported there. In addition, meaningful comparisons would need to incorporate the fact that the NSB population pyramids are heavily skewed to younger age groups.

The impacts of COVID-19 vary widely for Alaska Native villages. For example, Tuluksak, a village of around 500 residents in southwest Alaska, has infection rates of nearly a third of the population, the village is on lockdown and the school has been closed since October. In addition, a recent fire destroyed the water treatment plant, their only source of potable water and a case of water costs $61 to fly in. Residents of the community refuse to use the discolored water from the Tuluksak River as they feel it has been contaminated by an upriver gold mine. Their situation is precarious although a series of regional, state, and federal agencies are slowly working to replace the water treatment plant.

In contrast, the hub community of Kotzbue, mentioned earlier in this discussion, has vaccinated over half of their 3,300 multiethnic inhabitants and is closing in on herd immunity for their community. Not that achieving the 70% vaccination rate estimated to achieve herd immunity is going to be easy. Transporting vaccines to outlying communities is incredibly difficult given the refrigeration requirements of the vaccine (much colder than even an Alaskan winter). In addition, a good proportion of the regional population (~25%?) is reluctant to be vaccinated. And while the state of Alaska leads the nation in the proportion of first vaccine shots (16%), initial efforts at isolation could not be completely sustained and many small rural communities are suffering. Alaska Natives bore the brunt of the mortality in the 1918/1919 flu pandemic (~80%), mortality statistics indicate that currently 40% of the mortality is located in Alaska Native families, more than double the proportion of any other ethnicity (Lester 2021).

REFERENCES

APM Research Lab Staff. 2020. "COVID-19 Deaths Analyzed by Race and Ethnicity, 04–24–2020." APM Research Lab. American Public Media. August 18, 2020. https://www.apmresearchlab.org/covid/deaths-by-race.

Brown, C.L., N.M. Braem, M.L. Kostick, A. Trainor, L.J. Slayton, D.M. Funfola, E.H. Mikow, H. Ikuta, C.R. McDevitt, J. Park, and J.J. Simon. 2016. "Harvests and Uses of Wild Resources in 4 Interior Alaska Communities and 3 Arctic Alaska Communities." Technical Paper No. 426. Fairbanks: Alaska Department of Fish and Game Division of Subsistence. http://www.adfg.alaska.gov/techpap/TP426.pdf.

Callaway, Donald and Smith, Janell. 2008. "The Social, Economic and Dietary Components of Food Security for the Communities of Kiana and Buckland, Northwest Alaska." Institute for Circumpolar Health Studies, Alaska Department of Fish & Game, Division of Subsistence, Kotzebue Office, National Park Service and the Traditional Tribal Councils of Kiana and Buckland.

Campbell, Leah. 2020. "Native Alaskan Villages, Once Devastated by Spanish Flu, Are Taking Action against COVID-19. Direct Relief." May 6, 2020. https://www.directrelief.org/2020/05/native-alaskan-villages-once-devastated-by-spanish-flu-are-taking-action-against-covid-19/.

Clarion, Victoria Petersen Peninsula. 2018. "100 Years Ago, Spanish Flu Devastated Alaska Native Villages." *Peninsula Clarion*. June 22, 2018. https://www.peninsulaclarion.com/news/100-years-ago-spanish-flu-devastated-alaska-native-villages/.

Coleman-Jensen, Alisha, Matthew P. Rabbitt, Gregory A. Christian, and Anita Singh. 2017. "Household Food Security in the United States 2017." Washington, DC: United States Department of Agriculture.

Dau, Jim. 2005. "Two Caribou Mortality Events in Northwest Alaska: Possible Causes and Management Implications." *Rangifer* 25 (4): 37. https://doi.org/10.7557/2.25.4.1769.

Fall, James A. 2016. "Regional Patterns of Fish and Wildlife Harvests in Contemporary Alaska." *ARCTIC* 69 (1): 47. https://doi.org/10.14430/arctic4547.

Fall, James, and Marylynne Kostick. 2018. "Food Security and Wild Resource Harvests in Alaska." Alaska Department of Fish and Game Division of Subsistence. http://www.adfg.alaska.gov/static/home/subsistence/pdfs/food_security_whitepaper.pdf.

Figueroa, Robert, and Claudia Mills. 2001. Environmental Justice. In *A Companion to Environmental Philosophy,"* Richard Hofrichter and Michel Gelobter (eds.), 426–438. https://doi.org/10.1002/9780470751664.ch30.

Health Analytics Unit. 2018. *"Alaska Facts and Figures: 1918 Pandemic Influenza Mortality in Alaska."* Juneau: Alaska Division of Public Health.

Hofrichter, Richard, and Michel Gelobter (eds.). 2002. *"Toxic Struggles: The Theory and Practice of Environmental Justice."* Salt Lake City: University of Utah Press.

Inuit Circumpolar Council-Alaska (ICCA). 2015. "Alaskan Inuit Food Security Conceptual Framework: How to Assess the Arctic from an Inuit Perspective." Anchorage: Inuit Circumpolar Council-Alaska.

Lester, Caroline. 2021. "The Rural Alaskan Towns Leading the Country in Vaccine Distribution." *New Yorker*. https://www.newyorker.com/news/dispatch/the-rural-alaskan-towns-leading-the-country-in-vaccine-distribution.

Magdanz, James, Charles Utermohle, and Robert Wolfe. 2002. "The Production and Distribution of Wild Food in Wales and Deering, Alaska." http://www.adfg.alaska.gov/techpap/tp259.pdf.

Mallory, Conor. 2017. "How Will Climate Change Affect Arctic Caribou and Reindeer?" The Conversation. November 30, 2017. https://theconversation.com/how-will-climate-change-affect-arctic-caribou-and-reindeer–86886.

Nelson, Lucy. 2020. Proclamation of Additional Emergency Order. Office of the Mayor: Northwest Arctic Borough.

New York Times. 2021. "North Slope Borough, Alaska Covid Case and Risk Tracker." January 27, 2021, Sec. U.S. https://www.nytimes.com/interactive/2021/us/north-slope-borough-alaska-covid-cases.html?action=click&module=covid_tracking&pgtype=Interactive®ion=TableRowLink.

North Slope Borough (NSB) 2015 Economic Profile & Census Report. Alaska Borough: North Slope Borough.

North Slope Borough (NSB) 2019 Economic Profile & Census Report. Alaska Borough: North Slope Borough.

Sullivan, Cody. 2018. "2018 Arctic Report Card: Reindeer and Caribou Populations Continue to Decline" | NOAA Climate.gov. Climate.gov. https://www.climate.gov/news-features/featured-images/2018-arctic-report-card-reindeer-and-caribou-populations-continue.

Winfree, R., B. Rice, N. Fresco, L. Krutikov, J. Morris, D. Callaway, J. Mow, and N. Swanton. 2014. "Climate Change Scenario Planning for Northwest Alaska Parks: Cape Krusenstern and Bering Land Bridge. Natural Resource Report" NPS/AKSO/NRR—2014/830. Fort Collins, CO: National Park Service,.

Ziliak, James P., and Craig Gunderson. 2013. "Spotlight on Food Insecurity among Senior Americans: 2011." Alexandria, VA: National Foundation to End Senior Hunger.

6 Food Sovereignty for Food Security, Nutrition, and Climate Resilience

How Food Security Has Failed Haiti, and Why Peasants Want Food Sovereignty

Marylynn Steckley and Joshua Steckley

CONTENTS

INTRODUCTION

The Global Climate Change Risk Index 2019 tells us that Haiti is among the countries most vulnerable to both the recurrent annual impacts of climate change *and* the long-term impacts (Eckstein, Hutfils, & Winges 2018). The island nation is also infamous for its rural food insecurity, food import dependence, and malnutrition (WFP 2019). In the wake of the COVID-19 outbreak and pandemic, low-income developing countries, like Haiti, are particularly vulnerable and there is cause for concern that the pandemic and food chain disruption may increase vulnerability to food insecurity. In the case of Haiti, the vulnerabilities associated with COVID-19 come in the wake of a long line of disasters that have impacted food security and nutrition.

DOI: 10.1201/9781003014942-6

In this chapter, we illustrate that Haiti's contemporary food security, and climate vulnerability are rooted in rural development plans that have prioritized economic growth. Specifically, food security approaches to the hunger problem (i.e., increase food access) and mainstream and agricultural interventions (i.e., export-oriented production, monocropping, and expanded agrochemical access) run counter to climate resilience and disembody the connections between food, land, and the environment from people, nutrition, and health. Yet, since the 2010 earthquake, there has been talk of a new approach – food sovereignty. The key goals of food sovereignty dovetail nicely with broader Sustainable Development Goals of poverty elimination, nutritious diets, and ecological health, and as the world struggles with how to grapple with long-distance food supply chains in the midst of a pandemic, there is perhaps no better time to consider food localization and food sovereignty. At its core, food sovereignty asserts a revolutionary ontology of food – as biospheric, as democratic, as cultural...*all at the same time*" (Moore 2015, p. 289). Food sovereignty offers an integrative approach to the problems of food insecurity and climate vulnerability, envisions improved nutrition, and farmer goals of household food provisioning can be accomplished within community needs for environmental health. Our chapter illustrates that the Haitian state and bilateral organizations have made some movement toward food sovereignty in the post-earthquake period and recommends that continuing to build rural development policy based on peasant perspectives is the best path forward.

The 2030 Agenda for Sustainable Development (ASD) offers an integrative policy vision that conceptualizes human nutrition and well-being *amidst* environmental health and climate resilience. For the world's most vulnerable, this represents a hopeful paradigm shift, away from a growth at all cost mindset, and toward an integrative view of humans *with* nature. For countries suffering extreme poverty, hunger, and climate vulnerability, there is some urgency to understand how this international vision aligns with policies and social movements in local contexts. In this respect, the case of Haiti, where climate vulnerability, hunger, malnutrition, and poverty are rampant, is an important one. The history of food insecurity and climate vulnerability in Haiti not only illustrates that the integrated social, economic, and ecological approach of the Sustainable Development Goals is nothing new (Haitian peasants have had this vision of society for decades) but also sheds light on the connections between deepening poverty, hunger, and environmental problems and international and domestic policies that privilege market-oriented food security and poverty reduction through economic growth.

The Global Climate Change Risk Index 2019 tells us that Haiti is among the countries most vulnerable to both the recurrent annual impacts of climate change *and* the long-term impacts (Eckstein, Hutfils, and Winges 2018). These climate impacts are especially concerning for Haiti given its extreme rural food insecurity, high rates of poor nutrition, and food import dependence (WFP 2019). Over 50% of Haitians are food insecure. Over 50% are undernourished. One in five children is stunted as a result of malnutrition. And, 50% of women suffer from anemia (Global Hunger Index 2019). The country is also food import dependent and imports 60% of its food needs (IFAD 2019). As food prices have been consistently rising since 2010 (IFPRI 2019), it should come as no surprise that in 2019, Haiti continued to experience "serious" hunger problems, and ranked 111th out of 117 countries in terms of hunger severity. Yet, it is important to recognize that vulnerability to food insecurity is highly uneven within the country, with rural dwellers particularly vulnerable to the problems of climate volatility and food insecurity. Roughly 90% of rural dwellers live below the poverty line, and persistent extreme weather events often ravage agrarian landscapes, exacerbating food shortages. For example, in 2016, Hurricane Mathew – the strongest hurricane in 50 years – devastated Southwestern Haiti, affecting over two million people. That same year, Haiti was ranked the world's most affected by extreme weather (Eckstein, Künzel and Schäfer 2018). And yet, Haiti's disasters are not completely natural. Hurricane Matthew killed hundreds, and impacted over two million people, but disproportionately impacted the poor, and nearly 50% of the damage to the productive sectors was concentrated in agriculture (World Bank 2017).

Just like so-called *natural* disasters (i.e., earthquakes, hurricanes), the impacts of COVID-19 on Haitian experiences of food insecurity are likely to be highly uneven. On March 20, 2020, Haiti's first case of COVID-19 was confirmed and one month later the director for the Center for Global Health at Weill Cornell Medicine said that Haiti should expect tens of thousands of people to contract COVID-19 in Haiti (Porter and Dugan 2020). But, we expect that disease contraction and experiences of food security related to food systems disruptions will be very uneven. Specifically, it is likely that the wealthy will most likely be shielded both from the virus, and from food insecurity, while the poor will be hardest hit. With already poor health care, strong obstacles to social distancing and self-quarantine, rising cost of food while opportunities for remittances and employment are threatened, there is reason to believe that the long-term, market-based approach to food security has deepened COVID-related food insecurity for Haiti's poor, particularly for the urban poor. Obviously, it is difficult to predict the degree to which the COVID-19 pandemic will impact Haitian food security and nutrition, but we can look to Haiti's context and past disasters to provide some initial insights. In particular, we argue that Haiti's vulnerability to food insecurity in the wake of the 2010 earthquake, Hurricane Mathew, and following COVID-19 is a product of decades of domestic and international policies that failed to meaningfully address poverty, poor rural infrastructure, and resilience.

One objective of this chapter is to illustrate that there is nothing *natural* about Haiti's vulnerability to climate change or its food insecurity, and that the free market approach to food security has shaped programming for decades, and the continued pursuit of food security through economic growth is unlikely to move Haiti toward the Sustainable Development Goals of poverty reduction (SDG 1), hunger elimination (SDG 2), and climate resilience (SDG 13). The conventional narrative has been that increasing farmer incomes and integrating rural economies more deeply into markets will enable greater access to food and increase food security. But, it is now recognized that in many countries, food insecurity, and malnutrition have persisted *in spite* of economic growth (FAO 2019). In the context of Haiti, trade liberalization, the promotion of export orientation in agriculture, and the prioritization of market integration have done little to solve Haiti's hunger problems, or to bolster nutrition. Instead, this approach has deepened the rift between food, land, and the environment on one hand, and people, nutrition, and health on the other.

The second objective of this chapter is to highlight the recommendations of Haitian peasants' organizations, which suggest that there *is* an alternative. In this chapter, we draw from the perspectives of Haitian peasant leaders who argue that Haiti needs pro-poor framework that will provide nourishing food, dignified livelihoods, *and* climate resilience. This vision aligns with many of the integrative Sustainable Development Goals including the pursuit of human well-being through targets for zero poverty (SDG 1); zero hunger (SDG 2); decent work (SDG 8); and meaningful lives (SDG 3) *amidst* healthy environments, including sustainable agricultural systems (SDG 2), climate resilience (SDG 13) and ecosystem restoration (SDG 14). However, peasants are pushing for change *beyond* the ASD, which does not go far enough to address many conventional food system practices that underlie Haiti's persistent hunger and nutrition problems: long-distance food supply chains, energy-intensive production methods, power imbalances in agricultural decision-making, and unequal access to ecological resources (Windfuhr and Jonsén 2005). So, what is food sovereignty, and how does it push beyond the ASD?

A food sovereignty approach emphasizes the centrality of power relations to food insecurity and malnutrition (Bernstein 2014; Gordillo and Jerónimo 2013), and envisions those goals of poverty reduction, improved nutrition, and environmental health are best accomplished through democratic decision-making. This includes democratic decision-making over things like rural development agendas, agricultural subsidies, levels of market integration, food provisioning networks, and the pathways of achieving poverty reduction (Patel 2009; Walsh, Walford and McCarthy 2016). Food sovereignty also demands *localization* and increased (though not total) food self-sufficiency (Wittman 2015). The vision is for food systems that are ecologically, nutritionally, and culturally enriching. At its core, food sovereignty "asserts a revolutionary ontology of food–as biospheric, as democratic, as cultural…*all at the same time*" (Moore 2015, 289). For Haitian peasant organizations, food sovereignty is a more hopeful climate resilience framework that deserves financing and policy support in Haiti and beyond.

In this chapter, we begin with an outline of the core differences between food security and food, paying attention to Haitian peasant perspectives on both. Next, we illustrate that the free market approach to food security, and its focus on improving food access and availability, has continued to be an important component of Haiti's rural development agenda in the past ten years. However, in the final section, we argue that the growing integration of food sovereignty approaches in state policy is a hopeful indication that peasant perspectives are being considered.

METHODOLOGY

The research that informs this chapter is based on the authors' experience as support workers for the Haitian Food Justice Organization, Kore Pwodiksyon Lokal (Support Local Production) from 2007 to 2010, and our lived and ethnographic research experience in Haiti's Artibonite Valley from 2010 to 2013. The research phase included semi-structured interviews with over 100 peasant producers in three communities in Desarmes, and qualitative, key-informant in-depth interviews with leaders of national peasant organizations in Haiti, including Mouvman Peyizan

Papaye; Tèt kole Ti Peyizan Ayisyen; Mouvman Peyizan Nasyonal Kongre Papay; and Partenariat Developpement Local, among others. Our work is also informed by a content analysis of postdisaster, food security, and nutrition plans from 2010 to 2019.

FOOD SOVEREIGNTY AND FOOD SECURITY

> Food sovereignty and food security, these are totally different concepts. Food security is more widespread, but it means that food could be from anywhere, as long as we eat. But we need food sovereignty. Food sovereignty – Woy! – the big state authorities, they'll never talk about that! They'll always talk about food security. Instead of letting peasants produce, they would rather import it.
>
> *Peasant Leader, KOPAV*

Since the 1990s, poverty, hunger, and malnutrition in Haiti have mostly been combated with a modernist, free market approach to food security (Steckley and Weis 2017; Cohen 2013). Food security is a concept and approach to combating hunger that is said to be achieved when "all people, at all times, have physical and economic access to sufficient, safe and nutritious food" (WFS 1996). The goal is to improve food *availability* and food *access*. Put simply, the food security paradigm is about getting more people fed. And, in a country with high rates of hunger and malnutrition, who could argue with that? But Haitian peasants *do* take issue with food security. The free market approach to food security permits a dismissal of key questions that are central to a peasant vision of food systems: whether food is culturally appropriate, is locally sourced, or is produced with agrochemicals by large agribusinesses (Desmarais 2007; McMichael 2005).

In Haiti, the imposition of structural adjustment in the 1980s, and subsequent market liberalization in the 1990s, locked in the free market approach to food security. The Haitian government, international financial institutions, and international nongovernmental organizations have since prioritized the pursuit of comparative advantage both in low-wage factory work and in tropical commodity production. While it is widely recognized that export orientation and commodity dependence make countries more vulnerable to nutritional and food insecurity in the wake of both environmental disasters and economic downturns (FAO 2019), post-earthquake development plans in Haiti continued this logic, promoting the rehabilitation, expansion, and construction of free trade zones and export orientation in agriculture on the premise that exports would generate revenue, and wages would give Haitians the means to buy cheaper food imports. In concrete terms, this has meant that agricultural production has been geared toward export orientation (coffee, mangos, bananas[1]); yield gains (mechanization, subsidies for agrochemical inputs, growing farm sizes, and farm supports for mid-sized landholder, exporters, and agricultural enterprises); and land privatization and integrating rural folk into the wage economy (Steckley and Weis 2017).[2]

At the level of consumption, the idea has been that improving access to wages will enable households to purchase food, rather than grow it themselves. The model has been to improve food access by importing cheap food, and to address nutrient deficits (i.e., anemia) with imported "fortified" foods (i.e., fortified wheat biscuits, or peanut butter, like Plumpy'Nut®) that tend to be distributed by foreign NGOs (see Iannotti et al. 2016; Menon et al. 2007; Rice 2010). It is important to note that fortified foods are important in some contexts, and may indeed be essential in some circumstances. In Haiti though, it is hard to see the benefits of these nutrition programs, the problems of hunger, malnutrition, and anemia were recognized in the 1950s (Sebrell et al. 1959) and have persisted in spite of food aid and food fortification programs. One problem is that food aid is often resold in Haitian markets. Sometimes, the sales of fortified biscuits are worth more to the poor than the nutrients in them, and sometimes fortified food aid does not make it to those who need it most. For example, when we lived in the Artibonite Valley, a friend bought a World Food Program-fortified biscuit at the market and gifted it to our three year old. Needless to say, neither our friend nor our son was food insecure. Another day, a friend shared her fortified peanut butter pack with our son: she had received the pack through a food aid distribution program at her school. Again, this was not one of the most vulnerable schools in the area, and we frequently noticed that food aid was often allocated to sites near main roads, leaving those in the mountains, who tend to be the poorest, out of distribution chains.

Beyond food aid, Haitian markets are overrun with a whole host of imports: rice, beans, and chicken from the United States; eggs, corn flakes, and dried spaghetti from the Dominican Republic; and vegetable oil from China. Today, Haitian households spend over two-thirds of their income on food, and 80% report low levels of dietary diversity (Duvivier and Fontin 2017). While food is available in Haitian markets more than ever before, market integration has eroded household subsistence practices, undercut the prices of local crops, reduced dietary diversity, and tied food security to pocketbooks, increasing vulnerability to food price spikes at a time when food prices have become extremely volatile. Food price spikes and price volatility are pertinent issues as international food chains are disrupted by COVID-19 border closures and production disruptions. In Haiti, low levels of formal employment entail that many live hand to mouth, which entails that many feel compelled to continue work in spite of illness. This prevents prospects for self-quarantine, especially for the poor. It is also important to consider that border closure with the Dominican Republic will almost certainly impact the food supply, and fewer remittances from overseas will limit the ability of many households to purchase food. Again, it seems that the market-based food security approach has made Haiti more vulnerable to the food insecurity impacts of COVID-19.

But the failure of the free market to remedy malnutrition or food security is just the beginning. The free market approach to food security is also bound up in environmentally burdensome models of industrial agricultural that have been implemented in many low-income countries since the early 1980s. These are guided by the idea that yield gains, and efficiency will be the best way to reduce poverty and boost rural development. In agriculture, the long-distance supply chains, agrochemical-intensive production, and export orientation that have guided this approach are tied to a whole host of deleterious environmental consequences: agrochemical use has led to soil and water pollution; monocropping has reduced biodiversity and the proliferation of pests and "super-weeds" mechanization, and the growing need to service the transport of foods across great distances has spurred a growing dependence on petrol, and an increasing burden of agriculture on the climate in the form of carbon emissions. Importantly, industrial agriculture disembodied connections between food, land, and the environment from people, nutrition, and health. The bottom line is that the free market approach to food security is not climate friendly (Erickson 2008; Gonzalez 2004; McMichael and Schneider 2011; Weis 2007).

In Haiti, peasant producers are well aware of the shortcomings of the free market approach to food security, and various attempts to modernize agriculture have sparked protests from peasant producers (Steckley and Weis 2016). In 2010, for example, when Monsanto planned to donate 600,000 packs of hybrid seed sacks[3] to Haiti, over 10,000 Haitian peasants embarked on a protest march proclaiming, "long live native maize seed" and "Monsanto's GM [genetically modified] & hybrid seed violate peasant agriculture" (Via Campesina 2010). Peasants committed to burning Monsanto's seeds.[4] In 2013, peasants in Haiti's Artibonite Valley defended their land by blocking access to it from the coordinator of the mango exporter AgroTeknik, who had forcefully pushed them off their land two years earlier. National peasant organizations like Mouvman Peyizan Papay and Tét Kole Ti Peyizan Ayisyen assert that food *sovereignty* is the best way to resolve both the food and the climate crises (Steckley and Weis 2017; Via Campesina 2010).

As a conceptual framework, food sovereignty has gained global traction in the past 25 years.[5] While the meaning of food sovereignty is intensely debated, the core tenets are widely embraced:

- Agroecological production that prioritizes traditional seeds, biodiversity, ecosystem health, and local production for local consumption.
- Restructure food systems to ensure farmers and the poor have control over land, inputs, and the food and agricultural policies that govern them.
- Agrarian reform that focuses on gender inclusive, pro-poor land redistribution.
- Grow state control over agricultural trade, making sure that national trade policies respect local communities (i.e., giving states power to protect the nation from excessive imports).
- Social relations free of inequality (Via Campesina 2018).

It is important to emphasize that food sovereignty and food security are not antagonistic (FAO 2015). Food sovereignty includes food security objectives of improving food access and availability but pushes beyond these and asks us to see ecologies and nutrition as inseparable. Indeed, the ASD aligns with this vision in calls for both hunger reduction, improved nutrition, and sustainable agriculture. Yet, for peasants and food justice advocates, food sovereignty is a vision of food justice that challenges free market approaches to food security, and nutrition and sets out alternative policies that establish greater democratic control over food systems, and envisions food and agriculture, people and communities, and cultures and ecosystems as interdependent (Saturnino 2008). Food sovereignty advocates, for example, take issue with food import dependence, and nutrition programs that privilege imported fortified foods, instead advocating that nutritious diets are sourced from ecologically sound, diverse agricultural systems that contribute to both healthy communities and nutrition.

In Haiti, for example, national civil society organizations and peasant movements support fortified peanut butter produced by Haitian peasants and milled by Haitian collectives (Vansteenkiste 2017). At the same time, Haitian food sovereignty advocates reject imported peanuts; in 2016, the U.S. Department of Agriculture planned to ship 16,000 metric tons of peanuts to Haiti in a plan to stem malnutrition in school children, national peasant organizations demanded the cancellation of the shipment, articulating that it undermined Haitian peanut producers and food sovereignty (Bracken 2016; Kilhart 2016). Indeed, the advocacy of Haiti's peasant organizations is in tandem with the tenets of food sovereignty. In interviews, peasant leaders recurrently expressed this vision. For example, long-time leader of the Peasant Movement of Papaye described both concerns over modernist agriculture, and agrochemical inputs, and a vision for Haitian agriculture that embodies the important connections between population nutrition, farmer practices, and global environmental health saying:

Chemical fertilizer is a product of petrol. When there is no more petrol, there won't be any more chemical fertilizer. We have to look for an alternative. Tied to this, in high consuming societies, agriculture is killing the planet. Chemical fertilizer poisons the soil and destroys biodiversity. In terms of food security, countries like the United States are spending enormously to treat people who are sick because of poor food, they suffer because of obesity. That is because of food. We need to develop organic agriculture. This will allow peasants, Haitian people, to spend less money on diet-related illnesses *and* people will eat better. They will eat food that is simple and healthy, and the environment will be protected.

A leader of the organization Partenariat Developpement Local gives us insight into the limitations of the food security approach in Haiti and illustrates how food sovereignty necessitates meaningful government support of polyculture, and peasant-led food systems:

> I am working for peasants to have the food that they need, yes. For peasants to have, in quantity, what they need, and to produce to sell so that they have income to also meet their other household needs. But more than that, I am working – and I'm going to continue to work – for peasants to have ownership over their farming. For peasants to improve their understanding of the environment. To be able to grow their knowledge to manage the land even better and manage seeds to improve their lives. To practice polyculture that he is already doing, to be even better. Peasants can practice agriculture in a way that his family can live in good health in the long-term. that he can't do it by himself. If he could, he would have done it already.

A member of Tét Kole also expressed the need to take seriously a core dimension of food sovereignty in Haiti – agrarian reform and land security.

> In Haiti, there is no region that could not produce food for its people. If we used our land to produce food, it would permit us to have enough food. And even more – food for us to export to other countries! But the quantity of food that we have now is insufficient. This is because we don't have a state that will invest in our agriculture. And after the earthquake they say the country is open for business. Yikes! In the national budget you'll never find that they put in enough money to permit agriculture to be practiced

> in a way that will produce food. You will never see them subsidize agriculture for the producers, you will never see credit provision for farmers. If there is credit today, it is credit for industrial agriculturalists. We need agricultural credit for the peasants! To permit peasants to produce on their own land, to allow them to produce enough food for them to eat.
>
> *Tét Kole*

Food sovereignty has been used as a discourse, and approach by peasant and civil society organizations around the world to push back against the free market approach to food security, to contest trade liberalization, the influx of GM seed, and food dumping. In Haiti, until very recently, food sovereignty has been used distinctly by peasant movements and civil society organizations. However, since the 2010 earthquake, food sovereignty has featured more frequently in agriculture development plans. This is an exciting shift and is perhaps even more necessary in the pandemic period. More than ever before, the question of how food sovereignty is understood and practiced is central. How does the Haitian state, and bilateral organizations conceptualize food security and food sovereignty? Do state and international interpretations coincide or diverge from the visions of peasant organizations?

MORE OF THE SAME: FOOD SECURITY AND CLIMATE RESILIENCE PLANNING IN THE WAKE OF THE EARTHQUAKE

In large measure, Haiti's post-earthquake development planning has not diverted from the free market approach to food security. The tendency is for solutions to hunger and climate change vulnerability to be siloed. The dominant proposed solution to poor nutrition and hunger is to improve food access, and climate vulnerability is dealt with through environmental management (i.e., coastal protection, transportation infrastructure, and early warning systems). For example, the National Plan for Agricultural Investment (2010) and the Triennial Agricultural Recovery Program [Programme Triennal de Relance Agricole] (2013–2016) aim to improve food security by boosting economic growth and agricultural production around specific value chains. In tandem, the Ministry of Agriculture continues to focus on export-oriented growth sectors like coffee, cocoa, bananas, and mangos (Dieudonné 2015). Programs like the Enhancing and Building Capacity for Increased Food Security in Haiti (AKOSSA [Amelyorasyon Kapasite pou Ogmante Sekirite Alimantè an Ayiti]), which began in 2013, and the Program to Improve Food Security in Haiti [Programme d'Amelioration de la Securité Alimentaire en Haiti] (2013–2015), funded by the European Union and the FAO, seek to improve farmer revenue, integration into markets, and boost food *availability*. To be sure, Food Security is still critical for the development agenda – Haiti has a National Platform of Food Security (PFNSA [Plateforme Nationale de Sécurité Alimentaire]), a National Coordination of Food Security (CNSA), and a National Observatory of Food Security (ONSA [Observatoire National de la Sécurité Alimentaire]) – all lay out goals to improve food security by growing the economy and boosting household income with a focus on export orientation. Again, the World Bank has reiterated the importance of food security in the wake of the COVID-19 pandemic and has committed $9.5 million to address COVID-related food insecurity. This is the same drumbeat approach that has guided Haiti's agricultural plans for decades.

In terms of climate change, the Haitian government has demonstrated its concern about climate vulnerability and has emphasized the need for climate adaptation, but this discussion has largely been detached from a discussion of food security. For example, in 2017, the Government of Haiti ratified the Paris Agreement1[6] set out a National Action Plan on Climate Change Adaptation and established a National Climate Change Policy. In applied terms, there are also a range of climate resilience projects underway that focus on such things as disaster risk management and building coastal community resilience. One prominent example is the ten-million-dollar Inter-American Development Bank's Pilot Program for Climate Resilience (PPCR). The PPCR aims to better track geospatial data for storm impact and sea level rise. Still, the climate approaches put forth do little to tackle Haiti's underlying need for ecological regeneration and long-term climate resilience. In the area of reducing agricultural vulnerability, both the PPCR and Haiti's Strategic Program for Climate Resilience (SPCR) focus on disaster warning systems and hazard monitoring, collecting and managing climate data, and building climate-proof infrastructure to make sure that when bad weather hits, farmers can still get their products to the shipyards for export (PPRC). The climate mitigation projects are couched in broader objectives to "promote economic development by tapping socioeconomic potential" (CIAT 2013, 78).

Early warning systems, technology that improves rural access to weather reports, and improved infrastructure *are* indeed important in rural Haiti. So too are goals to reduce hunger. But Haiti's environment and hunger problems need to be conceptualized as integrated problems, and the question of who serves to benefit from climate resilience and agricultural solutions is paramount. Is the goal, for example, to support drought-resistant crops that are locally selected from traditional seed or to import hybrid and patented seed? To improve farm yields for home or international markets? To encourage poly-cropping with natural inputs, or monocropping agrochemical-intensive farming?

The leader of Haiti's most renowned peasant organization *Mouveman Peyizan Papaya*, Chavannes Jean-Baptiste, tells us that peasants must be wary of false solutions to the climate problem. A food security approach does not necessitate consideration of local ecologies, or long-term sustainable food systems, rural social relations, or the beneficiaries of agricultural value chains. In Haiti, this approach has done very little to abet hunger, reduces poverty, or improves climate resilience. Nearly 90% of Haitians are still poor; hunger still affects 50% of people in that country, Haitian farmers persistently suffer the full force impacts of environmental change, and food insecurity has increased since 2009 (WFP 2019).

GLIMMERS OF HOPE: FOOD SOVEREIGNTY(?) IN THE WAKE OF THE EARTHQUAKE

In 2010, the Action Plan for National Recovery and Development of Haiti (PARDN), the guidepost plan for Haiti's post-earthquake recovery, set out an important promise;

Haiti's environment would feature "in every decision" related to the nation's recovery and development (PARDN 2010). The Haitian government *is* very concerned about climate change and its food security impacts and there is some indication that the government, and international NGOs are beginning to see the links between environments, nutrition, and health. Some scholars, for example, are beginning to draw connections between malnutrition and national education and livelihood outcomes in Haiti and have found that improved nutrition for young mothers, and youth will improve productivity and improve workforce participation (Serigne et al. 2014). Similarly, the PARDN asserts in plain terms that agriculture has a significant impact on Haiti's environment and climate vulnerability, and there are glimmers of hope that some planning for rural Haiti aims to move past a vision that prioritizes market-based development models and instead seeks to build agrarian landscapes that are climate resilient and provide healthy communities and meaningful livelihoods.

For example, the Global Facility for Disaster Reduction and Recovery (GFDRR) and the Global Support Program of the Climate Investment Funds (CIF), financed by the World Bank, suggest that to prevent devastating impacts of climate change on Haitian agriculture, programming should be geared toward restoring soil quality and ecosystem health by integrating climate adaptations like planting drought-resistant seeds, growing crops that will stabilize and enrich soils, raising awareness of land conservation practices, developing a seed bank of drought-resistant and high-temperature tolerant varieties, and installing rainwater-harvesting tanks (GFDRR 2011). These align nicely with the SDG 15 objective to protect and restore ecosystems and halt land degradation. Both food security and food sovereignty advocates could get behind these ideas.

There has also been more concrete attention to food sovereignty specifically. In 2015, for example, Haiti's National Policy for Food Sovereignty, Food Security and Nutrition (PNSSANH) set objectives that align with a food sovereignty framework by doing such things as providing irrigation infrastructure, technical assistance, and subsidies to farmers and livestock producers and emphasized the need to promote Haitian products in the food baskets of Haitian households and institutions, all of which would increase farmer control over their production. On the consumption side, the Parliamentary Front against Hunger in Haiti is working to identify legal instruments to improve nutrition and support national agriculture (SUN 2019), and the PNSSANH outlines objectives for School Meals Programs to supply 50% of foods from local producers (Duvivier and Fontin 2017; PNSSANH 2015). The Government of Haiti also created an Artisanal Seed Producer Groups, the first of its kind in Haiti. The group produces, packages, and markets locally produced seed. Other NGOs and bilateral organizations also highlight the need to support local, sustainable food systems, build the capacity of rural associations (IFAD 2019), and improve smallholder resilience (WFP 2019). These projects resonate with the core goals of food sovereignty and indicate that some of the central aspirations of food sovereignty are being taken up in Haiti, a meaningful sign of change.

Still, it is important to be cautious of the ways that other core attributes of food sovereignty are being watered down or overlooked entirely. While food sovereignty is a significant part of the PNSSANH, the core objective to improve farmer food security by pursuing export-oriented economic growth remains explicit. For example, the PNSSANH goals to reduce wait times at customs, lower transport costs for agricultural products, and reduce fuel prices suggest that the export-oriented model is alive and well, with no recognition of the potential (or inherent) contradictions with food sovereignty. The government also continues to support the increased use of agrochemical fertilizers and has subsidized up to 80% of fertilizer to farmers since 2008 (Gustave et al. 2017). This diverges markedly from the kind of food sovereignty peasant organizations are calling for – agroecological practices free of chemicals. Most glaring in discussions of food sovereignty by the Haitian state and bilateral organizations is the omission of any objectives for agrarian reform, social relations free of inequality, or objectives for smallholder control over food systems.

Long-term climate resilience demands not just adaptation to climate change (building sea walls, fortifying transportation infrastructure, creating emergency warning systems), but bridging the social-ecological divide and taking seriously the power relations that impact climate vulnerability (Walsh, Wolford, and McCarthy 2016). Food sovereignty offers a framework for making sure that it is not just *any* agriculture producer that benefits from resilience policies, but small-scale producers in particular. That not just any seeds or inputs are subsidized, but that traditional, locally produced non-GM seeds, and local composting systems are supported. That not just *any* food is used to combat hunger, but that locally produced, culturally appropriate food is prioritized. Leaders of peasant organizations in Haiti demand that clear movement toward the principles of food sovereignty includes full policy and resource support. Peasants organizations agree with plans that call for agricultural extension programs but only those that support traditional seed and inputs. Peasant leaders support the idea that more food should be available to rural households but argue that we need to push beyond that so that food is healthy, locally produced, and grown in ways that dignify producers and enrich local ecosystems. Peasants argue that one of the central tenets of thriving rural food systems in Haiti is peasant land security, and the key here is for pro-poor redistributive land reform.

CONCLUSIONS

In this chapter, we illustrate that Haiti's food insecurity and vulnerability to climate change are tied up in the free market approach to food security that has been guiding Haiti's rural development planning since the 1980s. Haiti is still prone to malnutrition and poor yields, and the staccato blows of extreme weather are hitting Haiti harder every year. But there is nothing inevitable about Haiti's food insecurity, and there are meaningful ways that peasants are fighting for food sovereignty and climate justice. The uptake of food sovereignty would mark a radical change in Haiti's agricultural development agenda, and there are some indications that some aspects of food sovereignty are being integrated into Haiti's agricultural policy agenda. But in spite of the rhetoric, it is important to recognize that food sovereignty in Haiti is happening only in piecemeal, and many important components – agrarian reform, democratic decision-making, food systems free of inequality – are still off the agenda.

In interviews, leaders of peasant organizations emphasized that Haiti still can be a hopeful case, and there is perhaps no better place on earth to embrace and implement the core goals of food sovereignty. Indeed, Haiti is already part way there. Unlike its regional neighbors where land ownership is concentrated in the hands of wealthy few, in Haiti, customary practices have ensured that small-sized properties dominate the landscape, and most rural households have *de facto* access to land. Tied to this, Haiti has a large rural peasant population that are eager to improve their lives. As a leader of PAPDA says, "This is almost the last country where there are peasants. This is something very precious. Humanity must find another way of living, another relationship with the environment. Haitian peasants have answers." Examples from around the world show that there is a positive relationship between the number of workers on a unit of land and the level of agricultural output on that unit of land. Finally, it is heartening that Haitian agriculture is largely "organic" (Gustave et al. 2017). Only 30% of Haitian farmers rely on chemical fertilizers, meaning that has one of the lowest per capita uses of agrochemicals in the hemisphere. As COVID-19 tightens borders around the world, and as people aim to conceptualize a "new normal," Haitian peasants are advocating that the "new normal" is food sovereignty. Today, there is an opportunity to invest in Haiti's agrarian populations and landscapes, to attract the reserve army of labor in the overpopulated cities to the countryside, and to offer dignified work that increases national food provisioning, and supports nutritious, ecologically vibrant and culturally enriching food systems. As, the Haitian Agronomist, Talot Bertrand tells us, "It is the moment to revive the agricultural sector and enhance the Haitian peasantry in order to restore food sovereignty at the national level while putting Haiti on the path of the process of sustainable development" (Haiti Libre 2020).

RECOMMENDATIONS

In Haiti, experiences of disasters, like the 2010 earthquake and Hurricane Matthew of 2016, have revealed the acute vulnerability of the poor to food insecurity in post-disaster situations. In this chapter, we have illustrated how the historical emergence of the free market approach to food insecurity has amplified food insecurity, and we have highlighted Haitian peasant calls for food sovereignty as a new way forward. As we begin to consider how yet another disaster – the COVID-19 pandemic – will impact Haiti, the questions of how consumers access food markets (private car, or *taptap)*, where food is purchased (i.e., supermarkets, or the *maché* [outside, open-air markets]), and how food is stored (i.e., refrigeration) will likely all impact vulnerability to virus contraction and food insecurity. On the one hand, the Haitian elite and foreign NGO workers have private cars, the means to frequent high-end grocery stores with social distancing policies and free hand sanitizer, and the ability to store food in air-conditioned homes with refrigeration. On the other hand, for Haiti's majority poor population, there is no household electricity, which makes refrigeration very rare, and means it is necessary for people already living in densely populated areas to leave their homes and seek resources from the markets that are not only notoriously crowded but also where there is no running water, access to bathrooms, or places for hand-washing.

The COVID-19 experience in Haiti is likely to be another example of a disaster that exposes the same inequalities that were illuminated by the 2010 earthquake and Hurricane Matthew in 2016. In particular, the free market approach to food security – tying food security to people's ability to pay for food – makes the poor extremely vulnerable to food price spikes and food insecurity. Haitian peasants tell us that there is a better way.

There is much hope that the pursuit of food sovereignty in Haiti will lead to improved nutrition and climate resilience. As the Haitian state, and development practitioners continue to craft sustainable rural development and nutrition plans based on the core goals of food sovereignty, our hope is that this chapter illustrates that Haitian peasant leaders, and their calls for food sovereignty should guide the way. The Sustainable Development Goals are a meaningful place to start, and the ASD goals of hunger elimination, improved nutrition, and sustainable agriculture (SDG 2), improving climate resilience (SDG 13) and ecosystem restoration (SDG 15) dovetail nicely with the principles of food sovereignty. Yet, peasants also remind that power relations are important determinants of nutrition, food security, and environmental health. Haitian peasant leaders are clear that the dynamic problems of hunger, malnutrition, and climate vulnerability can best be solved by ensuring that goals to reduce inequality (SDG 10) include democratic decision-making around agriculture, equitable access to community resources, and that power lies with the Haitian people. With that in mind, we offer three recommendations to guide Haitian policy makers as they move toward the principles of food sovereignty.

Our first recommendation is for pro-poor redistributive agrarian reform. As one interviewee put it, "The first thing peasants need is land." While Haitian peasants maintain *de facto* land access in many parts of Haiti, there are glaring inequalities in Haiti's land ownership (Steckley and Steckley 2019), and in the past decade, peasants have continued to face threats to their land access, and in turn to their household food provisioning. A member of Tét Kole elaborated in concrete terms saying, "Peasants should not have to labour in fear. They should not constantly be turning their heads to protect their land from the elite. They should know that they are the masters of their own production." Pro-poor agrarian reform, including recurrent restrictions on land markets that could lead to land consolidation, is a hopeful mechanism to stem some of the trenchant rural class inequalities that have been deepened by the market imperatives of the export-oriented production model of the past century (Akram-Lodhi 2013). In the case of Haiti, pro-poor redistributive land reform can help meet some of the core SDGs of poverty reduction (SDG 1), improving rural livelihoods and dignified work (SDG 8), and supporting food security and sustainable agriculture (SDG 2).

Second, moving toward food sovereignty in Haiti requires state support for local, ecologically integrated agriculture, including markets to sell crops. Land reform will not be enough on its own; peasant producers need meaningful support to increase productivity through agroecology (i.e., low-tillage, diversified poly-cropping systems, and organic inputs). Peasants should be able to produce in consideration of soil and ecosystem health, and community nutrition, and this means being able to access affordable agricultural inputs (machinery, seeds, compost systems), water, and electricity. In concrete terms, this may include things like subsidies for locally produced, traditional Kreyòl seeds; support for domestic seed-saving cooperatives; and credit and agricultural extension services for small-scale producers. Peasants will also need access to markets where they can sell their crops at prices that reflect production costs. To start, the state must protect national production so that peasants are not competing with goods produced by global industrial agriculture and must support peasant production by privileging local food procurement for nutrition programs in hospitals and schools. State support for local, ecologically integrated agriculture is an important way for Haiti to move toward several SDGs.

Specifically, local, agroecological food systems are now widely acknowledged to be an important part of climate mitigation (SDG 13)[7]; just as productive as industrial agriculture (Tittonell 2014) but far more likely to sustain soil health and long-term land productivity (SDG 15); more labor intensive (McKay 2012), which means that this agricultural model will give more people work (SDG 8); and emblematic of nutrition-focused farming that are far better at ensuring healthy communities, particularly in terms of economic downturn and disaster (SDG 2) (Akram-Lodhi 2013; Ó Gráda 2009). The intention of this recommendation is for the Haitian state to support agroecological production systems that reflect Haiti's need for sustained or increased yields, rural ecosystem restoration, more secure farmer livelihoods, and enhanced food and nutrition. The leader of KOPAV urged that while peasants are committed, "Peasants cannot do it alone. We need a supportive state."

Third, and perhaps most challenging, peasant perspectives must be privileged in rural development decision-making. This must include meaningful participation of peasant organizations in determining state budgets on supports for agricultural enterprises, inputs, and farm types; decisions on how best to address trade policies that govern food imports; conceptualizing ecosystem health through rural food system services like seed sharing, local food policy councils, and rural market resources; and how best to mobilize knowledge on agroecology, climate adaptation to agriculture, and nutrition-focused production. Moving toward the core goals of food sovereignty demands addressing power imbalances and increasing peasant control over Haiti's food systems. One peasant producer expressed this in simple terms:

> When a peasant plants a sweet potato on his land, he'll take a bit of that sweet potato every time he goes and put it back in the ground to continue to grow - he controls when he can take it to eat even before he harvests formally. When he decides to formally harvest, *he* decides on the sale price, *he* negotiates, *he* brings it to market. And alongside the sweet potato he plants a whole host of other things, so any time he goes to his garden he'll leave with food. That is food sovereignty.

NOTES

1 For example, the Projet d'Amelioration de la Culture de la Banane, implemented in 2015 by the Haitian Ministry of Agriculture and the French Agency for Development (AFD), seeks to improve food security by increasing banana production to increase farmer income, and improve Haiti's trade balance by bolstering banana exports (Flecher 2015).

2 To offer some examples, the 2007 National Strategy Document for Economic Growth and Poverty Reduction DSNCRP aims to improve poverty by boosting economic growth. The 2010 National Plan for Food and Nutrition Security specifically aimed to improve food security (access and availability); 2010 National Plan for Agricultural Investment (PNIA) sought to improve value chains, and agricultural production; the 2012 National Nutrition Policy (PNN) seeks to improve nutrition measures and public

health; the 2013–2016 Triennial Agricultural Recovery Program sought to bolster food security by improving economic growth.

3 The seeds were treated with Thiram, a highly toxic chemical that the U.S. Environmental Protection Agency presents such an acute danger to agricultural workers, that in the United States they are legally required to wear protective gear when working with these seeds.

4 SDG 2, which sets out a vision for zero hunger, articulates the importance of preserving genetic diversity of seed. While this aligns with the interests of Haitian Peasants, there needs to be greater attention in the ASD to *seed sovereignty* in particular, which emphasizes seeds as open resources, highlights the need for public control over seed production, trade, and access, and again is concerned with democratic decision-making and control over biological resources. For Haitian peasants, seed sovereignty is a key part of food sovereignty movements, and local Kreyòl seeds in particular are an important part of culturally appropriate food provisioning, agricultural heritage, and sustainable rural livelihoods (Mazzeo and Brenton 2013).

5 Via Campesina introduced the term food sovereignty to the world at the World Food Summit in 1996 (Via Campesina 2007).

6 It should be emphasized that Haitians contribute very little to climate change. Per capita carbon dioxide emissions sit at a global low of 0.3 tonnes (UNDP 2019).

7 Agroecology production systems, for example, are more drought resistant, resilient to hurricanes, and have better soil and water holding capacity than industrial agricultural systems.

REFERENCES

Akram-Lodhi, A.H. (2013) Food Sovereignty: A Critical Dialogue. International Conference Yale University. September 14–15, 2013.

Bernstein, B. (2014) Food Sovereignty Via the "Peasant Way": A Skeptical View. *Journal of Peasant Studies* 41(6):1031–1063.

Bracken, A. (2016) The US Wants to Give Peanuts to Malnourished Haitian Kids. Why Is That a Problem? Public Radio International. https://www.pri.org/stories/2016-05-10/us-wants-give-peanuts-malnourished-haitian-kids-why-problem

CIAT (2013) Haïti Strategic Program for Climate Resilience (SPCR). Port-au-Prince, Haïti: Comité Interministériel d'Aménagement du Territoire. https://www.climateinvestmentfunds.org/sites/cif_enc/files/PPCR_SC.12_4_Strategic_Program_for_Climate_Resilience_for_Haiti.pdf

Cohen, M.-J. (2013) Diri Nasyonal ou Diri Miami? Food, Agriculture and US-Haiti Relations. *Food Security* 5:597–606.

Desmarais, A.A. (2007) *La Via Campesina: Globalization and the Power of Peasants*. Blackpoint, Nova Scotia: Fernwood Publishing.

Dieudonné, J. (2015) Haïti pourrait reconquérir sa souveraineté alimentaire. Le Nouvelliste. https://lenouvelliste.com/article/146791/haiti-pourrait-reconquerir-sa-souverainete-alimentaire

Duvivier, P and L. Fontin (2017) Building the Evidence Base on the Agricultural Nutrition Nexus. Haiti: Technical Centre for Agricultural and Rural Cooperation (CTA).

Eckstein, D., M.-L. Hutfils, and M. Winges (2018). Global Climate Risk Index 2019: Who Suffers Most from Extreme Weather-Related Loss Events in 2017 and 1998 to 2017. German Watch. https://germanwatch.org/sites/germanwatch.org/files

Erickson, P. (2008) Conceptualizing Food Systems for Global Environmental Change Research. *Global Environmental Change* 18(1):234–245.

FAO (Food and Agriculture Organization) (2015) Food Security and Sovereignty. Food and Agriculture Organizations of the United Nations. http://www.fao.org/3/a-ax736e.pdf

FAO (Food and Agriculture Organization) (2019) Haiti and FAO: Strengthening Food and Nutrition Security and Enhancing Rural Incomes. Rome: Food and Agriculture Organization of the United Nations. www.fao.org/3/a-az058e.pdf

Flecher, J. (2015) Le PACB pour Booster la Production de la Banane Plantain. Le Nouvelliste. https://lenouvelliste.com/article/149785/le-pacb-pour-booster-la-production-de-la-banane-plantain

GFDRR (2011) *Vulnerability, Risk Reduction, and Adaptation to Climate Change. Global Facility for Disaster Reduction and Recovery, Climate Investment Funds*. Washington, DC: World Bank.

Global Hunger Index (2019) Global Hunger Index Haiti. Haiti: Concern Worldwide and Welthungerhilfe. https://www.globalhungerindex.org/pdf/en/2019/Haiti.pdf

Gonzalez, C.G. (2004) Trade Liberalization, Food Security, and the Environment: The Neoliberal Threat to Sustainable Rural Development. *Transnational Law and Contemporary Problems* 14:419.

Gordillo, G., and M. Jerónimo (2013) Food Security and Sovereignty. Rome: Food and Agriculture Organization of the United Nations. http://www.fao.org/3/a-ax736e.pdf

Gustave, N.M., K. Karume, S. Vwima, and J. Francis (2017) The Agriculture-Nutrition Nexus in Haiti: CTA Technical Brief. Wageningen, The Netherlands: Technical Centre for Agricultural and Rural Cooperation. https://cgspace.cgiar.org/bitstream/handle/10568/100768/2012_PDF.pdf?sequence=1&isAllowed=y

Haiti Libre (2020) Haiti-Covid-19: The Agricultural Sector Needs Special Measures. https://www.haitilibre.com/en/news-30458-haiti-covid-19-the-agricultural-sector-needs-special-measures.html

Iannotti, L., S.J.-L. Dulience, S. Joseph, C. Cooley, T. Tufte, K. Cox, J. Eaton, J.R. Delnatus, and P.B. Wolff (2016) Fortified Snack Reduced Anemia in Rural School-Aged Children of Haiti: A Cluster-Randomized, Controlled Trial. *PLoS One* 11(12). https://doi.org/10.1371/journal.pone.0168121

IFAD (2019) Investing in Rural People: Haiti. https://www.ifad.org/en/web/operations/country/id/haiti

IFPRI (2019) Food Security Portal: Haiti. International Food Policy Research Institute. http://www.foodsecurityportal.org/haiti/indicators

Kilhart, K. (2016) Peanuts and Protest in Haiti Minimize US Surplus Dumping Scheme. Boston, MA: Grassroots International. https://grassrootsonline.org/blog/peanuts-and-protest-in-haiti-minimize-us-surplus-dumping-scheme/

Mazzeo, J. and B.P. Brenton (2013) Peasant Resistance to Hybrid Seed in Haiti: The Implications of Agro-Industrial Inputs through Humanitarian Aid on Food Security, Food Sovereignty, and Cultural Identity. In *Food and Identity in the Caribbean*, H. Garth, ed. Pp.123–137. New York: Bloomsbury.

McKay, B. (2012) A Socially-Inclusive Pathway to Food Security: The Agroecological Alternative. International Policy Center for Inclusive Growth Policy Research Brief. No. 23. http://www.ipc-undp.org/pub/IPCPolicyResearchBrief23.pdf

McMichael, P. (2005) Global Development and the Corporate Food Regime. In *New Directions in the Sociology of Global Development Volume 11 (Research in Rural Sociology and Development)*, F. Buttel and P. McMichael, eds. Pp. 265–299. Bingley: Emerald Group Publishing Limited. In *Bewildering Borders: The Economy of Conservation*, Werner Zips and Manuela Mairitsch-Zips, eds. Pp. 61–89. Münster: Lit Verlag and Wien.

McMichael, P. and M. Schneider (2011) Food Security Politics and the Millennium Development Goals. *Third World Quarterly* 32(1):119–139.

Menon, P., M.T. Ruel., C. Loechl, M. Arimond, J.-P. Habicht, G. Pelto, and L. Michaud (2007) Micronutrient Sprinkles Reduce Anemia among 9- to 24-Mo-Old Children When Delivered through an Integrated Health and Nutrition Program in Rural Haiti. *Journal of Nutrition* 137(4):1023–1030.

Moore, W.M. (2015) *Capitalism in the Web of Life*. London: Verso.

Ó Gráda, C. (2009) *Famine: A Short History*. Princeton, NJ: Princeton University Press.

PARDN (2010) Action Plan for National Recovery and Development of Haiti. Port-au-Prince, Haiti: Government of the Republic of Haiti. https://reliefweb.int/report/haiti/action-plan-national-recovery-and-development-haiti

Patel, R. (2009) Food Sovereignty. *Journal of Peasant Studies* 36(3):663–706.

PNSSANH (Politique Nationale de Souveraineté et Sécurité Alimentaire et Nutritionnelle en Haïti) (2015) The National Policy of Food Sovereignty and Food and Nutrition Security in Haiti. Port-au-Prince, Haiti: Government of the Republic of Haiti. https://faolex.fao.org/docs/pdf/hai209018.pdf

Porter, C. and I.J Dugan (2020) COVID-19 Trickles into Haiti: 'This Monster Is Coming Our Way'. *New York Times*. April. https://www.nytimes.com/2020/04/22/world/americas/coronavirus-haiti.html

Rice, A. (2010) The Peanut Solution. *New York Times*. September 2, 2010.

Saturnino, B.M., Jr. (2008) La Via Campesina and its Global Campaign for Agrarian Reform. *Journal of Agrarian Change* 8(2/3):258–289.

Sebrell W.H., S.C. Smith, E.L. Severinghaus, H. Delva, B.K. Reid, H.S. Olcott, J.Bernadotte, W. Fougere, G.Barron, G. Nicolas, K.W. King, G.L. Brinkman, and C.L. French (1959). Appraisal of Nutrition in Haiti. *American Journal of Clinical Nutrition* 7:538–584.

Serigne, D., E. Roberte, T. Kovac, M. Lêlio-Joseph, P. Moses, L. Oot, B. Ralph, K. Sethuraman, and A.E. Sommerfelt (2014). *Reducing Malnutrition in Haiti: Estimates to Support Nutrition Advocacy – Haiti PROFILES 2013*. Washington, DC: FHI 360/FANTA and Ministère de la Santé Publique et de la Population, Haiti.

Steckley, M. and J. Steckley (2019) Post-Earthquake Land Appropriations and the Dispossession of Rural Women in Haiti. *Feminist Economics* 25(4):45–67.

Steckley, M. and T. Weis (2016) Peasant Balances, Neoliberalism, and the Student Growth of Non-Traditional Agro-Exports in Haiti. *Canadian Journal of Latin American and Caribbean Studies* 41(1):1–22.

Steckley, M. and T. Weis (2017) Agriculture in and beyond the Haitian Catastrophe. *Third World Quarterly* 38(2):397–413.

SUN (2019) The Parliamentary Front against Hunger in Haiti Seeks to Refine the Draft Law on School Feeding. Scaling Up Nutrition (SUN). https://scalingupnutrition.org/news/the-parliamentary-front-against-hunger-in-haiti-seeks-to-refine-the-draft-law-on-school-feeding/

Tittonell, P. (2014) Food Security and Ecosystem Services in a Changing World: It Is Time for Agroecology. In *Agroecology for Food Security and Nutrition*. Proceedings of the FAO International Symposium. Pp.16–35. 18–19 September, Rome, Italy. http://www.fao.org/3/a-i4729e.pdf

UNDP (2019) Human Development Reports: Haiti. United Nations Development Programme. http://hdr.undp.org/en/countries/profiles/HTI

Vansteenkiste, J. (2017). Food Insecurity in Haiti: A Gendered Problem in the Making. Doctoral Dissertation. Guelph: University of Guelph.

Via Campesina (2007) Nyéléni Declaration. Forum for Food Sovereignty. Mali: Sélingué,.

Via Campesina (2010) Haitian Peasants March against Monsanto Company for Food and Seed Sovereignty. https://viacampesina.org/en/haitian-peasants-march-against-monsanto-company-for-food-and-seed-sovereignty/

Via Campesina (2018) Food Sovereignty Now! A Guide to Food Sovereignty. European Coordination via Campesina. https://viacampesina.org/en/wp-content/uploads/sites/2/2018/02/Food-Sovereignty-A-guide-Low-Res-Vresion.pdf

Walsh, M., W. Wolford, and J. McCarthy (2016) Rights for Resilience: Food Sovereignty, Power, and Resilience in Development Practice. *Ecology and Society* 21(2):11–20.

Weis, T. (2007) *The Global Food Economy*. London: Zed Books.

WFS (World Food Summit) (1996) Declaration on World Food Security. Rome: World Food Summit.

WFP (World Food Programme) (2019) Haiti Country Strategic Plan (2019–2023). https://www.wfp.org/operations/ht02-haiti-country-strategic-plan-2019-2023

Windfuhr, M., and J. Jonsén (2005) *Food Sovereignty: Towards Democracy in Localized Food Systems*. FIAN International. Chippenham: ITDG Publishing.

Wittman, H. (2015) From Protest to Policy: The Challenges of Institutionalizing Food Sovereignty. *Canadian Food Studies* 2(2):174–182.

World Bank (2017) Rapidly Assessing the Impact of Hurricane Matthew in Haiti. World Bank. Results Briefs. October 20th. https://www.worldbank.org/en/results/2017/10/20/rapidly-assessing-the-impact-of-hurricane-matthew-in-haiti

7 Constraints on Family Poultry Systems in Guatemala

Amy E. Snively-Martinez and Marsha Quinlan

CONTENTS

INTRODUCTION

Poultry rearing is an age-old practice, dating back at least 8,000 years (Alders and Pym 2009). Poultry husbandry systems are important small-scale production systems that provide income and food security for resource-poor households (Alders and Pym 2009; Alders, Bagnol, and Young 2010; Bagnol 2009; Conan et al. 2012; Thieme et al. 2014). Guatemala is a lower, middle-income Central American country with the highest poverty level in Latin America (FAO 2014). The COVID-19 pandemic has triggered a sharp increase in poverty levels as pandemic response measures resulted in decreased wage-earning opportunities while food prices increased due to decreased agricultural production and trade (FEWS NET 2020). In June 2020, the number of cases of acute malnutrition in children under five years of age (CU5) had doubled from June 2019 levels. Smallholder farmers, subsisting on less than 1.5 acres, manage 45% of Guatemalan land. Residents there have a deep history of poultry keeping, with Mayan turkey husbandry in Guatemala going back at least 2,300 years (Thornton and Emery 2015).

Family poultry systems continue to be important to households in Guatemala where up to 90% of smallholder households keep poultry (Mallia 1999; Pica-Ciamarra et al. 2011). They are primarily managed by women and are important for women's livelihoods because they provide direct access to cash income when needed

DOI: 10.1201/9781003014942-7

(Bagnol 2009; Mack, Hoffmann, and Otte 2005; Thieme et al. 2014). Access to direct cash is more important than ever to households during the COVID-19 pandemic, as they face reduced income opportunities (FEWS NET 2020). Women can easily manage fowl while raising children. And, women are more likely to reinvest the cash provided through poultry sales back into the household, most often spending on family health care needs.

Here, livelihood refers to a "combination of the household and production systems," including sociocultural values of production (Aklilu et al. 2008, 176). Livelihood systems target *food security*, or the ability of all people within a household to access nutritious and culturally appropriate foods at all times in order to lead an active and healthy lifestyle (Gunderson and Ziliak 2015; Holbin 2010). Poultry rearing as a part of rural livestock systems eases rural poverty because the birds provide extra nutrients and protein for households, and people can sell birds for cash in times of need, thereby contributing to household resilience (Guèye 2000; Mack, Hoffman, and Otte 2005; Wong et al. 2017).

We review data from ethnographic interviews conducted in two communities of the Monterrico Multiple-Use Reserve (*Reserva Natural de Usos Multiples de Monterrico* or RNUMM), located in the Pacific lowlands of Guatemala. The interviews come from a larger study conducted in 2014 and 2015 to understand the importance of family poultry systems to household food security and livelihoods and to understand poultry ethnoveterinary care. The principal outcomes of the study were (1) to model the constraints that local residents face in accessing appropriate care for poultry and (2) to understand nonprescriptive antibiotic use for poultry. This inquiry generally informs efforts related to SDGs 1 (no poverty), 2 (zero hunger), 3 (good health and well-being), 5 (gender equality), 13 (climate action), 15 (sustainable life on land), and 17 (partnerships for the goals) (UN 2015). Interviews were conducted with smallholder households located in the communities of Monterrico and La Candelaria, Guatemala, two of the ten villages forming RNUMM along the Chiquimulilla Canal (Godinez Orantes 2014; Hernandez Bonilla et al. 2011; Godoy 1992).

Poultry Systems in Low- to Middle-Income Countries (LMICs)

Poultry husbandry systems are relatively inexpensive: they require minimal land for production, and people can establish them with little time and monetary investment (Amos 2006; Conan et al. 2012; Mack, Hoffmann, and Otte 2005; Thieme et al. 2014). Low-cost investments in small-scale livestock provide women opportunities to contribute to household income and control a portion of it. This reduces gender inequality per Sustainable Development Goal 5, Promote Gender Equality and Empower Women and Girls (UN 2015). Women generally manage poultry in LMICs and managed birds provide important income sources for women who are otherwise tied to the household (Bagnol 2009; Mack, Hoffmann, and Otte 2005; Thieme et al. 2014). In addition, poultry is socio-culturally important for local ritual and celebration because cross-culturally, the meat generally has few taboos associated with consumption (Guèye 2000; Mack, Hoffmann, and Otte 2005); for example, the value of poultry in India where beef taboos are present (Mohana Devi et al. 2014);

poultry being acceptable in many Islamic areas with pork taboos; and poultry as part of postpartum diets in China (Koon, Peng, and Karin 2005).

In LMICs, "family poultry systems" involve free-ranging birds, raised under semi-intensive to nonintensive systems in both urban and rural areas (Thieme et al. 2014). Thieme et al. (2014) define four categories of family poultry units in which household production occurs: small extensive scavenging (up to five birds that scavenge for their food), extensive scavenging (5–50 birds), semi-intensive systems (50–200 birds that owners provision fairly routinely), and small-scale intensive production (over 200 birds). Each category indicates levels of breed diversity, provision of housing, feed inputs, and time required for poultry management.

Family poultry systems usually consist of a variety of intermixed species, of a range of ages, to ensure meat and egg production throughout the year. Chickens (*Gallus domesticus*) comprise up to 80% of poultry flocks in LMICs, while other species include ducks (*Cairina moschata domestica* and *Anas platyrhynchos domesticus*), turkeys (*Meleagris gallopavo*), guinea fowl (*Numida meleagris*), and geese (*Anser domesticus*) (Conan et al. 2012; Thieme et al. 2014). In small-scale systems, poultry interact closely with humans, livestock, and wild bird species. They are often free ranging and interbreed with neighboring flocks. Roaming may expose fowls to a variety of vermin, predators, and infectious diseases. Over generational exposure, locally bred poultry develops endemic protection from local climate conditions, and pests and disease, so locals often prize them over commercialized breeds (Wong et al. 2017). Therefore, locally developed poultry breeds can insure a more sustainable and viable food source for local populations per SDG 2 (end hunger) because they meet food security and nutrition needs (UN 2015). Specifically, SDG targets 2.4 and 2.5 address the maintenance of local sources' genetic diversity of seeds, plants, and domesticated animals to assure sustainable and resilient food systems. In this case, locally bred poultry are important because they tend to be better adapted to local conditions and ideally more resilient in the face of long-term climate change and worsening global food system crises, such as we have observed with COVID-19 pandemic (UN 2015).

With low rates of investment in family poultry flocks, however, high bird mortality is common, so the flocks often serve as secondary livelihood support. However, family poultry systems can provide sustainable sources of protein and nutrients for the household (Guèye 2000; Thieme et al. 2014; Wong et al. 2017). Scavenging-based poultry systems have the ability to transform plant and insect products, unsuitable for human consumption, in addition to food wastes from the household, into highly nutritious meat and eggs. A review by Wong et al. (2017) demonstrates that meat and eggs from family poultry provide essential protein, vitamins (A, B12, D, K, and riboflavin), and other micronutrients (iron, zinc, folate, and selenium). These nutrients are especially important for households with children. This reduces malnourishment per SDG targets 2.1 and 2.2, which call for an end to hunger and malnutrition through regular access to safe and nutritious foods (UN 2015). Malnourishment, coupled with persistent diarrhea as a result of unsafe drinking water and unsanitary living conditions, can cause a "double burden" on growing children resulting in stunted growth and impaired cognitive development (Guerrant et al. 2013). In addition, it has been found that these children are at greater risk of developing obesity later in life, thereby resulting in a "triple burden" for children that experience malnutrition coupled with persistent enteric infections throughout their childhood. Guatemala has one of the highest rates of stunting for children in the world and accounts for 56% of the cases of malnourished children in Central America (MSPAS et al. 2009; World Bank 2010 as cited in Chary et al. 2013). It is also critical to note that Indigenous populations there often suffer from malnourishment at much higher rates than non-Indigenous peoples.

BACKGROUND

The Monterrico Multiple-Use Reserve or RNUMM (Reserva Natural de Usos Multiples de Monterrico) or RNUMM) was established in 1977 with the goal to protect the natural wetland ecosystem of the southern Pacific region of Guatemala, while allowing traditional use of the wetland resources upon which local communities depend for subsistence. The entire wetland ecosystem covers about 4,000 hectares altogether; however, the RNUMM reserve only covers about 2,800 hectares. The maintained central canal, Chiquimulilla, was initially dredged in 1886 with the goal of connecting the area's various estuaries and increasing the flow of people and goods, runs the central length of this wetland ecosystem (Godinez Orantes 2014).

RNUMM consists of estuarine and coastal-marine mangrove habitats (García-Fuentes et al. 2013). The coastal lagoons and mangrove swamps serve as an important hatchery for crabs, mollusks, shrimp, and fish. The canal and wetland system provides a significant source of subsistence products for local communities. Many households consider fishing and hunting in the canal system their main subsistence activity.

Since the late 1970s, Monterrico has been a popular vacation spot for Guatemalan nationals and foreigners, with hotels appearing along with the first installations of the RNUMM reserve, including protected incubation areas for marine turtle eggs. RNUMM's sea turtle protection has had some international attention from tourists and nonprofit organizations. The establishment of the reserve coincided with an increased extraction of natural resources in the areas surrounding the Chiquimulilla Canal and the RNUMM reserve (Godoy 1992; Godinez Orantes 2014; Hernandez Bonilla et al. 2011). Households in Monterrico and La Candelaria are subsistence oriented and the majority are smallholders that participate in several livelihood activities which include animal husbandry, agriculture, fishing, and participation in the tourist economy. Smallholder households in this region raise primarily pigs, chickens, turkeys, and ducks. While women are the primary caretakers of the pigs and poultry, men dedicate themselves to fishing, crop farming, and wage labor.

Fishing by both locals and businesses from outside of the region has gradually intensified over the last three decades. RNUMM residents attribute overfishing of the canal system to illegal commercial fishing that especially depletes juvenile fish stocks as mature fish stocks have declined substantially. Residents note that they have had to adjust their nets to finer weaves to catch smaller fish, and that overall fish catches are decreasing in abundance (Snively-Martinez and Quinlan 2019). Many local men consider fishing their primary livelihood activity, so residents bemoan a persistent worried feeling over the dwindling canal resources.

Fieldwork in the communities indicates that householders feel the need to offset losses in fish catches with other activities. The purpose of the ethnographic research presented in this chapter is to understand poultry rearing as a livelihood activity for women (as an active and productive member of the smallholder household), in addition to understanding how approaches to poultry health may be shifting in relation to changing livelihoods, such as declining fishing outcomes. Therefore, the focus here is on poultry health and the actions householders take to improve it, with the underlying assumption being that people are actively exploring alternative livelihood supports (as indicated through ethnographic interviews).

In the RNUMM, most families live in a house compound (HC) that typically consists of the home and the surrounding area that may contain one or more outbuildings, including kitchens, eating areas, and latrines. HCs have either man-made or living fences of growing plants or trees that separate them from neighboring properties, but they are usually open to the street. The house itself consists of a two to four bedroom unit that opens to an outdoor kitchen and sitting area containing strung hammocks and a table for eating.

Animals are important sources of both direct and indirect income for households in RNUMM. Men work by fishing, farming (in fields away from the home), and wage labor. Women raise poultry primarily for household consumption and to sell for direct income in times of need. Home-raised swine are mostly under women's care until someone, usually the man, sells them at the market. Backyard animals therefore are essential components of a household's overall livelihood system, which primarily functions to assure a family's food security. Raising poultry and swine, well documented in the 1930s, has been an important traditional subsistence practice for area households (Hernandez Bonilla et al. 2011).

Livelihood Support and Poultry Systems' Sociocultural and Socioeconomic Importance in Guatemala

Almost three-quarters (74%) of householders involved in the original study indicated that women are the primary poultry caretakers (see Table 7.1), and 76% of women participants responded that they were solely tied to the home for livelihood purposes, indicating the importance of poultry systems to women's livelihoods in the study sites. Family poultry systems range from small units of a few mostly foraging/scavenging birds to holdings of greater than 50 birds. The majority of households that participated in the study (76%) indicated they rear from 6 to 25 birds composed mostly of chickens, with some ducks and fewer turkeys. Poultry roam freely outside and within the HC, including into and out of the kitchen, eating areas, and rooms for sleeping. In a few households, residents place gates closing the eating area off from the animals. The free-range nature of the birds is much easier for women to care for. Birds will roam into and out of neighboring HCs and are sometimes killed by passing cars; however, the overall savings in cost for poultry care are significant when considering housing and caging of birds. Participants said that costs for permanent poultry enclosures tend to be high and result in more work for the women who care for the birds. Hen housing often complicates women's work, requiring feed inputs and time in cleaning and upkeep of the hen house (Bagnol 2009). Managing hen houses can

TABLE 7.1
Socioeconomic Data for Monterrico and La Candelaria

	Monterrico No.	La Candelaria No.	Percent of Total
Household Heads			
Male	17	14	64%
Female	5	6	23%
Both	4	2	13%
Total	**26**	**22**	
Poultry Caretakers			
Male	6	1	17%
Female	17	20	74%
Family	3	1	9%
Total	**26**	**22**	
Livelihoods			
MALE			
Fishing/Agriculture	14	13	65%
Construction	3	0	8%
Shrimp hatchery	0	2	5%
Chalet guardian	0	2	5%
Other	5	2	17%
Total*	**22**	**19**	
FEMALE			
Home	17	17	76%
Food cart	5	3	18%
Commercial	1	1	4%
Fishing	0	1	2%
Total*	**23**	**22**	

* Totals indicate responses given for each question. "Livelihoods" represent the primary livelihood of each household head, as people often participate in several livelihood activities during the course of the year.

deter women from raising chickens at all due to the strain on already limited household resources and women's time.

All households consume the birds they rear to some extent. Besides food, flocks provide an important source of extra cash in needy times. And, it is women who manage this cash source. One participant, Madga Elena, expressed, "[The poultry] is for our benefit, if we need to eat, we can eat one, and if we need money, we can sell one."

Poultry is especially important for celebrations and holidays, including birthdays and Christenings. It is common to butcher one or more birds for a celebration, depending on the number of guests one expects. Women do the butchering and preparing of poultry in most cases. During Christmas and Holy Week, it is also common to butcher many birds at once for traditional feasts, as family members from out of town will come to visit for extended periods. Locals especially prize *Criollo* chicken, local heritage breeds, for making tamales, a regional dish made for Christmas celebrations. This is the time of the year that households will also sell much of their poultry, either to villagers who do not raise their own, or to out-of-towners (not from the village). Chickens therefore generally sell to out-of-towners for about Q75 (US$10) for butchering and, locally, a laying hen can sell for up to Q100 (US$13). Ducks sometimes fetch a high price for butchering, ranging from Q150 (US$20) to Q200 (US$27) for one bird.

Considering the average daily wage for agricultural and nonagricultural workers in Guatemala ranges between US$10 and US$15 (Gandara and Barrientos 2018), and that women's wages tend to be much lower, the sale of poultry can provide up to and beyond a day's wages in times of need for the household. It should be noted that it is rare for neighbors to sell the animals to one another at such high prices. The above prices reflected an average of what people charge to nonlocals. Many vacationers from Guatemala City come for holidays or the occasional weekend, when villagers take advantage to sell their birds. Most families have either direct or indirect access to poultry through a family member, so there is no need to purchase them for consumption.

Stressors and Constraints on Family Poultry Systems

The most frequent cause of death for poultry in RNUMM is disease. The most common poultry illnesses are locally known as *soco*, *peste/acidente*, and the less common *buba*. *Soco* is the general term that locals commonly use for a number of respiratory diseases, and *buba* refers to avian pox (Ceron et al. 2016; Merida Ruiz et al. 2016). *Acidente* and *peste* refer to a grim systematic or respiratory disease that can result in the sudden death of apparently healthy animals. Merida Ruiz et al. (2016) found that, in the Maya Biosphere Reserve located in the northern, tropical climates of Guatemala, *acidente*, and *peste* usually refer to Newcastle disease (Avian pneumoencephalitis, i.e., infection with virulent Newcastle disease virus [NDV]) (Merck 2016).

When asked about the difference between *acidente* and *peste*, respondents always said they were one and the same and, as such, I will hereafter only use *peste*, the more common of the terms. Respondents overwhelmingly noted that *peste* is, by far, the most fatal disease for poultry, especially chickens and ducklings, not affecting adult ducks nearly as often. Participants described the shocking sudden onset and death of apparently healthy birds. Ana remarked, "Once it comes, it doesn't leave me with anything! If one animal has it, the rest will get it and die. From one day to the next they die." In reference to the sudden nature of the disease, Magda Elena said that *peste* is terrible "because at night they will get up on their roost to sleep and be fine, and the next day they are dead."

Ethnographic interviews revealed that, in the face of poultry disease, a majority (66%) of respondents (n = 48), said that they use over-the-counter human antibiotics to treat their birds that appear to contract either *soco* or *peste*. One respondent, who had kept many birds in the past, said her family now only raises pigs. Poultry became too expensive due to yearly losses resulting from disease. Ethnographic data indicate that people in RNUMM resort to human antibiotics to treat their birds even though the pharmaceuticals are often not successful. In reference to the latest episode of *peste* that moved through La Candelaria, Lety explained, "…When the neighbor told me that her birds were infected, I started to put tetracycline in the birds' water, but it didn't do anything…they all died anyway." Indeed, if *peste* is the Newcastle virus, then antibiotics, whether human or veterinary, would not affect the virus, and might only tax the bird's condition.

Interviews indicated that village members perceive that episodes of infectious poultry diseases are increasingly common in the area. For *peste*, over half of participants attributed the disease to warmer, drier weather that comes in the summer. For *soco*, occurrences are associated more with cooler, wetter weather. Ceron et al. (2016) found that up to 95% of residents in Monterrico and Calendaria perceived climatic change to be a factor in animal ill health (poultry, swine, and ducks). In addition, about 40% of study participants perceived garbage or outside contamination as a source of infection. Participants noted that, as recently as about ten years ago, *peste* was not a regular problem, only showing up in the area about every two years. However, many participants noted that *peste* currently occurs once, even twice a year. Residents also noted that episodes of drought were more common in the last ten years.

Participants were aware of the difference between antibiotics for poultry and antibiotics for humans. However, 49% of participants in the ethnographic survey (n=35) believed that antibiotics for animals and those for humans work in similar manners and perceive human antibiotics as equally effective in treating poultry illnesses. Seventy-seven percent of participants believed that it is necessary to vaccinate their poultry. However, only 53% of people said they have access to money and appropriate transportation to purchase the veterinary medicines, leaving just under half the population unable to access appropriate veterinary immunizations or other medicines. Professional veterinary services for poultry are not available in proximity to the study communities. The biggest constraints to vaccination are opportunity costs in time away from work for traveling to a vet, and transportation difficulties (Snively-Martinez 2019; Snively-Martinez and Quinlan 2019). According to respondents, the closest professional veterinary services are located roughly 13 miles away from Monterrico, but travel to them requires a boat ride across the canal, then a bus ride into the closest town or to another urban center located roughly 16 miles from La Candelaria and about 18 from Monterrico. On public transit, these distances often result in a day's travel to and from both locations. Residents thus resort to post hoc and perceived prophylactic human antibiotics, which village general stores and pharmacies sell readily over the counter.

DISCUSSION

Guatemala has the highest rate of chronic child malnutrition in all of Latin America (Webb et al. 2016; World Food Programme 2017) and food prices continue to rise in response to the COVID-19 epidemic, resulting in disproportionate effects in low-income and Indigenous communities (FEWS NET 2020). In rural Guatemala, family poultry systems can provide a significant source of nutrition and food security, in addition to extra income for many households and may represent an alternative source of livelihood support as other, more traditional options like fishing and wage labor become ever less viable. Per SDG target 1.5 (end poverty: build resilience), poultry systems build resilience of these vulnerable groups and reduce their exposure to climate-related extremes, as well as social, economic, and environmental shocks (UN 2015). Waters-Bayer and Bayer note that "smallholders keep animals as a means to achieve a variety of aims, of which food production is only one" (1992, 6). Ethnographic studies of smallholder livestock keepers find that livestock are not only a form of wealth (as is common with pastoralists, e.g. Quinlan et al. 2016) but also function "as a savings account, producing offspring as interest" (Waters-Bayer and Bayer 1992, 7).

Poultry constitutes a substantial female contribution to subsistence and home upkeep in the RNUMM. A potential subsistence shift from reliance on fishing to reliance on poultry would also shift household gender roles away from men being solely responsible for all protein and income, to a more interdependent arrangement that benefits women. Similarly, in Africa and Asia, research has shown that poultry is important for increasing a household's access to food, schooling, and health services (Aklilu et al. 2008; Bagnol 2009). Across the developing world, women rear chickens for barter and for cultural purposes, and keeping chickens and other small livestock empowers women (Waters-Bayer and Letty 2010) and provides a primary source of income for female-led households (Aklilu et al. 2008; Bagnol 2009). Therefore, women's participation in decision-making activities in local villages, as well as their access to economic resources (including land ownership and control), is essential per SDG targets 5.5 and 5.A (UN 2015).

The biggest barrier to poultry rearing in the RNUMM reserve is disease and illness. In light of COVID-19, zoonotic infectious diseases that jump from animals to humans must also be considered. Further research is needed to verify the connection between resident's perceived increase in disease episodes in poultry with warmer, drier conditions. At this point, vaccination is essential to maintain flock health; however, accessibility of professional veterinarians and veterinary medications remains difficult with high opportunity costs (Snively-Martinez 2019). These costs increased in response to the COVID-19 pandemic, as a result of reduced transportation and wage-earning opportunities, along with higher overall costs of goods (FEWS NET 2020). Smallholder households therefore rely on readily available treatments for poultry illnesses. Those include human biomedicines and medicinal home remedies. If people feel there is a need to administer biomedicines to their poultry, they usually resort to purchasing human antibiotics.

Villagers are largely unaware of the implications of inappropriate antibiotic use, such as the risk of antimicrobial resistance or AMR development, which is an added burden to the poultry rearing systems. The process of natural selection selects for antimicrobial resistant bacteria in the guts of meat producing animals that are treated with antibiotics on a regular basis. Antibiotics used for human and animal consumption often come from the same class of antimicrobials, increasing the probability of crossover of resistant forms of bacteria in both humans and animals. Humans can potentially come into contact with AMR bacteria when they consume this meat.

While AMR is a global health concern, limiting access to antibiotics in regions like rural Guatemala would mean limiting access to these life-saving treatments for individuals who may otherwise not afford these medicines (Whyte 1992; Ramay, Lambour, and Ceron 2015), let alone the opportunity costs of their own doctors' visits. Therefore, health education campaigns are necessary to inform the public of the possible dangers of human antibiotic use in animals and the advantages of appropriate poultry vaccination. SDG target 4.7 calls for equal access to the knowledge and skills necessary to promote sustainable livelihoods and gender equality. This case study demonstrates that women should be directly targeted for education regarding poultry care, including for their own self-care in the COVID-19 climate. SDG target 3.B links with this as well; it calls for access to affordable and essential medicines and vaccines to live an active and healthy life.

Ethnographic research for this case study indicates that, in rural Guatemala, people often include veterinary biomedical treatments into one larger category without discernment between vaccinations, antibiotics, and vitamin treatments. The incursion of biomedicines into rural areas has occurred without proper guidance from biomedical practitioners (Ramay, Lambour, and Ceton 2015). Clifford et al. (2018, 662) state, "Poor-quality veterinary medicine as a contributor to antimicrobial resistance has been mentioned…Given the widespread use of antibiotics in animal husbandry and the persistent problems of drug quality in low- and middle-income countries, this is a significant oversight." The WHO (World Health Organization) has begun a Global Action Plan on Antimicrobial Resistance with an objective to optimize the use of antimicrobial medicines in human and animal health (WHO 2015), as demonstrated by this study and many others (Aklilu et al. 2008; Alders and Pym 2009; Alders, Bagnol and Young 2010; Bagnol 2009; Bagnol et al. 2013; Guèye 2000; Mallia 1999; Wong et al. 2017). In accordance with SDG 2.3 (increase agricultural productivity and incomes of small-scale food producers, especially women) and SDG 5 (promote gender equality and empowerment of women and girls), the WHO should aim toward women, particularly when considering household livestock rearing such as poultry (UN 2015).

LIMITATIONS OF RESEARCH

This project was conducted with the intention of understanding decision-making for poultry health in RNUMM; however, research revealed information regarding general family poultry systems in the RNUMM and their importance to women's work and household food security. As with any qualitative research, the generalizability of results from this study is limited due to geographical specificity and small sample sizes. However, findings of this study generally fall in line with what has been found elsewhere (see Eltayb et al. 2012; Heffernan 2001; Heffernan, Thomson, and Nielson 2008; Heffernan, Thomson, and Nielson 2011; Redding et al. 2013). More time investment at the field sites will increase rich information regarding poultry systems in RNUMM. Further research, therefore, is necessary to reveal the most effective approach to local education programs on poultry health.

We see that poultry systems link to the larger local food system through ancient tradition including turkey domestication and propagation of the local *criollo* chicken. Smallholder poultry farming also sustains families through women's participation in food – especially in protein acquisition, which prior reliance on male fishing had almost eliminated. On their own, Guatemalans have made cultural shifts inherent in various SDGs.

CONCLUSIONS AND RECOMMENDATIONS

At the study site, infectious poultry diseases are becoming increasingly common due to global processes of contact and exchange, and residents are responding by integrating human antibiotics into their local poultry treatment practices. Even though this study represents a limited geographical and cultural area, it is extrapolation worthy as results correspond to those found elsewhere regarding climate change, antibiotic use, and poultry and livestock treatment (Braykov et al. 2016; Caudell et al. 2017a, b; Ceron et al. 2016; Heffernan, Thomson, and Nielson 2008; Subbiah et al. 2020). It should be viewed as indicative of wider processes underway in areas where animal husbandry is important and access to veterinary care and medications is limited.

As women are the primary poultry health care providers in Guatemala, it is necessary to target health education messages appropriately to the poultry care and human health contexts in their villages. Family poultry systems are well established in rural Guatemala; therefore, extension programs that aim to improve animal health and increase household food security are needed to support the women who manage these systems. This tackles several interlinked SDG targets mentioned previously, including SDG 1 (end poverty) and 2 (end hunger), as well as SDG 4 (access to appropriate education) and 5 (gender equality).

Research has shown that village vaccination campaigns featuring local women as community vaccinators can significantly impact vaccination rates and make poultry rearing a valuable livelihood resource for those women (Alders et al. 2010; Bagnol et al. 2013). In RNUMM and across Guatemala, women should be provided an equal share in access to land, resources, knowledge, and financial services to support healthy poultry systems per SDG targets 2.3 and 5.A (increase agricultural productivity and incomes of smallholder farmers, particularly women, and increase women's access to ownership and control over land and other forms of property and natural resources). Shifting the focus of village vaccination campaigns toward women would, ideally, decrease the need for using human antibiotics on birds because vaccinated poultry would have increased resistance to disease, thereby decreasing the misuse of antimicrobials and associated risk for developing antimicrobial resistance. In addition, local (national and global) education regarding appropriate use of antimicrobials is needed, thus providing equal access to the knowledge and skills necessary to promote sustainable livelihoods per SDG 4.7 (ensuring knowledge to promote sustainable development) (UN 2015). Learning the smaller recommended doses for birds and confirming the inapplicability of antibiotic therapy for viruses (e.g. Newcastle virus) would reduce human and animal environmental antibiotic exposure.

Furthermore, adopting appropriate use of antibiotics for poultry would reduce families' overall household expenditures on unnecessary applications, thereby making poultry rearing more economically beneficial for households. With a lower disease burden afforded by vaccines, it is likely that women in RNUMM would worry less about saving eggs for flock reproduction. Consumption of more home-raised eggs would become an additional source of nutrients for households and serve to moderate the threat of the "triple burden" of malnutrition, infectious diseases, and chronic diseases (Guerrant et al. 2013). In addition, lowering flocks' disease burden would increase overall flock numbers for households, thus increasing the amount of income from their sale and available food resources per SDG targets 1.4 and 1.5 (build resilience of the poor and vulnerable, and ensure equal access to economic resources for men and women) (UN 2015).

The RNUMM area is a modest national and international tourist destination with small hotels and family homes dotted along the coast. Visitors frequent the RNUMM, presenting an opportunity for households to market their locally prized *criollo* breeds to the small-scale hotel industry there, and to visitors beyond the holiday seasons. However, when asked about the sale of chickens to area businesses, respondents indicated that it is rare. Local restaurants source their chicken meat elsewhere, presumably where they can buy more. Outsourced chicken farming requires relatively high-energy investments in fuel and transportation to get meat and eggs to these rural areas. SDGs 8 and 12 call for sustainable economic growth coupled with sustainable consumption in all areas of the world (UN 2015). Per targets 8.9 and 12.8, sustainable tourism should be promoted at local levels by making relevant information available and accessible to local people. Additionally, sustainable tourism has the potential to create jobs and income through the promotion of local cultural products. Poultry health education and vaccination campaigns could support more sustainable local food systems where there are enough chickens, and businesses feel secure in purchasing chicken meat from local smallholders. This would increase income possibilities and food security for community households while reducing local businesses' overall carbon footprints.

Poultry is important to smallholder households not only in Guatemala, but across Latin America. As research has shown from Africa and Asia, the information gained from this project indicates that family poultry systems at the RNUMM are similar to those found around the world. It is safe to assume, therefore, that the research presented in this chapter is applicable to other family poultry systems across Guatemala and Latin America. The information presented here should be taken into consideration when creating extension education programs for improvement of poultry systems. This fulfills SDG target 17.6 which focuses on national and international partnerships in science and technology and calls for the sharing of knowledge that in this case is directly referential to vaccine technologies to enhance protection against local poultry diseases and the possibility of future emergent zoonotic infectious diseases.

REFERENCES

Aklilu, H., Udo, H., Almekinders, C., & Van der Zijpp, A. (2008) How resource poor households value and access poultry: village poultry keeping in Tigray, Ethiopia. *Agricultural Systems 96*(1–3): 175–183.

Alders, R.G. & Pym, R. (2009). Village poultry: still important to millions, eight thousand years after domestication. *World's Poultry Science Journal 65*: 181–190.

Alders, R.G., Bagnol, B., & Young, M. (2010). Technically sound and sustainable Newcastle disease control in village chickens: lessons learnt over fifteen years. *World's Poultry Science Journal 66*: 433–440.

Amos, T.T. (2006). Analysis of backyard poultry production in Ondo State, Nigeria. *International Journal of Poultry Science 5*(3): 247–250. [Online] URL: http://www.docsdrive.com/pdfs/ansinet/ijps/2006/247-250.pdf.

Bagnol, B. (2009). Gender issues in a small-scale family poultry production: experience with Newcastle disease and highly pathogenic avian influenza control. *World's Poultry Science Journal 65*: 231–240.

Bagnol, B., Alders, R., Costa, R., Lauchande, C., Monteiro, J., Msami, H., Mgomezulu, R., Zandamela, A., & Young, M. (2013). Contributing factors for successful vaccination campaigns against Newcastle disease. *Livestock Research for Rural Development 25*(6). [online] URL: http://www.lrrd.org/lrrd25/6/bagn25095.htm.

Braykov, N.P., Eisenberg, J., Grossman, M., Zhang, L., Vasco, K., Cevallos, W., Munoz, D., et al. 2016. Antibiotic resistance in animal and environmental samples associated with small-scale poultry farming in Northwestern Ecuador. *MSphere 1*(1): e00021-15. https://doi.org/10.1128/mSphere.00021-15.

Caudell, M.A., Quinlan, M.B., Quinlan, R.J., & Call, D.R. (2017a) Medical pluralism and livestock health: ethnomedical and biomedical veterinary knowledge among East African agropastoralists. *Journal of Ethnobiology and Ethnomedicine 13*(7). https://doi.org/10.1186/s13002-017-0135-1.

Caudell, M.A., Quinlan, M.B., Subbiah, M., Call, D.R., Roulette, C.J., Roulette, J.W., Roth, A., & Quinlan, R.J. (2017b). Veterinary antibiotic use among agro-pastoralists in Northern Tanzania. *PLoS ONE 12*(1): e0170328. https://doi.org/10.1371/journal.pone.0170328.

Ceron, A., Ortiz, M.R., Alvarez, D., Palmer, G.H., & Cordon-Rosales, C. (2016). Local disease concepts relevant to the design of a community-based surveillance program for influenza in rural Guatemala. *International Journal for Equity in Health 15*: 69. [online] URL: https://equityhealthj.biomedcentral.com/articles/10.1186/s12939-016-0359-z.

Chary, A., Messmer, S., Sorenson, E., Henretty, N., Dasgupta, S., & Rohloff, P. (2013). The normalization of childhood disease: an ethnographic study of child malnutrition in rural Guatemala. *Human Organization 72*(2): 87–97.

Clifford, K., Desai, D., Prazeres da Costa, C., Meyer, H., Klohe, K., Winkler, A., Rahman, T., Islam, T., & Zaman, M.H. (2018). Antimicrobial resistance in livestock and poor quality veterinary medicines. *Bulletin of the World Health Organization 96*: 662–664. [online] URL: https://doi.org/10.2471/BLT.18.209585.

Conan, A., Goutard, F.L., Sporn, S., and Vong, S. (2012). Biosecurity measures for backyard poultry in developing countries: a systematic review. *BMC Veterinary Research 8*: 240. [online] URL: http://www.biomedcentral.com/1746-6148/8/240.

Eltayb, A., Barakat, S., Marrone, G., Shaddad, S., & Stålsby Lundborg, C. (2012). Antibiotic use and resistance in animal farming: a quantitative and qualitative study on knowledge and practices among farmers in Khartoum, Sudan. *Zoonosis and Public Health 59*: 330–338.

FEWS NET (Famine Early Warning Systems Network). (2020). Guatemala: Perspectiva de Seguridad Alimentaria. [online] https://fews.net/sites/default/files/documents/reports/FSO_GT_2020_06_final.pdf.

Food and Agriculture Organization (FAO). (2014). Country fact sheet on food and agriculture policy trends, Guatemala. [online] http://www.fao.org/3/a-i4124e.pdf.

Gandara, N. & Barrientos, M. (2018). Salario minimo 2019 en Guatemala queda sin aumento. *Prensa Libre.* Available at: https://www.prensalibre.com/economia/salario-minimo-2019-guatemala-publicado-en-el-diario-de-centroamerica/.

García-Fuentes, A., Castillo-Cabrera, F.J., Dávila-Pérez, C.V., Morales, A.S., Salazar-Mendias, C., Lendinez-Barriga, M.L., Torres-Cordero, J.A., & Ruiz-Valenzuela, L. (2013). Study of the vegetation in the multiple use natural reserve of Monterrico (Guatemala). *Plant Biosystems 148*(6): 1064–1074.

Godinez Orantes, R. (2014). Plan director de la población de Playa Negra 2015–2035 municipio de Taxisco, departamento de Santa Rosa. Universidad de San Carlos de Guatemala, Facultad de Arquitectura.

Godoy, J.C. (1992). Monterrico: A Reserve for Maximum Use. In: *Toward a Green Central America: Integrating Conservation and Development.* Valrie Barzetti & Yanina Rovinski, eds. Pp 88–99. Kumarian Press, West Harford, CT.

Guerrant, R.L., DeBoer, M.D., Moore, S.R., Scharf, R.J., & Lima, A.A.M. (2013). The impoverished gut – a triple burden of diarrhea, stunting and chronic disease. *Nature Reviews Gastroenterology and Hepatology 10*(4): 220–229.

Guèye, E.F. (2000). The role of family poultry in poverty alleviation, food security and the promotion of gender equality in rural Africa. *Outlook on Agriculture 29*(2): 129–136.

Gunderson, C. and Ziliak J.P. (2015). Food insecurity and health outcomes. *Health Affairs 34*(11): 1830–1839 [online] http://content.healthaffairs.org/content/34/11/1830.full.html.

Heffernan, C. (2001) Consumer preferences and the uptake of animal healthcare by the poor: a case study from Kenya. *Journal of International Development 13*: 847–886.

Heffernan, C., Thomson, K., & Nielsen, L. (2008) Livestock vaccines adoption among poor farmers in Bolivia: remembering innovation diffusion theory. *Vaccine 26*: 2433–2442.

Heffernan, C., Thomson, K., & Nielsen, L. (2011) Caste, livelihoods and livestock: an exploration of the uptake of livestock vaccination adoption among poor farmers in India. *Journal of International Development 23*: 103–118.

Hernandez-Bonilla, S., Lopez Alquijay, S., Pardo Villegas, P., & Gomez Conde, P. (2011). Dinámica socioambiental asociada a las áreas protegidas de Guatemala: el systema universitario de áreas protegidas-SUAP. Universidad de San Carlos de Guatemala, Dirección General de Investigación Programa Universitario de Investigación de Cultura, Pensamiento e Identidad de la Sociedad Guatemalteca, Centro de Datos para la Conservación, Centro de Estudios Conservacionistas, CECON. Available at: http://www.repositorio.usac.edu.gt/559/1/16_1187.pdf.

Holbin, D.H. (2010). Position of the American Dietetic Association: food insecurity in the United States. *Journal of the American Dietetic Association 110*: 1368–1377.

Koon, P.B., Peng, W.Y., & Karin, N.A. (2005). Postpartum dietary intakes and food taboos among Chinese women attending maternal and child health clinics and maternity hospital, Kuala Lumpur. *Malaysian Journal of Nutrition 11*(1): 1–21.

Mack, S., Hoffmann, D., and Otte, J. (2005). The contribution of poultry to rural development. *World's Poultry Science Journal 61*(1): 7–14.

Mallia, J.G. (1999). Observations on family poultry units in parts of Central America and sustainable development opportunities. *Livestock Research for Rural Development 11*(3). http://www.lrrd.cipav.org.co/lrrd11/3/mal113.htm.

Merck. (2016). *Merck Veterinary Manual.* Merck Sharp & Dohme Corp, Kenilworth, NJ. Available at: https://www.merckvetmanual.com.

Merida Ruiz, S.A., Guerra Centeno, D.S., Leonardo, E.L.B., Rohn, K., Kosters, S., & Kreienbrock, L. (2016). Participatory epidemiology at the neotropics: study of diseases of backyard livestock and description of hunting patterns in Uaxactún, Maya reserve biosphere, guatemala. *BMC Research Notes 9*(207). [online] https://bmcresnotes.biomedcentral.com/articles/10.1186/s13104-016-2009-3.

Ministerio de Salud Pública y Asistencia Social (MSPAS), Instituto Nacional de Estadística, Universidad del Valle de Guatemala, USAID, Agencia Sueca de Cooperación para el Desarrollo Internacional, CDC, UNICEF, UNFPA, PAHO, USAID/Calidad en Salud. (2009). *V Encuesta Nacional de Salud Materna Infantil 2008–2009.* Guatemala City: Ministerio de Salud Pública y Asistencia Social.

Mohana Devi, S., Balachandar, V., Lee, S.I., & Kim, I.H. (2014). An outline of meat consumption in the India population – a pilot review. *Korean Journal of Food Science 34* (4): 507–515.

Pica-Ciamarra, U., Tasciotti, L., Otte, J., and Zezza, A. (2011). *Livestock Assets, Livestock Income and Rural Households: Cross-Country Evidence from Household Surveys.* Food and Agriculture Organization, Rome, Italy. International School of Social Studies, The Hague, Netherlands. World Bank, Washington DC.

Quinlan, R. J., Rumas, I., Naiskye, G., Quinlan, M.B., & Yoder, J. (2016). Searching for symbolic value of cattle: tropical livestock units, market price, and cultural value of maasai livestock. *Ethnobiology Letters 7*(1): 76–86. [online] https://doi.org/10.14237/ebl.7.1.2016.621.

Ramay, B.M., Lambour, P., & Ceron, A. (2015) Comparing antibiotic self-medication in two socio-economic groups in Guatemala City: a descriptive cross-sectional study. *BioMed Central Pharmacology and Toxicology 16*: 11. https://doi.org/10.1186/S40360-015-0011-3.

Redding, L.E., Barg, F.K., Smith, G., Galligan, D.T., Levy, M.Z., & Hennessy, S. (2013). The role of veterinarians and feed-store vendors in the prescription and use of antibiotics on small dairy farms in rural Peru. *Journal Dairy Science 96*: 7349–7354.

Snively-Martinez, A. (2019). Ethnographic decision modeling to understand smallholder antibiotic use for poultry in Guatemala. *Medical Anthropology 38*(3): 295–310. https://doi.org/10.1080/01459740.2018.1550755.

Snively-Martinez, A. and Quinlan, M. (2019). Family poultry systems on the southern Pacific coast of Guatemala: gender, livelihoods, and food security. *Journal of Ethnobiology 39* (4): 493–509.

Subbiah, M., Caudell, M.A., Mair, C., Davis, M.A., Matthews, L., Quinlan, R.J., Quinlan, M.B., Lyimo, B., Buza, J., & Call, D.R. (2020). Antimicrobial-resistant enteric bacteria are widely distributed amongst people, animals and the environment in Northern Tanzania. *Nature Communications 11*:228.

Thieme, O., Sonaiya, F., Rota, A., Guèye, F., Dolberg, F., and Alders, R. (2014). Defining Family Poultry Production Systems and Their Contribution to Livelihoods. In: *Decision Tools For Family Poultry Development. FAO Animal Production and Health Guidelines NO. 16*. Rome, Italy: FAO. Pp. 3–8. Available at: http://www.fao.org/3/a-i3542e.pdf.

Thornton, E.K. and Emery, K.F. (2017). The uncertain origins of mesoamerican Turkey domestication. *Journal of Archaeological Method and Theory 24* (2): 328–351.

United Nations (UN). (2015). Sustainable Development Goals Knowledge Platform. Available at: https://sustainabledevelopment.un.org/sdgs.

Waters-Bayer, A. & Bayer, W. (1992). The role of livestock in the rural economy. *Nomadic Peoples 31*: 3–18.

Waters-Bayer, A. & Letty, B. (2010). Promoting Gender Equality and Empowering Women through Livestock. In: *The Role of Livestock in Developing Communities: Enhancing Multifunctionality*, F. Swanepoel, A. Stroebel, & S. Moyo, eds. Pp. 31–50. Technical Centre for Agricultural and Rural Cooperation (CTA), Wageningen, Netherlands.

Webb, M.F., Chary, A.N., De Vries, T.T., Davis, S., Dykstra, M., Flood, D., Rhodes, M.H., & Rohloff, P. (2016). Exploring mechanisms of food insecurity in indigenous agricultural communities in Guatemala: a mixed methods study. *BMC Nutrition 2*: 55. [online] https://bmcnutr.biomedcentral.com/articles/10.1186/s40795-016-0091-5.

Whyte, S.R. (1992). Pharmaceuticals as folk medicine: transformations in the social relations of health care in Uganda. *Culture, Medicines and Psychiatry 16*(2): 163–186.

Wong, J.T., de Bruyn, J., Bagnol, B., Grieve, H., Li, M., Pym, R., & Alders, R.J. (2017). Small-scale poultry and food security in resource-poor settings: a review. *Global Food Security 15*: 43–52. [online] http://www.sciencedirect.com/science/article/pii/S2211912416301043.

World Bank. (2010). Improving Health and Nutrition of Mothers and Young Children in Guatemala. World Food Programme. (2017). Guatemala, Rome, Italy. Available at: http://www1.wfp.org/countries/guatemala.

World Health Organization (WHO). (2015). Global Action Plan on Antimicrobial Resistance. Available at: http://www.wpro.who.int/entity/drug_resistance/resources/global_action_plan_eng.pdf.

8 Community-Led Change

Building Food Security, Gender Equity, and Climate Change Resilience in the Dry Corridor of Guatemala

Devon Wilson

CONTENTS

INTRODUCTION

Food security is a complex issue influenced by varying economic, political, and social factors as experienced in daily life for people across the globe. The United Nations defines food security as when "all people, at all times have physical and economic access to sufficient, safe and nutritious food that meets their dietary needs and food preferences for an active and healthy life" (IFPRI 2020). The UN 2015 Sustainable Development Goals (SDGs) outline measurable targets and indicators that address numerous key challenges to food security in developing countries. Global food security policy and programs are increasingly framed by SDG 1 (no poverty) and SDG 2 (zero hunger) and often incorporate interrelated factors such as gender equality,

DOI: 10.1201/9781003014942-8

access to employment and fair wage, and climate action (United Nations Statistics Division 2021). In the least developed countries, rural agrarian women often live in economic poverty, and as such are notably vulnerable to food insecurity. The ability to access secure sources of food for households is threatened by various factors such as informal employment, lack of access to education, health services, and vital subsistence resources such as land and water. Women whose families rely on household production of subsistence food are less likely to own land, make economic decisions, or hold active roles in community and political leadership (Oxfam 2019).

While the UN SDGs provide a conceptual framework from which governments and international development agencies may construct inclusive policy and programming, field ethnography demonstrates that climate-vulnerable groups hold valuable knowledge of the impacts of key challenges to food security in relation to climate events. This chapter presents a case study of a nongovernment organization's program initiatives and impacts toward achieving food security, women's equality, and resilience in a region highlighted as one of the most impacted by climate change on the planet – the Dry Corridor of Guatemala.

The Central American Dry Corridor (CADC) presents multiple challenges to rural communities in an increasingly unpredictable climate. The CADC stretches over a large geographic area, from south Mexico across central Guatemala, into Honduras, El Salvador, and Nicaragua, reaching northern Costa Rica and Panama (Quesada-Hernández et al. 2019; UN NEWS 2016). This arid, semi-forested region is defined by low annual precipitation, rocky soils, and increased exposure to severe flooding and droughts. The Dry Corridor's land placement between the Caribbean and Pacific Oceans makes the region particularly susceptible to droughts during El Niño Southern Oscillation (ENSO). ENSO brings atmospheric warming of the Pacific Ocean surface, resulting in measurable alterations in precipitation every two to seven years to the region (Stanke 2013; Briones 2017; Rojas, Li, and Cumani 2014). During an ENSO rotation year, subsistence farmers in Guatemala's Dry Corridor report less precipitation and drought conditions that destroy the agricultural crops essential for survival.

The geography of Guatemala places the area consistently in the top 15 vulnerable countries in the world to climate change (Eckstein et al. 2018). Increasingly unpredictable fluctuations in the Dry Corridor's precipitation levels have resulted in climate shocks that reduce subsistence crop yields for millions of rural Guatemalan households (FAO 2015). Of the 16 million inhabitants of Guatemala, 60% reside in economically impoverished rural areas and engage in rain-fed subsistence agriculture as the basis for survival (Lastarria-Cornheil 2003), making a high portion of the population especially vulnerable to climate pattern variations. Within these rural communities, 76% of the population live in poverty, with 39% percent living in extreme poverty, rates that have nearly doubled from 2000 to 2014 (INE 2015; IFAD 2018). Most recently, the additional impact of losses to employment income from the COVID-19 pandemic led directly to a food security crisis (FEWS Net 2021).

Guatemala has the fourth-highest level of chronic malnutrition on the planet, and the highest in Central America and the Caribbean (USAID 2019). Rates of poverty are highest in the majority Indigenous Maya population, with 79% of Indigenous families living in poverty or extreme poverty, earning less than $2 US per day (WFP 2019).

Many of these families call the Dry Corridor home. During the Spanish Colonial period, colonization of the Americas marginalized Indigenous communities, heavily restricting access to land, political structures, formal education, and community infrastructure such as roads, potable water, and health programming (Diccionario Geográfico de Guatemala 1976). The resulting socioeconomic inequality remains today. Particularly, Indigenous women continue to suffer the consequences of land tenure, lack of human rights, decision-making, male household, and state control, and access to education and fair employment (Project Harvest 2020).

This chapter will reflect on multivariate influences on food security for rural agrarian populations in the CADC region of Guatemala, demonstrating how challenges may be addressed through community-driven strategies for local food production, women's empowerment, and climate resilience.

METHODS

This case study presents the actions and results to date of a Canadian-Guatemalan nongovernmental organization, Project Harvest/*Proyecto Cosecha*, whose work within the most isolated and economically impoverished communities of Guatemala's Dry Corridor demonstrates measurable, replicable, and synergistic impact. *Proyecto Cosecha* focuses on empowering beneficiaries to become drivers of their own culturally appropriate, localized community development through women's leadership, employment, and skill-building programs that addresses human rights discrepancies, specifically facilitating the socio-political voice of women to access healthy, nutritious food. Research presented here was self-funded and completed in partnership with Project Harvest. Data were synthesized from field visit observations and interviews with the Canadian Project Harvest Founder, the Guatemalan in-country Director, and beneficiaries from 2016 to 2019. Data were also sequestered from 2015 to 2019 project activity reports written by the Guatemalan in-country Women's Formation (leadership) Officer. Questions for the interviews were constructed based on field observations and climate change research focusing on the Dry Corridor of Guatemala.

The two pillars of Project Harvest's work are (1) the development of household vegetable gardens to immediately address family food and nutrition security and (2) to build community resilience through women's community-driven leadership and empowerment programming. Targets aim to support beneficiaries' ability to identify and construct meaningful local resilience strategies that increase their family and community's food security, health, and nutrition as well as address Indigenous and gendered social inequities. Project Harvest initially began work in response to a request from local small-scale agricultural cooperatives to provide training and irrigation technology for beneficiaries in rural areas. Women arose as key purveyors of project activities as men in the community often travel for some months for cash crop employment. This resulted in women designing social structures of self-education and governance called "Formations," led by female community Boards of Directors (*Junta Directivas*). *Junta Directivas* are community-elected women assigned to various leadership roles that are responsible for organizing Project Harvest activities. The *Junta* also arranges monthly workshops for women that promote discussion of human rights, self-esteem, and gender-based political equality. Workshops are supported by Project Harvest's Formation Leader, a position reserved for a Guatemalan woman who specifically holds understanding of and education in issues experienced by socially and politically isolated Guatemalan Indigenous women. Over the years of operation, Project Harvest's women's leadership formation participants consistently report increased ability to organize within their community, engage in their human right to access nutritious food, and define their own adaptive community plans to address food insecurity that responds to climate change (Project Harvest 2020).

CLIMATE CHANGE AND FOOD SECURITY IN THE DRY CORRIDOR

> We believe the rain will come. But we do not know exactly when, or for how long.
>
> *Project Harvest participant*

The Dry Corridor's annual weather patterns correspond with seasonal fluctuations in temperature and precipitation in Central America. Rains arrive in the warmer months from April to October, followed by the dry, cooler season between November and March (INSIVUMEH 2018).

Guatemalan weather station data show an increase in overall annual rainfall and higher overall temperatures since 1971 (INSIVUMEH 2018). However, increasing variability in the arrival and amount of precipitation is connected to warming temperatures brought on by both climate change and the El Niño Southern Oscillation, resulting in droughts and flooding that lead to recurring food crises in the region (FEWS 2016). Droughts of more than 20 days result in subsistence crop failure. Otherwise, strong rains result in flooding in the steep hills of Eastern Guatemala, washing crops away (Leary et al. 2019). Families are often left with significant food losses, resorting to other methods of survival such as reducing daily meals or migrating to seek employment. The last major drought of 2014 influenced by the ENSO system lasted for two years, resulting in over 3.5 million people in Guatemala, Honduras, and El Salvador requiring humanitarian aid (FAO 2016). Even in a normal weather year, the Dry Corridor residents will reach a crisis level of food security during the rainy season, known locally as the "lean" season, typically between May and October (FEWS 2020).

To supplement subsistence crops, most male heads of families in the Dry Corridor find informal work in export crop field labor for 4–6 months during the dry season, from late October to early April (Leary et al. 2019). Droughts, flooding, and rising temperatures also negatively impact the harvests of rain-fed export crops such as coffee, a widespread export crop that offers seasonal employment to thousands of rural workers (FEWS NET 2016). Losses to coffee crops result in significantly decreased employment opportunities, reducing household purchasing power to meet daily food basket caloric needs. During the long and devastating drought of 2014, warmer air temperatures linked to the El Niño system contributed to the spreading of *La Roya* coffee rust fungus to higher altitudes (Project Harvest 2020). La Roya infected and destroyed thousands of coffee plants, leading to significant reduction in seasonal employment for field laborers, causing the government to announce a national

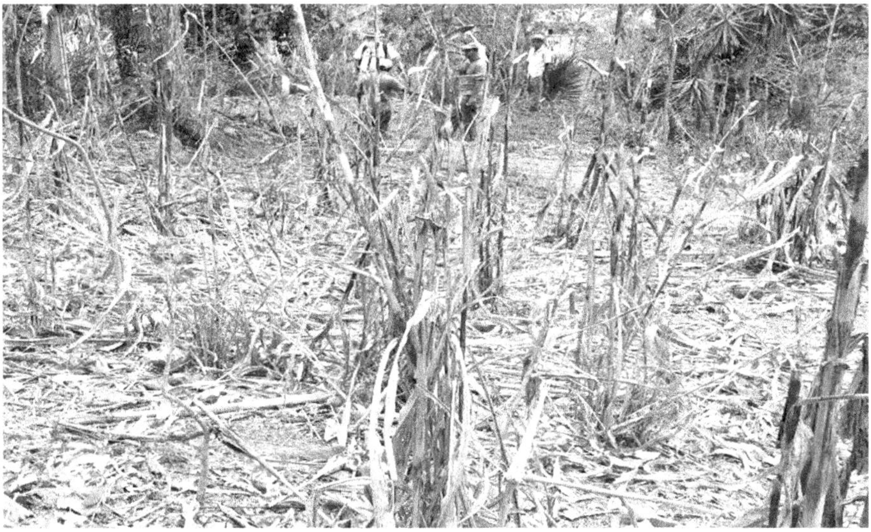

FIGURE 8.1 Dried maize crops in rural Chiquimula.

emergency. This phenomenon has been indicated as a key influence on the increase of Guatemalan migration to the United States (Leary et al. 2019). The number of Guatemalan families apprehended at the United States border doubled between 2017 and 2018 and again quadrupled in 2019 (US Customs and Border Protection 2020) (Figure 8.1).

Recent studies increasingly shed light on the intersectionality of poverty, food security, health, and climate vulnerability for Guatemala's rural population (Martinez et al. 2017; Beveridge Whitfield, and Fraval 2019; Metz 2001; Hellin et al. 2018). The Guatemalan government has responded to challenges by framing the UN SDGs within the 2014 presentation of *Plan Nacional de Desarrollo K'atun: nuestra Guatemala 2032*, or the National Development Plan: Our Guatemala 2032 (Guatemala 2014). Baseline data from 2014 on poverty, health, and food security were used to declare national targets such as halving the national level of poverty by 2032 (Ibid).

International organizations have been important actors in establishing humanitarian aid and long-term food security programs in the Dry Corridor in response to continuing poverty, malnutrition and health, and climate emergencies. The World Food Programme (WFP) has been operating food aid programs in Guatemala since 1974 (WFP 2019; Martinez et al 2017). Responding to the 2014–2016 drought, the WFP initiated a two-year project designed to build community resilience to climate shocks (WFP 2019). Beneficiaries were provided with agricultural training including flood prevention through reforestation of land, and vegetable garden installation and training to boost food production. Additionally, in 2017, the US Agency for International Development's (USAID) Office *Food for Peace* provided over 20 million USD in annual funding directly to the Save the Children and Catholic Relief Services for immediate food aid cash transfers and training programs in agricultural methods, financial literacy, and prevention of malnutrition, with the aim of sustainably enhancing resilience to climate shocks that affect food sources (USAID 2019). Many other organizations and agencies are active in the region, each with independent yet overlapping goals and programs. As a result of Project Harvest's success in the Dry Corridor, organizations have reached out to consult on methodology and practices that have resulted in notable impacts.

RURAL ECONOMY, GENDER ROLES, AND FOOD SECURITY IN THE DRY CORRIDOR

Rural populations in the Dry Corridor often identify as one of Guatemala's distinct Indigenous Maya groups, from the Spanish-speaking *Ch'orti* in the east to the *Ki'che'* culture encountered in the western highlands. The population typically relies on traditional methods of planting and harvesting subsistence crops according to annual rainfall cycles. Families intercrop maize (yellow and white corn) and black beans throughout the rainy season on small rented plots of land, consuming or selling the harvest in local markets. About 70% of families supplement subsistence food harvests with income from informal agricultural export crop labor, such as coffee and sugar cane, and with income from various other small business ventures, such as the sale of handmade goods, livestock tending, or chopping and selling firewood (INE 2015; Dary, Elías, and Reyna 1998). For example, over the 4–6-month harvesting cycle, sugar cane processing work earns a family an estimated Q4,000–Q5,000 (Leary et al. 2019). This marginal income pays for household costs such as rented land plots, small adobe homes, and household materials. There is little remaining money for additional costs such as health care, education, or potable water. Many families subsist on three meals of corn tortillas with salt per day, and in times of work, add beans and fruits. Between May and November, with reduced access to informal employment and as stored crops run low, families often reduce their consumption to one or two meals of tortillas and salt per day. Thus, this time of year is referred to as the "lean season" (FEWS Net 2020). The lean season began early in 2021 after a challenging COVID-19 pandemic year that resulted in low employment and high food prices, as markets fluctuated with availability. These multivariate pressures on food security have driven communities in the Dry Corridor into early food security crises (FEWS Net 2021).

High rates of poverty, large family sizes, and lack of reliable employment for rural families within the Dry Corridor result in food, nutrient, and health deficiencies. A sample of eastern and western regions in the Dry Corridor shows that child growth stunting is found in up to 62% of children under five years old (Pereyr et al. 2015). The majority of children aged 6–23 months were found to have insufficient diets (Ibid). National government health programs that would address health and nutrition-related issues notoriously lack funding in rural areas. As one example, the Expansion of Coverage Program was dismantled under allegations of government corruption in 2015 (Martinez et al. 2017), yet to be revived. Extensive government corruption at the national level led CICIG to arrest the President, Vice President, and many officials in Guatemala (Cuffe 2020). The national development plan that included proposed extension of health services to areas outside of Guatemala city, the

Plan Nacional de Desarrollo K'atun: nuestra Guatemala 2032, was penned by this former government, adding to general skepticism that community improvement will ever be facilitated as so often promised.

CHALLENGING GENDER NORMS TO ADDRESS FOOD SECURITY

In Guatemala, gender disparity, or the measurable inequality in power, access, and political influence for men and women, ranks high in Central America (WFP 2019). In traditional Mayan Indigenous culture, men have access to houses and land, and greater access to employment opportunities (FAO 2020; Leary et al. 2019; Cook, Grillos, and Andersson 2019). National data state that about 33% of females over 15 years old are employed, whereas the employment rate for males in the same age group is 66% (ENEI 2018). As of 2014, 59.2% of rural women did not have incomes of their own. The division of labor in the home is typically gender based. Women contribute to family income by selling goods at local markets like handmade weaving, tortillas, and products such as chickens, eggs, vegetables, and beans. Often, women remain at home with younger children during the months when men and older sons migrate for work, managing daily food and water procurement and protecting household assets. Although women experience high levels of responsibility in the home, many lack opportunity to significantly contribute to household income, and are traditionally excluded from education and decision-making (FAO 2020; Leary et al. 2019).

Rural women's participation in building climate change resilience strategies is vital for multiple reasons, as emphasized in the UN SDGs 1 and 2 framework and targets. Women are often the most vulnerable to climate change impacts in rural traditional communities, as they are typically home throughout the year and therefore responsible for household family diet and health (Dankelman 2010). At the same time, women have substantial knowledge of local seasonal and climatic effects on food and water sources due to their gendered roles that define them as primary caretakers of the household. The women involved with Project Harvest know which streams are available for water acquisition, what months the water begins to reduce in the dry season, and how to harvest and store subsistence crops. Women have extensive capacity and valuable knowledge to contribute to regional food security planning and policy formation, but the expressions of their knowledge and creative ideas are often boundaried by culturally embedded male hegemony or lack of formalized organization (Oxfam 2019).

Allowing safe spaces for the expression of women's knowledge around food and water security is pivotal to developing resources and synergizing local with national and international targets. Recognizing both the socially inherent gender inequity in Guatemala and the potential of women to build food security resilience in their community, Project Harvest structures its work around women. The typical style of community gathering to engage in discussion around food security challenges involves men sitting at the forefront of the group, talking and conceptualizing actions to respond to challenges. If women attend, they typically sit behind the men and generally do not speak unless addressed (Project Harvest 2020). The creation of various administrative positions for local women, including group leaders through

Junta Directivas, agricultural promoters (*promotoras agrícolas*), and community links (*enlaces*), structures safe spaces where gendered issues and solutions can be expressed. Administrative roles held by women at Project Harvest allow for structured leadership, with women driving the organization of discussions and workshops on current issues, such as accessing nutritious food, fair employment, and equal human rights at all levels, from family units to federal agencies. Monthly workshops are often facilitated by Project Harvest's female national Guatemalan Formation Officer. Workshops are half-day gatherings with targeted learning outcomes, where women feel safe to speak, be heard, organize, learn skills, and create solutions to food insecurity.

CASE STUDY: WOMEN ORGANIZE FOR CHANGE IN PITAHAYA, CHIQUIMULA REGION OF THE DRY CORRIDOR

Background

Project Harvest grew out of the founder's work in improving subsistence crop irrigation in the Totonicapán Department of Guatemala, located in the western highlands of the Dry Corridor. A member of a Guatemalan NGO who heard of their success requested assistance for the small, rural community of Pitahaya, nestled in the steep mountains of the eastern Dry Corridor in the Municipality of Camotán, Chiquimula Department. A long drought in 2012 related to an ENSO rotation year resulted in a widespread food crisis by May 2013 with significant losses to subsistence crops. Answering the request for assistance, the Guatemalan Project Harvest Coordinator traveled to Pitahaya to facilitate community discussions around methods for reconstructing food security and irrigating crops.

The isolated town of Pitahaya was experiencing a food crisis at a time when many male members of the household were away for export crop field work. As a result, the Project Harvest Coordinator assisted women who had remained in the community in writing requests for immediate food aid. Transportation was arranged for a group of four women to travel to Guatemala city to present their aid request to international and national organization's head offices. The results were mixed, with some refusals and a few offerings to sponsor food aid for the community. The women came up with an idea for sustainable change; that beneficiaries would, as a stipulation to receiving aid, implement a vegetable garden on a small plot of land on each household. The women returned to Pitahaya, feeling relief and excitement with the positive results. Upon arriving home with the news of incoming aid, the women were hailed as local heroes by everyone in the community. This bolstered their motivation to organize local meetings where they would plan the implementation of the vegetable gardens, including identifying beneficiaries based on need, location of the gardens, types of seeds preferred, and when participants would attend training.

On their return to the town, male members of the Pitahaya community celebrated and supported the gardens by constructing terraces that would collect rainwater and prevent damaging runoff, a traditional method used in Mayan agriculture (Dary et. al 1996, 98). The women continued to hold meetings, soon naming their group *Forjadoras de Desarollo*, or "Shapers of Development." The group identified key

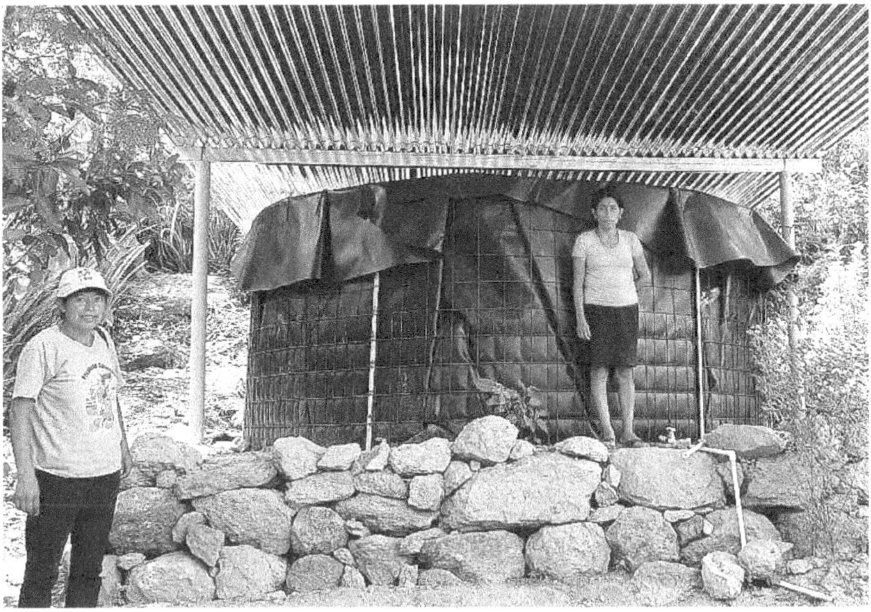

FIGURE 8.2 SCAL rainwater irrigation unit with agricultural promoter and beneficiary.

administrative roles that would manage the leadership committee, or *Junta Directiva* (Board of Directors). The women gathered regularly to learn about vegetable garden production, including types of seeds, planting depth and distance, and making compost tea to replace lost soil nutrients in the dry landscape. They discussed their rights to secure food through self-driven actions, which led to the request for support to identify ways to irrigate the gardens during the dry months, as access to water requires walking long distances to small streams. Project Harvest responded by obtaining local, affordable materials to design and construct a rainwater catchment system, known in Spanish as *Sistemas de Captación del Agua de Lluvia* (SCAL). The women determined whose household would first receive a SCAL based on the availability of a small plot of land adjoining the house. Project Harvest community *enlaces* purchased the materials and learned how to build the SCAL following a diagram. They taught beneficiaries how to clear the land and install the SCAL. Women assisted in the construction of the SCAL system and continue to monitor and report on its efficacy (Figure 8.2).

Project Expansion

Requests for assistance from nearby communities came when others saw the success of the Pitahaya gardens, which were bursting with fresh, healthy vegetables. Project Harvest *enlaces* assisted in the expansion into 12 communities within the Dry Corridor. In response to interest in expanding knowledge of human rights and exploring topics like self-esteem and personal power, Project Harvest created a

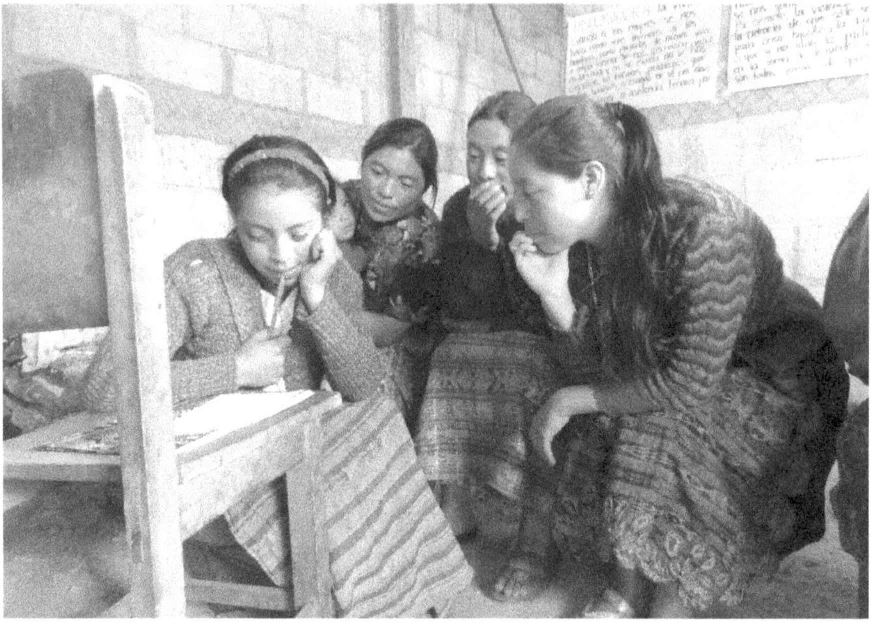

FIGURE 8.3 SCAL women reflect on addressing inherent power structures and discrimination.

national position of Formation Officer, a key role filled by female Guatemalans who demonstrated a keen understanding of social and political systems, power relations, and human rights. The Formation Officer travels extensively across the Dry Corridor, selecting topics for workshops, providing workshop materials, and leading sessions with intended goals and results evaluation (Figure 8.3).

Participants in the Project Harvest program grow family vegetable gardens to supplement food stores, diversify nutrition, and earn additional income by selling excess crops. Table 8.1 details the planting, growing, and harvesting months as well as earnings for participants. For most months of the year, household diets can be supplemented with healthy, organic vegetables. The women add the produce to soups or beans. Most vegetables are harvested every 2–3 months, though radish can be harvested every month (Project Harvest 2020; Leary et al. 2019). Unexpected variances in the annual climate cycle that reduce subsistence crop yields (maize and beans) can be buffered by growing vegetables that utilize rainwater catchment units during the dry months.

Project Goals

1. Reduce food insecurity and chronic malnutrition by increasing access to and consumption of nutritious food through the production of household vegetable gardens, promote incorporating vegetables into diets.
2. Reduce extreme poverty by supplementing household income from excess vegetable crop sales in local markets.

TABLE 8.1
Annual Climate, Income, and Food Availability in Eastern Guatemala

Month	Avg. Rainfall[a]	Crops Planted[b]	Crops Harvested	Food Available	Income Source
Jan	5 mm	Vegetables	Vegetables[c]	Vegetables + beans	Sugar cane + coffee labor
Feb	2–5 mm	Vegetables	Vegetables	Vegetables	Sugar cane + coffee labor
Mar	2–10 mm	Some vegetables	Some vegetables	Vegetables	Sugar cane labor
Apr	10–20 mm	80% Maize, 20% beans, some vegetables	None	Vegetables	Sugar cane labor
May	50–100 mm	80% Maize, 20% beans, some vegetables	None	Lean season as crops in growth stage; reduce daily meals depending on maize harvest and food storage	Small income from selling products like weavings, chickens, eggs, firewood; pastoral or other local manual labor
Jun	50–300 mm	Vegetables	Vegetables		
Jul	50–160 mm	None	Vegetables		
Aug	45–170 mm	Vegetables	Vegetables		
Sep	48–200 mm	100% Beans	Maize + vegetables	Maize, beans, vegetables	
Oct	45–120 mm	Vegetables	Maize + vegetables	Maize, beans, vegetables	
Nov	20–45 mm	Vegetables	Beans + vegetables	Maize, beans, vegetables	Sell 80% of bean harvest; sugar cane + coffee labor
Dec	7–42 mm	Vegetables	Beans + vegetables	Maize, beans, vegetables	Sugar cane + coffee labor

Source: INSIVUMEH 2018.
[a] Rainfall 1971–2010.
[b] Source: Leary et al. 2019.
[c] Vegetables from Project Harvest gardens include cabbage, celery, radish, onion, cilantro, broccoli, and coriander.

3. Improve annual garden productivity by constructing new rainwater irrigation units (SCAL) to provide water to vegetables during the dry season.
4. Improve nutritional content and increase vegetable growth by promoting use of strong seeds and enhancing soil nutrients through compost training. Training and monitoring are community-driven by *enlaces* and agricultural promoters.

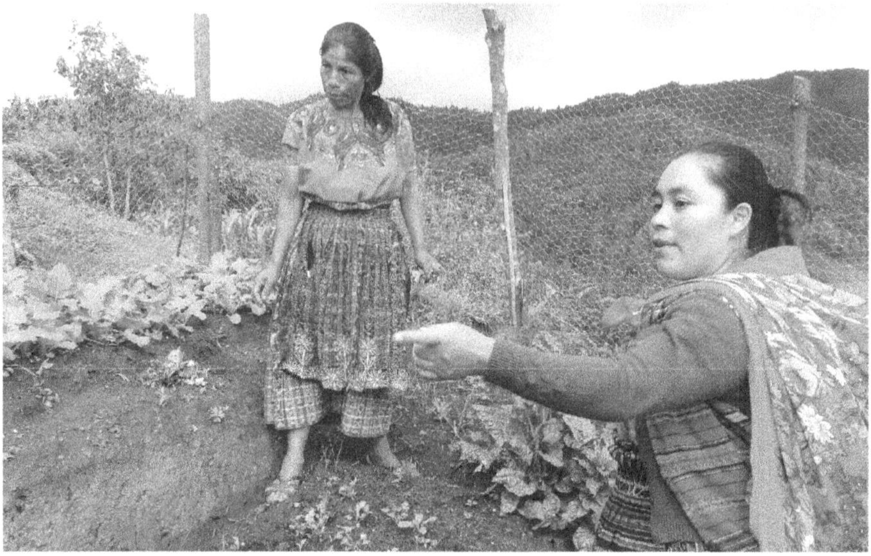

FIGURE 8.4 An Agricultural Promoter consults with a woman on terracing and composting.

5. Continue to build on women's organizational and leadership capacity through supporting group roles, workshops, and activities that result in women creating and acting toward community self-development plans.
6. Expand the food security program into more isolated communities in the Dry Corridor (Figure 8.4).

Quantitative Project Results

Project Harvest officially began its work in 2013 in five communities in two departments located in the Dry Corridor; the isolated villages of Pitahaya and Guayabo in the Chiquimula Department in the east, and Vásquez, Casa Blanca/Xecajá, and Cuesta del Aire towns in the western highlands within the Totonicapán Department. As of 2019, Project Harvest members are active in 12 communities in the two regions of the Dry Corridor, with a total of 527 participants.

A snapshot from 2017 to 2018 (Figure 8.5) demonstrates results of participatory Project Harvest actions, where participants within ten rural communities in the two Dry Corridor departments reported:

- 57 pounds of vegetable seeds distributed
- 121 tons of vegetables produced
- 165,000 pounds of fertilizer distributed
- 1.4 million liters of rainwater harvested
- 75 agricultural workshops completed
- 12 women's formation leadership workshops completed

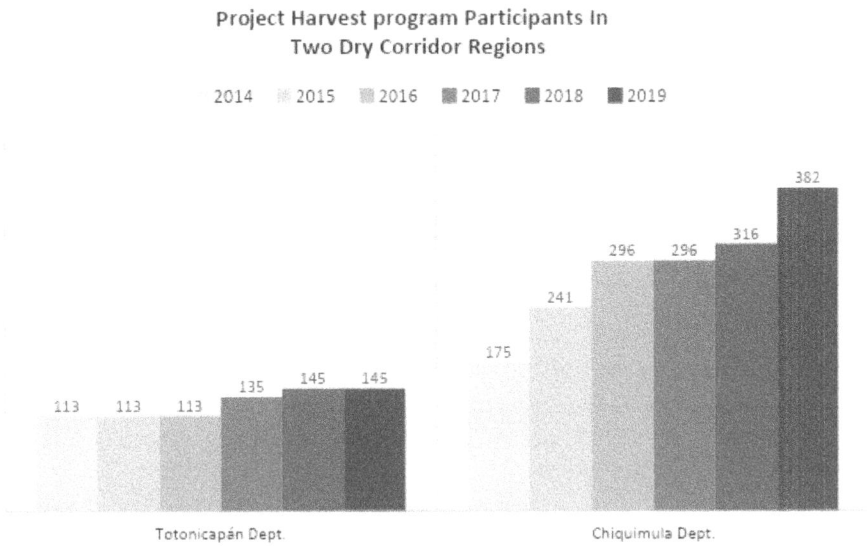

FIGURE 8.5 Snapshot from 2017 to 2018 of Project Harvest participants.

- The first *Encuentro de Comunidades* occurred: a regional meeting of communities to discuss food and nutritional aspirations and future collaboration opportunities

Implementing vegetable harvesting and rainwater catchment irrigation has resulted in increased vegetable yields for consumption and sale in local markets; average annual income from additional vegetables produced per family = $575 CDN.

Qualitative Project Results

Through informal discussions with participants, interviews with Project Harvest staff and reviewing data in reports written by Project Harvest staff reveal the following quantitative observations of note:

1. Participants have increased their knowledge of human rights, specifically the right to access diverse, nutritious food and clean water, gender equity in society, and the right to share thoughts and ideas in the community and greater political sphere.
2. Participants developed skills in accounting, organizing, and administering meetings by holding leadership positions with key responsibilities.
3. Participants completed actions on increasing household access to nutritious food, addressing challenges like pest management and irrigation.
4. A handful of participants developed proposals to present to municipal government officers regarding solving issues around food and nutrition security, potable water, and household electricity.

5. Some female children of participants who engaged in workshops, observing their mothers' participation in leadership activities, have now reached adulthood and fulfilled leadership roles in community food security projects.
6. To date, one women's group leader was elected to local municipal government, where she proposed and implemented a potable water station in her community.

In the women's leadership workshops, it was observed that participation and engagement varied by month and between communities. The key factors observed by the Project Harvest's Formation Officer that affect participation and engagement by participants are as follows: annual climate variations affecting immediate needs, whether other projects were present in the area, seasonal availability of women's time to participate as a result of women working in agricultural labor (coffee) or local maize cultivation periods, and cultural default to men's leadership is notably stronger in some communities than others.

CONCLUSIONS

As subsistence food access systems are reliant on rain-fed crops and are supplemented with tenuous low-income employment in informal export crop field labor, the cycle of poverty and malnutrition for millions of people continues in the Central American Dry Corridor. Temperatures are predicted to rise, and rainfall patterns will become increasingly variable in Guatemala in the coming decades (INSIVUMEH 2018, 124–129; Porter et al. 2014). In the 2016 FAO Situation Report, impacts caused by climate variance "exceeds the capacities of a single organization or government and requires strategic partnerships amongst the international community" (FAO 2016). Project Harvest as well recognizes the need for collaboration: "stakeholders must synergize their efforts" (Leary et al. 2019). With Project Harvest actions showing positive results in empowering local communities to drive the stabilization of food security and increase household nutrition, partnerships would bring greater potential to scale up impacts within and outside the Guatemalan Dry Corridor.

Strengthening leadership skills in rural populations can allow vulnerable people to develop synergistic, effective actions to enhance immediate and long-term food and nutrition security and expand connected, gender-equal communities. In supporting locally driven actions by a network of female community leaders and project promoters, organizations can facilitate gender-equal ideas that respond to climate-based food shocks. Women's leadership structures and roles in a community drive collaborative reflection define solutions and resilience-based strategies in response to varying conditions at the local level.

With a growing number of gender-balanced voices and the skills to formulate and present citizen's needs to international food security organizations and governing bodies, and ultimately developing the ability to lead and govern at the departmental level, resilience to future food crises through actions has the potential to be effective. As the Guatemalan Ministry of Agriculture, Livestock and Food (MAGA) recently ratified the first gender-equality policy in food security and nutrition (FAO 2020), it is possible that better opportunities will come for rural women living in the Dry

Corridor to present their ideas on food and nutrition security and climate change resilience at the regional and national level.

RECOMMENDATIONS

Often in the field, we observed that nongovernment and international organizations, academics, and local cooperatives complete independent analyses and design programs driven by specific SDG targets relating to their mission, which is sensical given limited organizational resources. At times, lack of communication with other organizations working in the area resulted in confusion; for example, during a SCAL installation in 2016, an international aid agency unexpectedly delivered household water buckets, interrupting the Project Harvest training activity. As the Dry Corridor climate is expected to increase future challenges to food security with increasing droughts and floods that have devastating consequences on food supplies and informal export crop labor, it is vital that organizations and all levels of government synthesize data from beneficiaries to build strategies based on changing local needs. Attention should be paid to variances in beneficiary participation, as noted previously, and ideas from within the community on how to better engage beneficiaries should be considered. Both women and men in Dry Corridor communities must feel empowered to reflect on and voice their observations, ideas, and varying needs. Additionally, technology would support traditional monitoring of programs by filling the gaps between surveys and organizations. For example, if women had access to reliable cell phones and solar electricity, they could report weather, crop, and other environmental observances in their community to organizations and academics.

Project Harvest's Guatemalan Director stresses the valuable concept of synergy. A conjoined report by the WFP, IFAD, and FAO in 2019 outlines the value of working in partnership in highly vulnerable regions (FAO, IFAD, and WFP 2015). It is recommended that all stakeholders working toward sustainable food security structure cross-organizational communications to share knowledge, ideas, and important feedback on climate resilience strategies. The efforts within the 2015 development framework of stakeholders in presenting local data around contributing factors to seasonal hunger, malnutrition, and migration, such as climate change and gender equity, can inform national policy and programs that incorporate all voices. By establishing relationships between community members, local NGOs, intragovernment and international development organizations, the potential exists to broaden transformative change for rural subsistence families to address the widespread and ongoing effects of poverty, gender inequity, climate change, and food insecurity.

REFERENCES

Beveridge, L., Whitfield, S., Fraval, S. et al. 2019. Experiences and Drivers of Food Insecurity in Guatemala's Dry Corridor: Insights from the Integration of Ethnographic and Household Survey Data. *Frontiers in Sustainable Food Systems* 3. https://www.frontiersin.org/articles/10.3389/fsufs.2019.00065/full

Briones, F. 2017. How Did Central America Cope with El Niño 2015–2016? Lessons and Challenges. https://www.researchgate.net/publication/321038131_How_did_Central_America_cope_with_El_Niño_2015-2016_Lessons_and_challenges.

Cook, N.J., Grillos, T., and Andersson, K.P. 2019. Gender Quotas Increase the Equality and Effectiveness of Climate Policy Interventions. *Nature Climate Change* 9: 330–334.

Cuffe, Sandra. n.d. “Guatemalan Officials Arrested for Corruption after Leaving Office.” Accessed April 25th, 2020. https://www.aljazeera.com/news/2020/1/16/guatemalan-officials-arrested-for-corruption-after-leaving-office.

Dankelman, I., ed. *Gender and Climate Change: An Introduction. 2010.* London: Earthscan.

Dary, C., Elías, S., and Reyna, V. 1998. *Estrategias de sobrevivencia campesina en ecosistemas frágiles: los ch'orti' en las laderas secas del oriente de Guatemala.* Guatemala: FLACSO.

Diccionario Geográfico de Guatemala. 1976. Instituto Geográfico Nacional de Guatemala, TOMO I, Segunda edicion. Guatemala: Instituto Geográfico Nacional de Guatemala ,, 735–745.

Eckstein, D., Hutfils, M.-L., and Winges, M. 2018. *Global Climate Risk Index 2019: Who Suffers Most from Extreme Weather Events? Weather-Related Loss Events in 2017 and 1998 to 2017.* Bonn, Germany: Germanwatch e.V.

ENEI Instituto Nacional de Estadística (Guatemala). 2018. Encuesta Nacional de Empleo e Ingresos 2–2018. Guatemala City: INE. https://www.ine.gob.gt/sistema/uploads/2019/07/05/publicacion_ENEI_2_2018.pdf.

FAO. 2015. Disaster Risk Programme to Strengthen Resilience in the Dry Corridor in Central America. El Salvador-Guatemala-Honduras-Nicaragua: Food and Agriculture Organization of the United Nations. http://www.fao.org/fileadmin/user_upload/emergencies/docs/Corredor_Seco_Breve_EN.pdf.

FAO Dry Corridor. 2016. Central America Situation Report – June 2016. Rome: Food and Agriculture Organization of the United Nations. http://www.fao.org/emergencies/resources/documents/resources-detail/en/c/422097/.

FAO. 2020. Giving Women in Guatemala a Voice in Food Security and Nutrition. Rome: Food and Agriculture Organization of the United Nations. http://www.fao.org/in-action/gender-equality-guatemala/en.

FAO, IFAD and WFP. 2015. Strengthening Resilience for Food Security and Nutrition: A Conceptual Framework for Collaboration and Partnership among the Rome-Based Agencies. http://www.fao.org/resilience/resources/resources-detail/en/c/335336/.

FEWS Net. February 2020. Central America and the Caribbean Food Security Outlook Update: Limited Food Stocks and Early Market Dependence Mark the Beginning of the Lean Season. https://fews.net/central-america-and-caribbean/guatemala/food-security-outlook/february-2020.

FEWS Net. November 2021. Staple Grain Prices Remain High Despite the Flow of National Harvests. https://fews.net/central-america-and-caribbean/guatemala Field Discussions with Coffee farmers in De la Gente Cooperative. Discussions with author. 2015 & 2017. Guatemala: Huehuetenango and Antigua.

FEWS Net Washington. 2016. Guatemala Livelihood Zones and Descriptions. https://fews.net/sites/default/files/documents/reports/Consolidated%20GT%20LZ%20document_Jan%2031%202017.pdf.

Gobiernoa de Guatemala2014. Consejo Nacional de Desarrollo Urbano y Rural. Plan Nacional de Desarrollo K'atun: Nuestra Guatemala 2032. Guatemala: Conadur/Segeplán, vii, 502 p. il; 28 cm. Anexos. Guatemala: Gobierno de Gualtemala.

Hellin, J., Ratner, B.D., Meinzen-Dick, R., and Lopez-Ridaura, S. 2018. Increasing Social-Ecological Resilience within Small-Scale Agriculture in Conflict-Affected Guatemala. *Ecology and Society* 23(3): 5. https://doi.org/10.5751/ES-10250-230305.

IFAD. Latin American and the Caribbean Division, Programme Management Department. 2018. Republic of Guatemala, Country Strategy Note. https://www.ifad.org/documents/38711624/40077965/Guatemala_Country%20Strategy%20Note_2018-2020_09july2018/9528714e-e6e2-4c28-a168-e5ec58ca0343.

IFPRI. 2020. Food Security. Washington, DC: International Food Policy Research Institute. https://www.ifpri.org/topic/food-security.

INSIVUMEH (El Instituto Nacional de Sismología, Vulcanología, Meteorología e Hidrología) (Guatemala). 2018. Variabilidad y Cambio Climático en Guatemala. Guatemala: INSIVUMEH.

Instituto Nacional de Estadística (INE) (Guatemala). 2015. Encuesta Nacional de Condiciones de Vida, 2014: principales resultados. Guatemala City: INE. https://www.ine.gob.gt/index.php/encuestas-de-hogares-y-personas/condiciones-de-vida.

Lastarria-Cornheil, S. 2003. Guatemala Country Brief: Property Rights and Land Markets. University of Wisconsin-Madison, Land Tenure Center.

Leary, N., Conde, C., Kulkarni, K., Nyong, A., and Puljin, J., eds. 2008. *Climate Change and Vulnerability*. London: Earthscan. Interview with Project Harvest Country Director. Interview by author. September 25, 2019.

Martinez, B., Flood, D., Cnop, K., Guzman, A., and Rohloff, P. 2017. Improving Infant and Young Child Nutrition in a Highly Stunted Rural Community: A Practical Case Study from Guatemala. In *Handbook of Famine, Starvation and Nutrient Deprivation: From Biology to Policy*, ed. Preedy, V. and Patel, V.B., 1–19. Cham: Springer. https://link.springer.com/referenceworkentry/10.1007%2F978-3-319-40007-5_52-1.

Metz, B. 2001. Politics, Population, and Family Planning in Guatemala: Ch'orti; Maya Experiences. *Human Organization* 60(3): 259–271.

Oxfam. 2019. Gender Inequalities and Food Insecurity: Ten Years after the Food Price Crisis, Why Are Women Farmers Still Food-Insecure? Oxford, Great Britain: Oxfam GB for Oxfam International https://www.oxfam.org/en/research/gender-inequalities-and-food-insecurity.

Pereyr, D., Ibargüen, J., Walter, G., McDonald, C. Juárez, G., and García, M. A. 2015. Nutrition, Mortality, Food Security, and Livelihoods Survey based on SMART Methodology: Western (Livelihood Zone 5) and Eastern (Livelihood Zones 7, 8, and 9) Regions of Guatemala's Dry Corridor. Washington, DC: United States Agency for International Development Famine Early Warning Systems Network (FEWS NET).

Porter, J.R., Xie, L., Challinor, A.J., Cochrane, K., Howden, S.M., Iqbal, M.M., Lobell, D.B., and Travasso, M.I. 2014. Food Security and Food Production Systems. In *Climate Change 2014: Impacts, Adaptation, and Vulnerability*. Part A: Global and Sectoral Aspects. Contribution of Working Group II to the Fifth Assessment Report of the Intergovernmental Panel on Climate Change [Field, C.B., Barros, V.R., Dokken, D.J., Mach, K.J., Mastrandrea, M.D., Bilir, T.E., Chatterjee, M., Ebi, K.L., Estrada, Y.O., Genova, R.C., Girma, B., Kissel, E.S., Levy, A.N., MacCracken, S., Mastrandrea, P.R., and White, L.L. eds.]. Cambridge and New York, NY: Cambridge University Press, 485–533.

Project Harvest. 2020. *Resilience* Winter 2020–2021. https://www.projectharvest.org/wp-content/uploads/2020/12/Resilience-2020.pdf.

Quesada-Hernández, L.E., Calvo-Solano, O.D., Hidalgo, H.G., Pérez-Briceño, P.M., and Alfaro, E.J. 2019. Dynamical Delimitation of the Central American Dry Corridor (CADC) Using Drought Indices and Aridity Values. *Earth and Environment* 43: 627–642. https://doi.org/10.1177/0309133319860224.

Rojas, O., Li, Y., and Cumani, R. 2014. *Understanding the Drought Impact of El Niño on the Global Agricultural Areas: An Assessment Using FAO's Agricultural Stress Index (ASI)*. Rome, Italy: Food and Agriculture Organization of the United Nations.

Stanke, C., Kerac, M., Prudhomme, C., Medlock, J., and Murray, V. 2013. Health Effects of Drought: A Systematic Review of the Evidence. *PLoS Currents* 5. https://doi.org/10.1371/currents.dis.7a2cee9e980f91ad7697b570bcc4b004.

UN News. November 2016. Nicaragua's 'Dry Corridor' to Benefit from UN-Backed Sustainable Agriculture Project. https://news.un.org/en/story/2016/11/546542-nicaraguas-dry-corridor-benefit-un-backed-sustainable-agriculture-project.

United Nations Statistics Division, Development Data and Outreach Branch. 2021. The Sustainable Development Goals Report 2021. https://unstats.un.org/sdgs/report/2021/.

USAID. 2019. Food Assistance Fact Sheets: Guatemala. https://www.usaid.gov/guatemala/food-assistance.

US Customs and Border Protection. 2020. U.S. Border Patrol Southwest Border Apprehensions by Sector Fiscal Year 2020: Southwest Border Unaccompanied Alien Children (0–17 yr old) Apprehensions. https://www.cbp.gov/newsroom/stats/sw-border-migration/usbp-sw-border-apprehensions.

World Food Programme. 2019. WFP Guatemala Country Brief November 2019. WFP/Library. https://docs.wfp.org/api/documents/WFP-0000111516/download/.

9 Food Security and the Viability of Yucatec Maya Sustainable Traditional Subsistence Strategies

A.L. Hopkins, C. Gibbes, A.F. Inurreta Díaz, D. Pastrana Cervantes, K. Rodríguez Ruz, C. Owens, D. Rawandoozi, and J. Jiménez-Osornio

CONTENTS

INTRODUCTION

Globally, there has been a positive trend in food security in recent decades until the COVID-19 pandemic. However, the current intersection of climate change, policy, and shifting economic centers is putting this positive change at risk. This risk is especially pressing for the Indigenous peoples internationally, as they are more vulnerable to these crises due to high levels of poverty. While many of these Indigenous communities have been adapting to neoliberal policy changes and shifting economic centers for the past three decades, the effects of climate change over the last several years are now contributing to issues related to food security in these communities. This study further extends our understanding of food security by uncovering how the Yucatec Maya, an Indigenous group in Yucatan, Mexico, are experiencing the added effects of the intersections of policy, economic changes, and climate change, and are experiencing heightened vulnerability to food insecurity as a result of that intersection.

The concept and associated definition of food security have morphed from one focused on food supply and the production at regional and global scales to one that currently acknowledges the temporal dynamics in access to food, as well as the range

DOI: 10.1201/9781003014942-9

of scales – from the individual to the household to global – at which food insecurity can manifest. More recent framings for food security reduce the centrality of production and the market and instead highlight the role of social factors that shape food access and consumption. One commonly cited definition from the FAO (2002, 2003) defines food security as a "situation that exists when all people, at all times, have physical, social, and economic access to sufficient, safe, and nutritious food that meets their dietary needs and food preferences for an active and healthy life." Thus, by extension food insecurity occurs when physical, social, or economic access to food is limited and does not meet dietary and food preference needs. Although consensus does not exist regarding thresholds at which individuals or households are categorized as food secure/insecure, Smith and Subandoro (2007) suggest that vulnerability with regard to food insecurity is present when 75% or more of income is spent on accessing and obtaining food, while moderate to high levels of insecurity begin when 50% of income is allocated to accessing food. Vulnerability to food insecurity, as described in recent definitions of food security, is dynamic and changes over time in response to short- and long-term variations in factors such as poverty, conflict, and climate change.

Food sovereignty has similarly taken on different definitions over time which, although more complex to clearly track, has included tenants which refer to the right to shape food policy, and emphasizes the needs of food producers, distributors, and consumers (Patel 2009; Campesina 2007; PFSN 2002). Core to food sovereignty is the refocusing of food narratives and systems from global to local. This refocusing is proposed to address social inequalities and environmental degradation associated with the globalization of food trade (Wittman, Desmarais, and Wiebe 2010). Although food security and food sovereignty were initially defined in two different arenas – food policy and peasant movement respectively – both concepts contribute to the debate of how best to address continuing issues of hunger (Clapp 2014).

Food sovereignty, security, and production are impacted by global processes and phenomena, not the least of which are changes in global climate. Climate change impacts food production by extension of food security and arguably sovereignty both directly and indirectly. Direct impacts of climate change are already observed in regard to the role of changing environmental conditions – temperature and precipitation – on crop yields. For example, Lobell et al. (2011) used country-level FAO data for large commodity crops to demonstrate that precipitation and temperature are dominant drivers of variability in crop yield. Indirect impacts of climate change include both the effect of climate variability on food prices (tied to crop yield) and the role that these changes (crop yields and food prices) have on regions and populations dominated by agricultural livelihoods. The influence on agricultural livelihoods will not be evenly distributed spatially or socially and could manifest increases in already existing inequalities, particularly for poorer countries where agriculture can play a significant economic role at both the individual and national levels (Hertel, Burke, and Lobell 2010). Furthermore, climate changes are expected to yield increased occurrences of extreme weather events which produce sudden, and large in magnitude, impacts on crops. Extreme events including COVID-19 pandemic and economic crises may further challenge agricultural producers, and consumers, to rapidly adapt to contrasting conditions, such as flood and drought, thus presenting multiple climate stressors in a short period of time (see, for example, Brida, Owiyo, and Sokona 2013). Such compounding effects of climate change and crises will be temporally and geographically varied and yield differential effects on communities.

This spatial and temporal variation is further intensified through changes in global dynamics, including health crises such as the COVID-19 pandemic, economic conditions, and resource variability. Rising prices and declining per capita cultivated land have threatened food security across many communities over the last two decades (FAO 2007). It is anticipated that climate change will continue, and exacerbate, food security reductions around the world in the coming decades (Brown and Funk 2008). As noted above, variations in the impact of climate change will result in varied food security stressors. This is combined with variations in market policies at the national level, and household characteristics – such as diversification of livelihoods, access to land, and access to remittances – which already contribute to uneven food security at the local level. The most pronounced impacts of climate change and pandemics, such as COVID-19, on food security will be experienced in spaces where food policies emphasize imports thus creating import dependencies, and where individuals and households lack power over resources, such as land, needed to produce food. This reduction in food sovereignty is closely tied to trade agreements, such as NAFTA and the United States–Mexico–Canada Agreement (USMCA), which have marked impacts on the agricultural markets, and also to local and regional processes such as migration patterns which result from the intricately intertwined relationships between food production, policy, and changing environmental conditions (Warner and Afifi 2014). For example, migration of family members may result in an increased buffer to the impacts of climate change and disasters on food security due to increased availability of capital; however, local and regional migration from rural food producing areas to urban centers can have a negative impact on food security where potential to produce food for subsistence is decreased and simultaneously the access to lower quality food increases.

The remainder of this chapter offers an introduction to an interdisciplinary research agenda that seeks to investigate the intricacies of food security and sovereignty through the examination of how policy, economic change, and climate change are experienced by the Yucatec Maya and the corresponding insecurity that arises as a result of these experiences.

METHODS

In an effort to understand the complexities related to food security among the Yucatec Maya, the research team developed a context-appropriate survey instrument using a participatory process with academic and local community members, which is complementary to the existing Mexican government data related to the United Nations Sustainable Development Goals (SDGs).

The first step in developing the survey instrument was to review the SDGs, Targets, and Indicators at the international level and the existing Mexican data at the national, state, and municipality levels. Then open-ended questions were developed to capture aspects of each indicator that are not addressed by the existing data at the municipal level. Additionally, questions were added to help define from a local

TABLE 9.1
Subset of Questions from the Interview Schedule

Question	Aim	SDG Relevant Goal
"What foods and drinks did your family have yesterday?"	Understand current food consumption	Goal 2: Zero hunger
"What food and drinks do your family like to consume?"	Elicit food preferences	Goal 2: Zero hunger
"What are the conditions necessary to achieve well-being?"	Understand the role of food in well-being	Goal 1: No poverty Goal 3: Well-being
"What changes in agricultural production have you noticed over time?"	Identify changes in local food production	Goal 2: Zero hunger
"What changes in forest harvest have you noticed over time?"	Identify changes in local resources integral to the tradition of practicing agroecology	Goal 15: Life on land

perspective critical terms such as hunger, sustainable agriculture, and poverty, which are used in the SDGs and relate to food security. Next, a group of regional research experts, along with graduate students and local community members, revised the questions collaboratively. The result was an 18-page interview schedule written in both English and Spanish. A subset of questions were used to obtain the data analyzed in this chapter and are shown in Table 9.1. The survey instrument along with additional consenting materials was then approved by the TAMU IRB.

Mexico was selected as an appropriate country to carry out this research as there is SDG data publicly available. Additionally, there are stark regional disparities in poverty and malnutrition (Fuentes and Montes 2004), and as such, this region exemplifies the regional variation common in other countries as well. The southern states and Indigenous groups in Mexico tend to have worse outcomes in education, infrastructure, poverty, and gender equity. Thus, the state of Yucatan, which is located in south-eastern Mexico, has one of the largest Indigenous populations in the country at 65% (INEGI 2015) and is apt as the regional focus. Additionally, the Yucatec Maya have a 3,000-year tradition of practicing agroecology for their subsistence in this area. However, the adoption of neoliberal policies in Mexico over the last 30 years has disrupted their ability to depend solely on their own production for subsistence. Three communities in the Yucatan, Tabi, Tixmehuac, and Tahdziu, were selected as the specific research sites because they fall in the lowest tertile for development based on the available MDG data in 2015 (See Hopkins et al. under review for more details) and the researchers already had established relationships with community members in these places.

A community research assistant carried out 20 interviews in Tabi and two graduate students from Universidad Autónoma de Yucatán administered nine interviews in Tixmehuac and ten in Tahdziu. The participants were primarily recruited through existing contacts; however, efforts were made to recruit a demographically broad sample to increase the potential for a diversity of responses. The participants ranged in age from 19 to 79 years with an average age of 47. Approximately three-quarters

(74%) of the participants were women heads of household and the remainder were men in the same role. They ranged in the amount of formal schooling they completed from none through high school with the majority completing elementary school. Households ranged in size from 1 to 12 people with most people having four people living in their household.

The data analysis process began with the research team compiling the data into an Excel spreadsheet. The responses to each question were then analyzed qualitatively by several team members by coding them for themes across all respondents using the method of item-level analysis (LeCompte and Schensul 2016). More specifically, team members grouped like responses through a collaborative and iterative process, which resulted in multiple themes for the responses to each question. Once the themes were defined, representative quotes were identified to illustrate what types of responses fell into each theme. Additionally, the frequency of responses in each was determined and variations in theme patterns based on major demographic variables like age, gender, and location were noted.

RESULTS

To get a sense of the types of foods consumed in each household participants were asked to respond to the question: "What foods and drinks did your family have yesterday?". For breakfast, they primarily ate bread and crackers (42%) followed by eggs (26%) and black beans (16%). Coffee was commonly drunk coffee (61%) and in some cases milk (21%). Similarly, black beans (29%) sometimes with pork (8%) and eggs in different forms (24%) were also common for lunch. However, a greater variety of dishes were reported for lunch than breakfast, including chicken with vegetables, roasted, and as mole (21%), dishes made with squash seeds and different kinds of meat (11%), and pork prepared without black beans (11%). Tortillas occasionally complemented dishes (13%), although likely many did not mention them given the ubiquity of consuming tortillas with the main meal in this area. Soft drinks (34%) followed by horchata, a rice-based drink (24%), and lemonade or natural juices (11%) were drunk during lunch. Dinner was reminiscent of breakfast with bread and crackers (42%) and coffee (34%) as most frequently reported along with eggs (13%), black beans (11%), and milk (11%). Leftovers from lunch were also commonly consumed (13%) and often in the form of *panuchos*, a Yucatecan taco (11%), or as nachos (5%). Soft drinks were another beverage consumed at dinner (18%). In Tahdziu and Tixmehuac, fewer respondents reported consuming foods between meals, and in Tabi, the foods that were consumed were primarily fruits.

Participants were also asked "What food and drinks do your family like to consume?" to determine how closely what people are consuming aligns with food preferences. In regard to beverages, participants reported preferring juices (50%), such as watermelon and orange. Lemonade (23%) was a popular juice of choice that was often mentioned separately from other juice beverages. Soft drinks (25%) were also prominently featured in beverage responses. Coffee (8%) and milk (5%), which were commonly reported in what was actually consumed, had low presence in preferences. In regard to meals, participants reported different kinds of dishes that are common to the region including black beans with pork (13%), soups (20%), and lots of fruits (33%) and vegetables (35%). For meat, the preference leaned toward chicken (20%). Eggs were mentioned on their own (15%) or as part of a dish with tomato (8%), which is less than what was reported as being consumed. There was little mention of bread (5%), cookies (0%), and crackers (0%), which were prominent in the reports of what was actually consumed.

The responses given to the question: "What are the conditions necessary to achieve well-being?" suggest that food security is not a given in these communities with over a third (41%) of the participants responding "Food," along with "Money" (Figure 9.1). "Work" and "Health," which were mentioned by half of the sample (51%), were the only conditions provided more frequently, and both of which are related to food. One participant from Tabi describes this relationship between food and work in his definition of well-being: "Someone's work to get money to buy something to eat."

The recognition of the importance of food was even greater when participants were asked to define poverty (Figure 9.2). Over half of respondents (59%) reported that "Not having enough food" as well as "Not having enough money" were the most important features in defining poverty. "Not enough work" was part of the definition

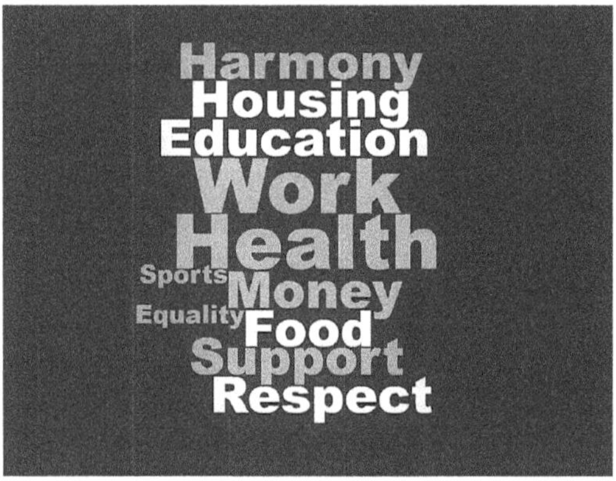

FIGURE 9.1 Local definitions of well-being.

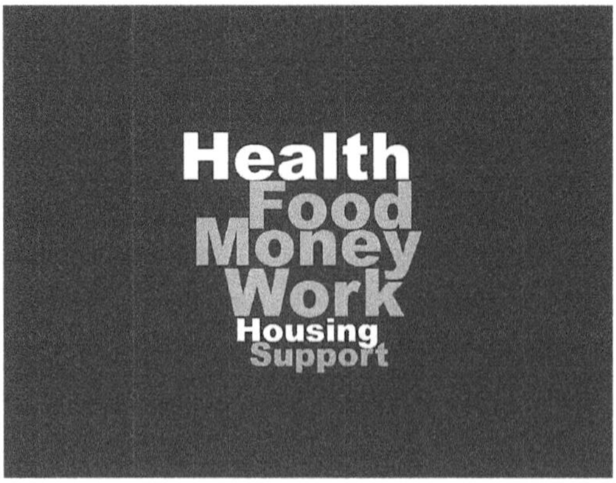

FIGURE 9.2 Local definition of poverty.

of poverty for a little over a third (38%) of participants. The relationship between food, money, and work was often included in participants' definitions of poverty, such as the case of another participant from Tabi who said: "Not having money, not having to eat, not having a job." The emphasis of food along with work and money in both well-being and poverty definitions suggests that it is no longer possible to acquire all of one's food from subsistence agriculture for participants.

The responses by participants to the question: "What changes in agricultural production have you noticed over time?" also indicates that strictly subsistence agriculture is no longer viable in these communities. Over 90% of participants reported a perceived negative change in agricultural production (Figure 9.3). Many respondents described the negative changes in general terms, as exemplified by this participant from Tabi's response "It is no longer the same production as in previous years." Others focused on crop loss and/or weather-related changes, which another participant from Tabi connects in her statement: "Everything that was sown was produced long ago and now it is not. It used to rain on time and it wasn't so hot." Only 8% of the participants noticed no changes in the production. No one perceived positive changes in agricultural production.

Participants were also asked about changes in harvest of forest products since these products play an integral role in their subsistence. The SDGs separate forest products from agriculture by putting them under Goal 15 (Life on Land), instead

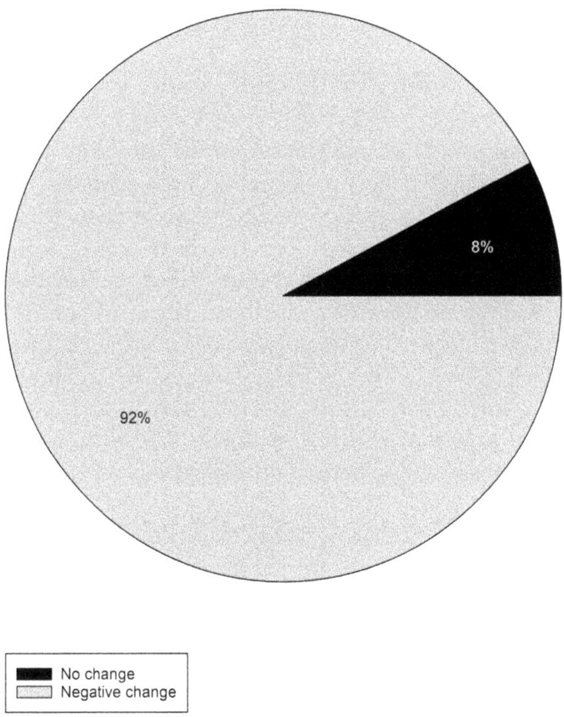

FIGURE 9.3 Perceived changes in agricultural production.

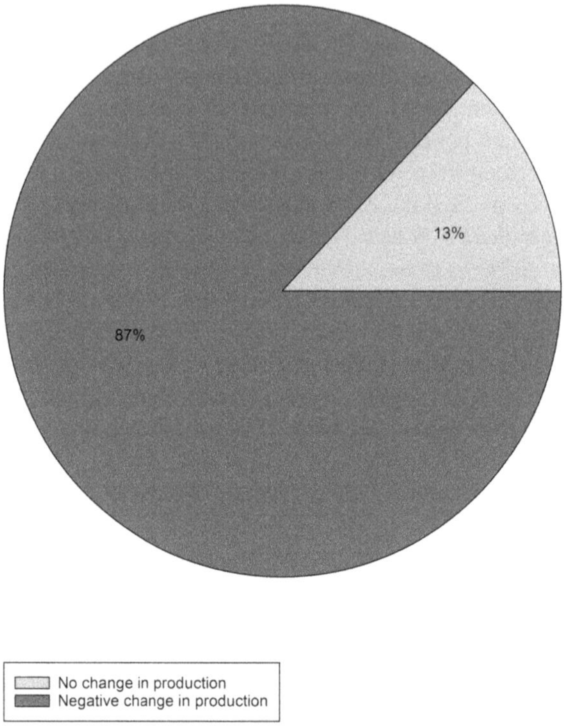

FIGURE 9.4 Perceived changes in forest harvest.

of Goal 2 (Zero Hunger). It became clear from the similarity in responses to the agricultural questions that for most participants, forest products were not a salient category separate from agricultural production. A little under 90% of participants reported negative changes in harvest of forest products (Figure 9.4) with qualitative responses very similar to agricultural production. However, there were a handful of participants that focused on firewood, which was not mentioned in the agriculture section. Several of them focused on the scarcity of the resource, like in this example from Tahdziu, which also relates this to forest damage: "Before there was a lot of firewood, now there is almost none. The forest is low." One participant from Tixmehuac emphasized the change in the quality of the food: "The wood comes thinner now." The remaining participants (13%) noticed no change, and no one observed any positive changes.

As for the causes of changes in agricultural production, a majority of the participants (61%) perceived them to be the result of weather changes, such as hotter temperatures and less predictable rainfall (Figure 9.5). A little over a quarter (26%) blamed damage to the forest. The remainder (13%) cited general misuses of the environment, including contamination.

The response for perceived causes of changes in forest harvest was again similar to agricultural production with a little over half reporting weather changes

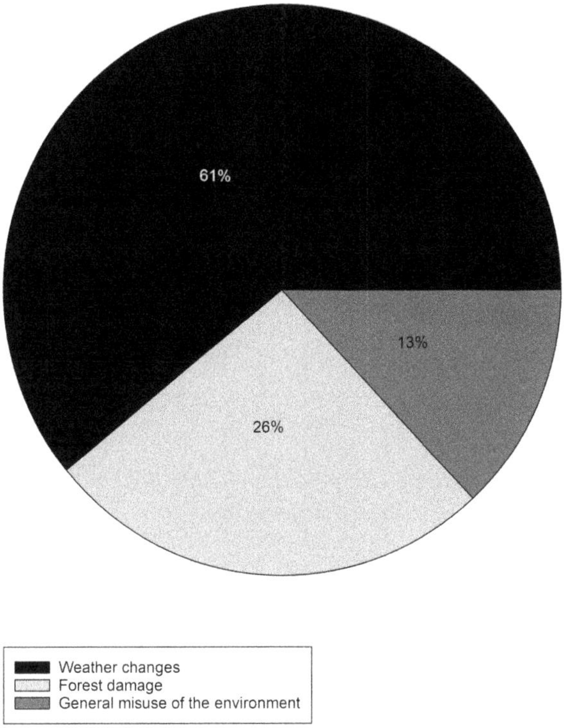

FIGURE 9.5 Perceived causes of change in agricultural production.

(52%) (Figure 9.6). Many spoke of those changes in general terms, like this participant from Tabi: "due to weather changes." However, others focused more specifically on rain-related changes: "The rain is late, it does not rain on time and who knows what causes it. There are a lot of storms and that affects it." describes one participant from Tabi. Still, others emphasized the heat-related changes, as did this participant from Tixmehuac in her comment: "The overheating." Forest damage was also a common response (37%), with this Tahdziu respondent helping us to understand why forest product harvest and agricultural production are not separate salient categories: "Because many people cut down the forest to sow." A few participants from Tabi (7%) cited general misuse of the environment as the cause with these statements: "we don't care for the environment" and "because of the chemicals." Lastly, one participant emphasized decreased soil fertility.

Eighty percent of the participants live in households that have chosen to supplement their subsistence agricultural practices with one or two members of the family participating in a regular low-paying wage labor job (Figure 9.7). The rest of the families do not have anyone in the household in a regular salaried position, although they may have someone that works irregularly for wages. When participants were then asked how the money from the wage labor jobs is spent, 90% responded with

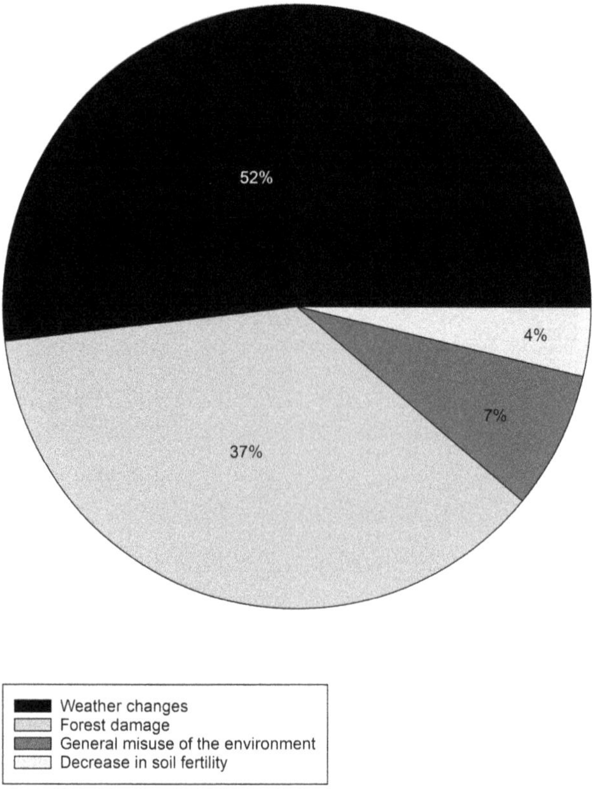

FIGURE 9.6 Perceived causes of change in forest harvest.

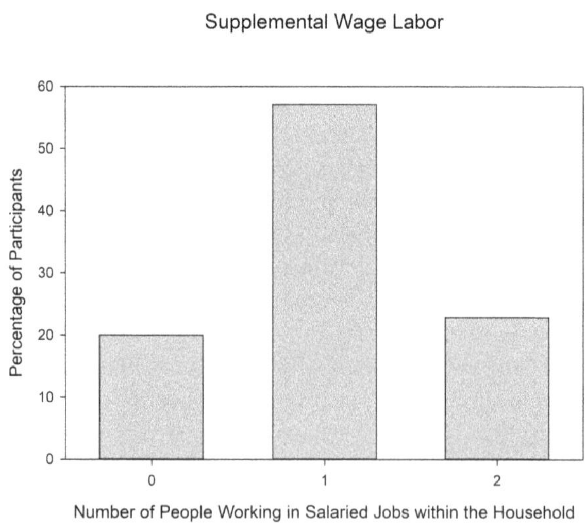

FIGURE 9.7 Supplemental wage labor.

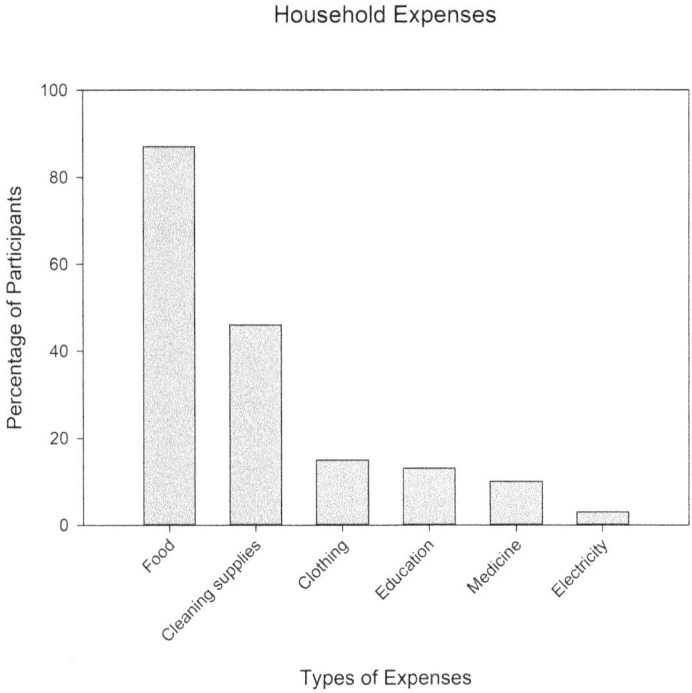

FIGURE 9.8 Household expenses.

food (Figure 9.8). This provides further evidence of the inability of the participants to rely solely on subsistence agriculture for food.

DISCUSSION

Mexico's Consejo Nacional de Evaluación de la Política de Desarrollo Social (CONEVAL) data on food security present a varied picture at multiple socio-political scales (municipality, state, national) (CONEVAL 2015). Comparison of the 2010 and 2015 data on food access indicates a decrease in percentage of the population lacking access to food in Sotuta (−21.9%) and Tahdziu (−64.2%) but almost a doubling in the percentage of the population lacking access to food in Tixmehuac (+15.8%). These changes signify a dramatic improvement in access to food within Tahdziu, a more moderate improvement within Sotuta, and a worsening in Tixmehuac. The decreases in food insecurity observed in Sotuta and Tahdziu are notably larger than changes in food insecurity measured across a similar time period (2010–2016) at the state and national level (see Table 9.2). The data indicate a 2.1% decrease in the percentage of the population experiencing food insecurity within the Yucatan state and a 4.7% decrease nationally. The CONEVAL data present an understanding of food security derived from the complementary and publically available Mexican government data on the SDGs. While this portrayal of food insecurity is a valuable starting point and offers the potential to explore temporal changes, our study adds to the understanding

TABLE 9.2
Consejo Nacional de Evaluación de la Política de Desarrollo Social (CONEVAL) and UN-SDG Sustainability Indicators for the Proportion of the Population with Moderate or Severe Food Insecurity by Geographical Unit in 2010 and 2015/2016

Geographical Unit	% of Population with Moderate or Severe Food Insecurity	
	2010	2015/2016
Mexico	24.8	20.1
Yucatan State	21.4	19.3
Sotuta	41.7	19.9
Tadziu	70.9	60.7
Tixmehuac	16.8	32.6

of food security through a presentation of the lived experience associated with these changes in food security.

Our findings suggest that despite measured declines in the lack of access to food within two of the three study locales, food vulnerability continues to be part of the lived experience in these places. For example, the participant responses regarding the definitions and conditions for poverty and well-being heavily emphasized food. This is also evident in the lack of inclusion of food in measures of well-being for highly developed countries (CDC 2018). When people with food security are asked similar questions, they do not mention food as it is treated as a given, as opposed to a daily concern that they associate with well-being. What this implies is that the participants are still very much concerned with where they are getting their food.

The substantial differences in participant food preferences and what they are actually eating suggest that food sovereignty may also be an issue in these areas. This is particularly evident in that the preferred foods emphasized fresh fruits and vegetables and animals that were traditionally produced by subsistence farmers in these areas and consumed by their families (O'Connor and Anderson 2017) and are being replaced by processed foods like coffee, bread, cookies, and crackers. A decline in food sovereignty is common for subsistence food producers that are shifting away from diverse agroecological systems and are becoming increasingly reliant on the market economy (Altieri and Toledo 2011; Altieri, Funes-Monzote, and Petersen 2012; Prevost et al. 2017). The local reliance on the market economy is evidenced with four-fifths of the families supplementing subsistence farm activities with one or more family members working in a wage labor position. Additionally, the prominence of money in the responses to the definitions for well-being and money also support this connection to the market.

In addition to the previous evidence of food insecurity and lack of sovereignty, participants almost unanimously articulated a decline in their agricultural production in recent times. The perceived causes for the decline in production by the participants were climate-centered with an emphasis on increasing temperatures and decreasing predictability of rainfall. This is in line with recent changes in climate data for the region. The maximum temperatures recorded in May 2019 were the highest temperatures recorded since January 2009 (WWO 2019). Meanwhile, in June 2019, the Yucatan experienced 490.3 mm of rainfall, which is also the highest amount recorded since 2009. An increase in variation in rainfall was also evident in the data over the last ten years.

Participants also emphasized the impact of the overuse of the forest, which leads to a reduction in soil fertility for farmers who are practicing slash-and-burn agriculture. If climate change is negatively affecting farmers' yields, this places the participants who are relying on these crops for food and income in an increasingly vulnerable economic position. A common strategy for reducing vulnerability among subsistence farmers is by diversifying the crops that they produce (Cunningham 2001). However, the diversifying strategy in this area has now extended to include wage labor employment in growing regional urban centers, such as Merida and Cancun. This can lead to a decline in food security as individuals earning low incomes cannot purchase the same quality of food that they can produce in a diverse agroecological system (Prevost et al. 2017; Herforth and Ahmed 2015; Bharucha and Pretty 2010; Reardon and Berdegué 2002), as is traditionally utilized by the Yucatec Maya.

Epidemics can also complicate the ability of this extended diversification strategy to help with food insecurity, as has become evident with the COVID-19 pandemic. For example, in rural areas of the state of Yucatan, many communities have restricted access making it difficult or impossible for family members working in urban areas to get food resources to their rural dwelling counterparts. Additionally, many of the urban workers, especially those in the service and construction industries, are experiencing at least a temporary loss of employment and a decline in income. This job loss has resulted in many individuals attempting to return to their home communities and reentering the agricultural sector through working on their families' farm plots; however, this is only possible when the communities are willing to grant them access.

When a pandemic is coupled with weather-related disasters, the compounding impacts further threaten food security. For example, in the first five days of June in 2020 amidst the COVID-19 pandemic, tropical storms Amanda and Cristobal deposited 635 mm of rain across the Yucatan Peninsula (NHC 2020), which is approximately half of the total average annual rainfall (Duch Gary 1988) for our study area. This resulted in extensive loss of crops in the rural areas thereby further magnifying food insecurity in the communities that primarily rely on subsistence crop production. Some local governments, including the municipalities where this research took place (J.C.P.K. 2020) and nonprofit organizations, like Agencias de Desarrollo Humano Local Alianzas (Lendechy Grajales et al. 2020), are stepping in and providing food and temporary jobs to those most affected by the pandemic and the tropical storms. Yet, even institutions with substantial economic and network resources are finding it difficult to acquire basic food supplies for households in need as the COVID-19 pandemic intersects with disastrous weather-related events.

While climate change is currently the most pressing influence on crop production for the participants, there are still other intersecting factors influencing their food security and sovereignty (Ebel et al. 2018). Much of this is a result of living in a complex globalized society. For example, while individuals identify climate changes as impacting their ability to produce food, this might be further impacted by economic changes within the community resulting from pandemics like COVID-19 or otherwise. Our results indicate that in addition to concerns about environmental conditions, economic shifts are present in the minds of community members as they consider poverty and well-being. Metaphorically, changes in the environment, social or natural, affect communities in waves. Each issue acts as its own wave, with peaks and troughs of intensity at varying points in time. However, their impact is compounded as they coalesce making the individual impact difficult to ascertain and the integrated impact potentially more detrimental. Indigenous people, such as the Yucatec Maya, are more vulnerable to waves of change, because they are historically socioeconomically disadvantaged, and thus tend to have limited resources and power accessible to them to protect themselves from the compounding impacts of changes in climate and the economy as is evident with the COVID-19 pandemic.

These multiple and intersecting threats to food security, and recent global events such as the COVID-19 pandemic, highlight the need for policies and programs at multiple scales that contribute to the formation of resilient and adaptive food systems. Systems that are grounded in local need yet able to respond to global change processes, which may be sudden and overlapping. Additionally, policies and programs must consider the urban–rural relationships necessary to support resilient food systems, and how such relationships will be impacted by internal and external disturbances, such as epidemics and extreme weather events.

CONCLUSION AND RECOMMENDATIONS

We demonstrate that felt food insecurity and lack of sovereignty by our Yucatec Maya participants are coupled with declines in agricultural production perceived to be caused primarily by climate change. Many families are coping with this increased vulnerability by incorporating low-wage employment in regional urban centers into the traditional mix of livelihood strategies.

These findings contribute to the burgeoning body of scholarly work on subnational development and the localization of the SDGs by providing evidence of local perspectives on food security that are complementary to existing regional and national data. Ultimately, this work has the intended practical application of providing a guide for the development of locally appropriate interventions and evaluations to improve food security among the Yucatec Maya. In particular, this research offers a basis for evaluating interventions from the perspective of the individuals for whom the interventions are intended to work. Evaluation that integrates statistical analysis (as is possible with the CONEVAL data) and understanding of the lived experience of individuals and communities holds the potential to provide a more robust and multidimensional assessment of efforts to address food insecurity. This research is also broadly situated in research related to sustainable development and Indigenous peoples as a part of efforts to reverse the loss of Indigenous food sovereignty that have accelerated with the expansion of neoliberal policies throughout the developing world.

The work presented here is the result of the first phase of a long-term research project designed to explore sustainability and food-related issues from local perspectives within the Yucatan. Limitations of this work relate to the testing and design of the context-appropriate survey instrument. Our research agenda emphasizes the participatory process necessary to ensure a strong link between research and policy (Thomas-Hughes 2018). Through the participatory and iterative process of developing the survey instrument, we recognize that the current version of the instrument presented opportunities for participants to speak to some topics and not others. For example, future improvements in the instrument will provide an increased opportunity for participants to reflect on the role of policy. Although questions regarding change in production provided a space for discussion of policy, the version of the survey instrument used at this phase of the research did not adequately integrate question redundancy to increase reliability around this construct. Results presented here are from the first implementation of our collaboratively designed research instrument. As such, our initial findings serve to generate hypotheses for future research phases and to orient the direction and design of follow-up studies. For example, further examination of the role of climate change and its intersections with policy will be addressed using a confirmatory study design within the next phase of research. The following phases of the research project are designed to be reflexive and integrate knowledge gained from previous phases. New findings from future research hold the potential to provide more nuanced and even different understandings of food security as experienced in the Yucatan. In this chapter, we present the findings of a nascent research endeavor and offer an understanding of the context within which individuals are navigating food security and related sustainability issues. This chapter, and also future research, aims to respond and contribute to the call for an expanded understanding of the ways in which the complexity and dynamic nature of food security are integrated into research and policy-making.

ACKNOWLEDGMENTS

We would like to thank the people of Tabi, Tahdziu, and Tixmehauc who participated in this research endeavor. We are also very grateful for the financial support from the Yucatan Initiative, an agreement between the State of Yucatan and Texas A&M University, the Texas A&M University Liberal Arts Seed Grant, and the University of Colorado Springs Global Intercultural Research Center (GLINT), that made this research possible.

REFERENCES

Altieri, Miguel A., Fernando R. Funes-Monzote, and Paulo Petersen. 2012. "Agroecologically efficient agricultural systems for smallholder farmers: contributions to food sovereignty." *Agronomy for Sustainable Development* 32 (1):1–13. doi: 10.1007/s13593-011-0065-6.

Altieri, Miguel A., and Victor Manuel Toledo. 2011. "The agroecological revolution in Latin America: rescuing nature, ensuring food sovereignty and empowering peasants." *The Journal of Peasant Studies* 38 (3):587–612. doi: 10.1080/03066150.2011.582947.

Bharucha, Zareen, and Jules Pretty. 2010. "The roles and values of wild foods in agricultural systems." *Philosophical Transactions of the Royal Society B: Biological Sciences* 365 (1554):2913–2926.

Brida, Ange-Benjamin, Tom Owiyo, and Youba Sokona. 2013. "Loss and damage from the double blow of flood and drought in Mozambique." *International Journal of Global Warming* 5 (4):514–531. doi: 10.1504/IJGW.2013.057291.

Brown, Molly E., and Christopher C. Funk. 2008. "Food security under climate change." *Science* 319 (5863):580–581.

Campesina. 2007. "Declaration of Nyéléni." Forum for Food Sovereignty. https://nyeleni.org/spip.php?article290.

Centers for Disease Control and Prevention. 2018. "Well-Being Concepts." U.S. Department of Health & Human Services, National Center for Chronic Disease Prevention and Health Promotion, Division of Population Health, accessed January 31, 2020. https://www.cdc.gov/hrqol/wellbeing.htm.

Clapp, Jennifer. 2014. "Food security and food sovereignty: getting past the binary." *Dialogues in Human Geography* 4 (2):206–211.

CONEVAL. 2015. "Medición de la pobreza, Estados Unidos Mexicanos, 2010–2015, Indicadores de pobreza por municipio." editado por CONEVAL (Consejo Nacional de Evaluación de la Política de Desarrollo Social). http://agenda2030.mx/ODSopc.html?cveCob=31&lang=es#/geocov.

Cunningham, Anthony B. 2001. "Conservation behaviour, boundaries and beliefs." In *Applied Ethnobotany: People, Wild Plant Use, and Conservation*, edited by Anthony B. Cunnigham, 222–263. London: Earthscans Publication Limited.

Duch Gary, J. 1988. *"La conformación territorial del estado de Yucatán: los componentes del medio físico."* México: Universidad Autónoma de Chapingo: Centro Regional de la Península de Yucatán.

Ebel, Roland, María De Jesús Méndez Aguilar, and Heather R. Putnam. 2018. "Milpa: one sister got climate-sick. The impact of climate change on traditional Maya farming systems." *International Journal of Sociology of Agriculture & Food* 24 (2):175–199.

FAO. 2002. *The State of Food Insecurity in the World 2001*. Rome: Food and Agriculture Association.

FAO. 2003. *Trade Reforms and Food Security: Conceptualizing the Linkages*. Rome: Commodity Policy and Projections Service, Commodities and Trade Division, Food and Agriculture Organization of the United Nations.

FAO. 2007. *The State of Food and Agriculture 2007: Food Agriculture Organization of the United Nations*. Rome: Food and Agriculture Organization of the United Nations.

Fuentes, Ricardo, and Andres Montes. 2004. "Mexico and the millennium development goals at the subnational level." *Journal of Human Development* 5 (1):97–120.

Herforth, Anna, and Selena Ahmed. 2015. "The food environment, its effects on dietary consumption, and potential for measurement within agriculture-nutrition interventions." *Food Security* 7 (3):505–520. doi: 10.1007/s12571-015-0455-8.

Hertel, Thomas W., Marshall B. Burke, and David B. Lobell. 2010. "The poverty implications of climate-induced crop yield changes by 2030." *Global Environmental Change* 20 (4):577–585. doi: 10.1016/j.gloenvcha.2010.07.001.

Hopkins, Allison L., Cerian Gibbes, Armando F. Inurreta Diaz, and Juan Jimenez-Osornio. Under review. Sub-national variation in internationally recognized sustainability goals in Yucatan, Mexico. *Journal of Human Development and Capabilities*.

INEGI. 2015. "Encuesta Intercensal 2015." Instituto Nacional de Estadística y Geografía (INEGI), accessed October 27, 2018. http://www.beta.inegi.org.mx/app/areasgeograficas/?ag=31.

J.C.P.K. 2020. "Dan apoyos y empleos." *Diario de Yucatán*, 29 de Mayo 2020, Yucatan. Accessed June 26, 2020. https://www.yucatan.com.mx/yucatan/dan-apoyos-y-empleos.

LeCompte, Margaret D., and Jean J. Schensul. 2016. *Analysis and Interpretation of Ethnographic Data: A Mixed Methods Approach*. 2nd ed, *Ethnographer's Toolkit*. Lanham, MD: Rowman & Littlefield.

Lendechy Grajales, Manuel Triay Peniche Ángel, Victor Manuel Ávila Pacheco, Margarita Zarco Salgado, Juan José Jiménez Osornio, Mariana Pacheco Ortiz, and Terecita del Socorro Solís Gasca. 2020. Informe de Entrega de Ayuda Alimentaria a Familias en Situación de Vulnerabilidad por COVID-19. Mérida: Agencias de Desarrollo Humano Local (ADHL) Alianzas.

Lobell, David B., Wolfram Schlenker, and Justin Costa-Roberts. 2011. "Climate trends and global crop production since 1980." *Science* 333 (6042):616–620. doi: 10.1126/science.1204531.

NHC. 2020. "BULLETIN: Tropical Storm Cristobal Intermediate Advisory 20A from June 6, 2020". Miami, FL: National Oceanic and Atmospheric Administration, National Weather Service, National Hurricane Center (NHC), accessed 6-30-20. https://www.nhc.noaa.gov/archive/2020/al03/al032020.public_a.020.shtml?

O'Connor, Amber M., and Eugene N. Anderson. 2017. *K'oben: 3,000 Years of the Maya Hearth, Rowman & Littlefield Studies in Food and Gastronomy*. Lanham: Rowman & Littlefield.

Patel, Raj. 2009. "Food sovereignty." *Journal of Peasant Studies* 36 (3):663–706. doi: 10.1080/03066150903143079.

PFSN. 2002. "People's Food Sovereignty Statement." People's Food Sovereignty Network (PFSN). https://nyeleni.org/IMG/pdf/Peoples_Food_Sovereignty_Statement.pdf.

Prevost Otero, David Enrique, Francisco Delfin Gurri, Ramó Mariaca Mendez, and Francisco Guizar Vazquez. 2017. "The inclusion and increase of the industrialized foods supply in the diets of households and their relationship with the abandonment of the self-subsistence system in the rural Mayan communities of Yucatan, Mexico." *Cuadernos De Desarrollo Rural* 14 (80):16. doi: 10.11144/Javeriana.cdr14-80.iaoa.

Reardon, Thomas, and Julio A. Berdegué. 2002. "The rapid rise of supermarkets in Latin America: challenges and opportunities for development." *Development Policy Review* 20 (4):371–388.

Smith, Lisa C., and Ali Subandoro. 2007. *Measuring Food Security Using Household Expenditures Surveys*, Food Security in Practice Technical Guide Series. Washington, DC: International Food Policy Research Institute (IFPRI).

Thomas-Hughes, Helen. 2018. "Ethical 'mess' in co-produced research: reflections from a UK-based case study." *International Journal of Social Research Methodology* 21 (2): 231–242.

Warner, Koko, and Tamer Afifi. 2014. "Where the rain falls: evidence from 8 countries on how vulnerable households use migration to manage the risk of rainfall variability and food insecurity." *Climate and Development* 6 (1):1–17. doi: 10.1080/17565529.2013.835707.

Wittman, Hannah, Annette Aurelie Desmarais, and Nettie Wiebe, eds. 2010. *Food Sovereignty: Reconnecting Food, Nature and Community*. Halifax: Fernwood.

WWO. 2019. "Yucatan Monthly Climate Averages: 2009–2019." accessed January 28, 2020. https://www.worldweatheronline.com/lang/en-us/yucatan-weather-averages/oaxaca/mx.aspx.

10 Agrochemicals, Health, and Environment on the Coast of Oaxaca

The Role of Agriculture in Climate Change

Anna Batet Figueras

CONTENTS

INTRODUCTION

With agricultural modernization initiated in the 1940s, it was intended to achieve growth and agrarian development by increasing food production, introducing mechanization, chemical fertilizers, high-yield seeds, and transgenic crops, among others. The Green Revolution (GR) was conceived in Mexico[1] and from there the importation of the "technological package"[2] began, intended to increase cereal production and productivity in poor countries through intensive use of land. Those who emphasize the advantages of the GR rely on the neutrality of science and technology and appeal to increased production[3] to solve the problems of hunger and development in rural countries, but this discourse has proven to be invalid when we find millions of hungry people in a world where food is produced for far more people (Vivas 2014).

DOI: 10.1201/9781003014942-10

The monumental failure of the world food system starts from one of its foundations: the industrial agricultural model, characterized by high consumption of fossil energy, overproduction of food through the intensive use of chemical fertilizers, the incorporation of high-tech seeds with its agrochemicals, and free trade. This agricultural model offers the raw material of a long agrifood chain that converts food into industrial goods that are processed, stored, frozen, and transported, consuming in the process a large amount of energy,[4] generating greenhouse gasses and contributing to the destruction of local markets. If we add all this together, there is a loss of agrobiodiversity implicit in the industrialization of the agrifood system, and we can affirm that the global food model contributes significantly to climate change (GRAIN 2011; Montagut and Vivas 2009).

Global warming highlights the failure and unsustainability of the world agrifood system. Organizations such as the FAO, PAHO, WHO, and IAASTD[5] have incorporated new arguments in their reports that relate food security to climate change and sociopolitical conflicts. Among other things, they claim that direct and indirect climate-related impacts have a cumulative effect on food insecurity and malnutrition and have repercussions on water and sanitation, with health implications and disease risks (FAO et al. 2018). So, whether we like it or not, food is and will be at the center of this ongoing climate crisis (GRAIN et al 2009, 7).

We know that the causes of food insecurity are not due to insufficient food produced,[6] but, on the other hand, we also know that achieving food sufficiency does not ensure healthy and nutritious food, nor good quality and safe food. The meaning of *food safety*, the consumption of toxic-free food, is closely related to notions such as *environmental risk and suffering* through the correlation between contamination of the environment and the forms of production (environmental risk) and the contamination that moves within the body through food (food risk). We know that chemical contamination can take different meanings depending on the sociocultural context, and despite the fact that the notion of risk is not specific to a given context, its manifestations and perceptions are (Gracia 2002).

In this chapter, chemical contaminants (pesticides, fertilizers, growth hormones, etc.) take the leading role in the social and individual perception of food risk. Focusing on the use of agrochemicals in agricultural activity, I wonder what collateral consequences they have on people's health and the environment, with the main objective of knowing how this model of intensive agricultural production influences the perception of risk for farmers' health, and how this perception of risk is articulated in discourse and practices in favor of a more sustainable and environmentally friendly agriculture.

The research setting for this work is located in the state of Oaxaca, Mexico, specifically in the coastal strip of the municipality of Villa de Tututepec de Melchor Ocampo (hereinafter Tututepec), including the communities of Santa Rosa de Lima, San José del Progreso, Rio Grande, El Renacimiento, San Miguel, Playa Vieja, Camalotillo, Charco Redondo, Chacalapa, La Luz, San Vicente, Santa Cruz, and Santiago Jocotepec. Oaxaca ranks as the second poorest state in the country, and according to OECD[7] welfare indicators, it ranks second to last in access to services, income, and education. The third largest municipality in the state and the largest in the coastal region is Tututepec, which is classified with a high degree of marginalization and a medium degree of municipal delay[8] by the Ministry of Social Development of Mexico (SEDESOL). It is estimated that 51.2% of the population of Tututepec experiences food shortages related to food access (CECIPROC and ECOSTA 2018; CONEVAL 2015; INEGI 2015).

In Mexico, news reports,[9] studies, and proposals demanding greater food safety are taking center stage (Arellano et al. 2009; Díaz-Barriga 1996; García Hernández et al. 2018; Karam et al. 2004; Ortega-Ceseña, Espinosa-Torres, López-Carrillo 1994), especially if we consider that highly dangerous pesticides are used in the country, which are prohibited in other countries. The General Directorate of Epidemiology of the Ministry of Health of Mexico (2013) reported that there had been 67,711 cases of pesticide poisoning throughout the country between 1995 and 2012, mainly in the working age population (60%) and among males (71.02%), which indicates that this exposure constitutes a high risk[10] in work-related activity.

Sustainable Development Goal (SGD)[11] 8.8 refers to the protection of labor rights and the promotion of a safe work environment, yet, in the study area, the personal protective equipment required during the handling and application of pesticides is not used. Safety regulations[12] are systematically breached by the farmers themselves but also by the employers. The causes of noncompliance are diverse: from deficient protective equipment or its poor condition that the employer offers to their workers, to ignorance of the risks involved in not using protection by farmers, or the extreme heat and humidity of the area that discourages anyone from putting more layers of clothing on their skin. As noted by the indicators related to SDG 8.8, compliance with national legislation regarding labor rights should be strengthened, both by employers and by farmers themselves, increasing on the one hand the training of different actors in the use and management of agrochemicals, including women, Indigenous people, and other groups that are in vulnerable situations, and on the other hand, technologically improving production processes through the use of environmentally friendly technologies and the preservation of natural resources.

Today, we have a large number of scientific arguments on the sustainability of traditional agroecological practices to face challenges related to food security, but these solutions are extremely difficult to implement due to the threat they represent to the sales and profitability of the powerful food industry. Let us remember that the industrialization of agriculture is an imposition of the conventional food marketing and distribution system (ODELA 2018) rooted in the capitalist logic of the search for maximum profit. Olivier de Schutter, United Nations Special Rapporteur from 2008 to 2014, gave scientific arguments on how peasant and organic agriculture could end food crises and address the challenges linked to poverty and climate change, overcoming forms of production based on chemical fertilizers (Schutter 2010).

The aim of this study is to share the voice of farmers and their perceptions of food security and to demonstrate how discourse on the perception of pesticide risk is articulated, or not, with initiatives in favor of more sustainable and healthy agricultural production models. This study also seeks to contribute to critical debates on manufactured risks, the distribution of socio-ecological conflicts, and capitalist forms of production within the framework of environmental justice. In the field of medical anthropology, the contribution of the study is framed in anthropological analysis on health, development, and the environment, taking the concept of risk as a central theoretical element (Martínez-Hernáez 2011; Larrea Killinger and Martínez Mauri 2012).

METHODOLOGY

The methodology used in the present work is qualitative with an ethnographic basis. Techniques used included semi-structured interviews and direct observations. The units of analysis were agricultural parcels and the social actors within those units. This involved farmers who work directly in the field, agricultural technicians, organizers of communal or ejidal lands,[13] representatives of agricultural land, and civil associations that promote the defense and recovery of the natural and sociocultural heritage. A total of 43 interviews (20 farmers, 15 authorities, and 8 members of civil associations) were conducted between January and April 2018. All contacts and appointments with informants – with the exception of 6 cases – were facilitated by ECOSTA.[14]

The project participants, mostly men between 36 and 55 years of age, are distinguished into three groups: (a) farmers; (b) technical, medical, or political authorities[15]; and (c) activists and civil associations. The distinction between the three interviewee profiles is in response to the recognition of the multiplicity of actors involved in the meaning of social structures, incorporating a relational approach in ethnographic analyses (Menéndez 2009).

RESULTS

Food Risk and Environmental Risk

The United Nations recommends two divergent definitions for evaluating the toxicity of chemicals: one focused on probability, understanding *risk as a statistical concept*, and the other focused on *utility properties*, where benefit enters the risk equation treating safety as a measure of the acceptability of a certain degree of risk (Douglas 1996). As an objective of the Sustainable Development Goals (SDGs), there is an intention to double the agricultural productivity and income of small-scale food producers (SDG 2.3), measured by the volume of production per unit of work, according to its type and size. Although target 2.4 proposes to increase productivity through resilient agricultural practices, the indicator proposed for its evaluation does not guarantee a decrease in the use of pesticides. If, in addition, according to the Codex Alimentarius,[16] the analysis of risks related to the health and safety of food should consider the economic consequences and the viability of the options for managing these risks, then we can understand that the minimization of pesticide risk is approached from the perspective of risk as a *calculation of probabilities* subject to economic benefits. In order to consider the cost of pesticides to human health and the environment, we have to put aside crop yield and economic profitability and begin to assess the long-term productivity potential of agroecological systems. This is one of the criticisms that Hilal Ever presents in an analysis of the question of risk, addressing it from the right to food, a right that should not endanger either human health or the environment (A/HRC/34/48 2017). And, it is clear that the right to food referred to by the United Nations Special Rapporteur is not simply the right to a minimum calorie ration but the right to "adequate food," also referring to quality and its appropriate character according to the cultural or physiological aspects of the person (FAO 2017).

Considering a brief review of the contribution of anthropology on the study of risk, Douglas and Wildavsky's (1983) cultural theory starts from the idea that risk is a social construction, where each culture creates and represents its risks based on a system of values and beliefs, depending one's social and personal position within society (Gracia 2004). Conversely, the theoretical approaches defended by Beck (1998, 2002), Giddens (1994), and Bauman (2001) on risk in society put the emphasis on the (macro) structural aspects of the economic and political organizations and in the *manufactured risks* that characterize them (Gracia 2004). Lupton (1999) combines the symbolic-cultural perspectives of risk by Douglas with that of risk in society by Beck and Giddens, to show how risk is a culturally, politically, and socially constructed phenomenon (ODELA 2018).

Entering into the conceptual development of food risks, these can be grouped into three areas: those related to the forms of consumption; those related to sanitation, hygiene and microbiology; and the *risks related to the forms of production*. The latter is the object of study in this work.

Chemical contamination of food may be due to the presence of residual phytosanitary products (pesticides, herbicides, growth hormones, etc.) applied systematically during production, the lack of environmental controls, or the inappropriate use of certain technologies (biomodification) or agrochemicals. In this sense, the risk is associated with dangers related to food quality and chemical poisoning, moving into the body and constituting a silent risk due to the accumulation of synthetic chemical substances at small doses over a long period of time. Investigating the social perceptions of this type of risk and the meanings about internal contamination and toxic corporeality have been reviewed by Begueria (2016), Larrea-Killinger and Mauri (2012), and Porta et al. (2002). According to Beck (2002), the environmental risk is latent, has negative socio-environmental effects, and is a global phenomenon that must be analyzed and discussed locally. When this materializes in environmental disasters, the dimensions of the social vulnerability of the population and the environment in which they live are manifested (Alfie 2017).

Another key theoretical question is how we conceptualize nature and how we understand the relationship between humans and nature.[17] The separation between society and nature has led to the adaptation of the natural world to the needs of the social world to guarantee the sustainability of capital accumulation (Busqueta et al. 2017). The theory of *socio-ecological metabolism*[18] (Küster 2016; Toledo 2013) would become an example of overcoming the society–nature dichotomy, since it allows us to analyze agrifood systems considering both the social sciences and the natural sciences.

From the perspective of critical medical anthropology, I consider Menéndez's (1981) work on *transaction systems* in the Mexican sphere to be useful, since it describes the forms of exploitation, domination, and hegemony of the elites over the subordinate classes and becomes a valuable tool of denunciation against the hegemonic system that conditions the framework of farmers' needs, determining the economic, political, and ideological dimension of their way of life (Martínez-Hernáez

2011). In this sense, we can understand pesticides as a form of domination used by the agribusiness elites as well as other power structures over the peasants of the Oaxaca coast, and this, more than anything, is what needs to be transformed.

The Process of Agrarian Modernization: The Use of Pesticides in Mexico

The municipality of Tututepec has a long agricultural history that has undergone important changes in recent decades, causing impacts on natural resources, genetic material, farming practices, and food consumption of the communities (Lara and Reyes 2010). Agriculture, which represents 55% of the productive sectors of the municipality, is mainly industrial that is combined with some elements of traditional agriculture, such as the use of slash and burn[19] and *milpa*.[20]

As is well known, the objective of industrial agriculture is to improve the performance and efficiency of the production system, and for this, a large number of fertilizers and agrochemicals are applied, some of which are considered highly dangerous (Bejarano et al. 2017; Díaz-Barriga 1996; Karam et al. 2004). The momentum of the GR, combined with the neoliberal governments of the last decades in Mexico, has favored the development of a set of public policies to support agroindustry, betting on export agriculture and leaving aside small farmers. The most notable events that have favored the current Mexican scenario are, on one side, the enactment of the Free Trade Agreement with North America (United States and Canada) (NAFTA), which caused changes[21] in the mechanisms for setting domestic prices, affecting national agricultural production (Montagut and Vivas 2009), and conditioned the regulatory framework for pesticides. On the other side, the financial, energy, and food crisis of 2008 had a negative impact on world food security, causing a series of momentous events to be unleashed in Mexico that would modify the scenario of federal policy on food security: the national program *Mexico without Hunger 2014–2018* (Urquía-Fernández 2014). This included the PROAGRO subsidy, which is basically received in the form of transgenic seeds, fertilizers, and agrochemicals.

Government authorization for the sale and use of pesticides in Mexico is made by the Federal Commission for the Protection against Sanitary Risks (COFEPRIS) based on the toxicological, environmental impact, and biological effectiveness studies of a pesticide as required by the R-PLAFEST regulation (2014). However, the evaluation carried out by state agencies does not guarantee that there are no unacceptable risks to health and the environment when it comes to including a pesticide in the catalog of authorized products here is a legal gap in risk assessment (it is not a legal obligation under the same regulation), and consequently, the precautionary principle does not apply in the denial or revocation of a registration. Furthermore, pesticides authorized before 2005 have an indefinite validity and those registered after this date do not require additional information to update the registry, which for practical purposes translates into a majority of authorized pesticides (80.7%) with an indeterminate validity in the country (Bejarano et al. 2017). For example, in the 2016 COFEPRIS catalog of pesticides, we found that 183 active ingredients are highly dangerous, of which 34.43% present high acute toxic effects on human health, and of these, 140 are prohibited or unauthorized in other countries (ibis).

Social Representation of the Risk of Agrochemicals

All interviewees' discourse revolves around market pressure, the need for inputs to produce, the increase in pests, and the decrease in soil productivity. There seems to be no alternative to the industrial agricultural model.

> We use conventional agriculture because we all want quantity, to produce more. We saturate the trees with fertilizers.
>
> *(OCS, Municipal Agent of Santa Rosa de Lima)*

> You must use fertilizer, otherwise there is no yield.
>
> *(MMR, Commissariat of Communal Assets)*

They also reveal to us the experience of the socially marginalized peasants vis-à-vis large industrial farmers, when subsidies and agrarian policies are mainly aimed at transnational corporations that market agricultural products.

> The subsidy for the producer is going to be given with the priority of increasing productivity or increasing market competitiveness, and these subsidies are being monopolized by the strongest, the largest.
>
> *(FB, Activist)*

Focusing on the subject of study, we can observe the ambivalent situation in which pesticides position us on the risk/benefit scale, generating simultaneously opposite and contradictory feelings, both in the environmental field and in the health of the person (Widger 2014). In general, they are accepted as *dangerous products* with a wide range of health and environmental afflictions but also as promoters of agriculture and social and economic development. Thus, the majority of informants working in the field (81.5%) continue to use agrochemicals despite the high perception of risk.

> For me it would be a necessary evil. It is helping you, but in the long run it will change you.
>
> *(MMR, Authority)*

> I hear that there is a lot of cancer and I think that it could be all the chemicals applied to the fruit.
>
> *(JLT, Farmer)*

According to Beck (1998), the expansion of risks goes hand in hand with capitalist development, which on the one hand increases productivity and on the other causes diseases. In today's society, the immediate need created by the capitalist system competes with the known risk, and for farmers, the choice between perceived wealth and imperceptible risks will be won by the former. This paradox is precisely due to the invisibility of risks, its economic exploitation of dangerous situations, and social and environmental vulnerability.

> We do not know the risk, because we do not see it, and see the crop benefits. You do not see the damage, you don't even know that got you're sick.
>
> *(PAP, Authority)*

In general, the risk of agrochemicals is perceived in the form of acute poisoning, putting aside sickness and chronic diseases, and even deaths attributed to the pesticide. Misinformation about the dangers of chemicals creates uncertainty, but the commercial approach to agriculture is so ingrained that discourse in favor of reducing agrochemicals in the field contradict the need to keep the fields "clean" (sociocultural factors) or are discarded due to the entangled difficulties by the sectors that operate at the macrostructural level.

Beyond these generalities, analysis of the discourse allows us to understand what the social representation of risk is for the three informant profiles. Starting with *farmers*, the uncertainty and confusion manifested toward the toxicity of agrochemicals are remarkable and often directly admitted. If we also add the lack of "habit" in the use of personal protective equipment (PPE) – 71% of farmers do not use them – we are in a situation of notable social vulnerability.[22] This uncertainty about the danger of the agrochemical products itself is transferred and influences the exposure factors, the mitigation measures adopted, and the chosen therapeutic route.

The most notable feature of the discourse analysis is the presence of the concepts of *lazy* (vago) and *weak*, understood as sociocultural factors that condition the social perception of the risk of agrochemicals. Being *lazy* is related, on the one hand, to the presence of bush or undergrowth on the plot, which in turn is linked to the presence of pests and low yield of the crop. Having the field *clean* is synonymous with being a worker and if you have weeds it means that you are *lazy* and this is cause for scorn. On the other hand, *lazy* is also related to the substitution of the traditional way of working the field: "now the peasant has become lazy, before you did not detach yourself from the machete" (JRA, farmer). This second meaning is used mainly by organic farmers, who have not replaced the machete with the *liquid*.[23] The concept of *weakness* is related to the construction of male identity and the belief in subjective immunity from physical harm or disease when facing the risk of agrochemicals: only those who are weak are poisoned. The construction of masculine identity is nourished by social conventions related to the way in which a "man" should act, such as being strong, hardworking, having the obligation to provide for their family, facing the consequences of heavy labor, and hiding discomfort and suffering. In this way, masculinity symbolically distances itself from everything related to care (self-care) and attention. Males socialize their suffering and painless, and this means that if they suffer any illness during work, they tend toward therapeutic inaction, overconfidence, and the minimization of harm. Being weak is not appropriate for men, and for this reason, agricultural laborers in Sonora (Mexico) attribute disease to weak blood (Calvario 2007).

Therefore, both *lazy* and *weak* have pejorative connotations that discredit, stigmatize, and influence the perception and exposure to the risks of agrochemicals used in productive activity.

The group of technical, medical, and political *authorities* place more emphasis on the risk related to bad practices in the productive sphere and the incorrect handling of agrochemicals than on the dangerousness of the product itself. It would be in the case of *activists* and/or members of civil associations where we can see that the health risk is related to both acute poisonings caused by agrochemicals and the increase in diseases that have occurred in the area in recent years,[24] perceiving the risk beyond the present moment. The association between risk, health, and food quality includes the production environment but also food consumption and the state of environmental degradation. The link between environmental health and human health is especially relevant among the group of activists, although farmers also differentiate and classify chemicals between those that harm the land (less fertility, salinization, and soil degradation) and those that do not. For some informants, the effects on the environment are seen in a more comprehensive way, such as lack of water, impact of the food chain, or contamination by residues associated with the use of agrochemicals. In others, environmental health is subordinated to the needs of the market (soil productivity) and detaches itself from human health.

Nature is related to the meaning of *pure, good and of the earth* (ODELA 2018, 65), and all people link health with nature. Thus, there is a socially shared perception that products of chemical origin are dangerous, although this perception is culturally modeled. In the present investigation, organic farmers, who represent 18.5% of the total of interviewees, relate organic products to health and environmental benefits. On the other hand, the rest of the farmers believe that organic agriculture is more expensive to work, they must have specific knowledge to manage pests, and also, there is no market for organic produce in Mexico because it is not considered to be of quality.

So, from this perspective, food security is understood as the provision of enough food for everyone and the agrochemicals as the guarantor of this. Only organic farmers understand food security as a broader concept, incorporating notions related to the concept of food sovereignty:

> Food security is to have our seed to be able to cultivate and preserve our culture.
>
> *(EPM, Farmer)*

Food sovereignty is related to the right of individuals or communities to define their own food and their own model of food production, as well as to determine to what degree they want to protect domestic production and regulate trade in order to achieve sustainable development (ODELA 2018). This concept was developed by the social movement of peasants and citizens known as La Vía Campesina, affirming that food sovereignty is the precondition for achieving authentic food security.[25]

La Via Campesina emerges as a protest against the neoliberal agrofood model (which damages local and sustainable production systems, local markets, and squanders natural resources) and advocates comprehensive land reform. With the adoption of the neoliberal paradigm in the 1980s, the Mexican government's food policy opted for commercial exchange as the mechanism to guarantee the availability of food, an act that according to Rodríguez Gómez (2007), has placed the country of Mexico in a state of increasing food vulnerability. The long-awaited agrarian reform should consider the food system as the central object of the new food and nutrition security policies, and at the same time, these should be elaborated within the framework of the right to food; in addition, it is necessary to prepare a food sovereignty law that guarantees equal access to quality food for all Mexicans (Rodríguez Gómez 2007). These proposals are in accordance with SDG 2.3, 2.4, and 2.B, and the Mexican government has already begun to draft a general law initiative for the right to food and food sovereignty,[26] which aims to stimulate and increase national food production, preferably through family, agroecological and peasant production, and guaranteeing their due safety.

Scientific Evidence

Discourses on the perception of health risk are interspersed with the experiences of oneself, family, and/or acquaintances with sickness and diseases that are the consequence of interactions between agrochemicals and the human body. Starting from this premise and leaving aside acute poisonings, *experts*[27] associate agrochemicals with cases of dermatitis, conjunctivitis, allergies, chronic headaches, diseases that affect the immune system, pregnancies without an embryo (the testes are an area where the toxicants are easily absorbed), various cancers, and depression.

The recognized multicausality of diseases can no longer obviate the presence of industrial and agricultural toxicants within our bodies and in the biosphere, leading researchers to coin new expressions such as "toxic bodies" or "environmentally obese" (Porta 2009; Porta nd). There is no doubt that what farmers pour into the field, doctors end up finding in the human body. Dr. Porta, in a study carried out in Almería in 2008, concludes that most of the agricultural products analyzed present contamination by pesticides, and as they are substances that act as endocrine disruptors, and are persistent and bioaccumulative, the legal limits established by the regulations do not guarantee the protection of public health (Porta et al., 2008).

Other studies on the effects of pesticides on health and the environment say that exposure to pesticides can lead to the role of active ingredients in different metabolic, developmental, reproductive, lung toxicity, neurotoxic or carcinogenic diseases (Calderón-Garcidueñas et al. 2018; Castillo-Castañeda et al. 2016; Suárez-Jacobo et al. 2017; Giulivo et al. 2016; Fénichel and Chevalier 2017; Loomis et al. 2015), or in neurodegenerative diseases, autism, asthma, metabolic syndrome, and fertility problems (Pelallo Martínez 2010; Quintanilla 2017; Xiao, Clark, and Park 2017). In the case of Mexico, one of the most recent studies on the risk of pesticides in vegetables is that of Pérez, Navarro, and Miranda (2013), which highlights the presence of unauthorized[28] or prohibited pesticides in certain crops, as well as the presence of pesticide residues in more than 50% of the evaluated samples of vegetables and fruits. In a study carried out in Veracruz, Mexico, 150 individuals were sampled to detect the levels of organochlorine residues in adipose tissue. All of them presented residue levels associated with the consumption of contaminated food.

The effects of pesticides not only endanger human health but also impact the environment,[29] as shown in studies such as those by González (2010) on environmental effects and ecological receptors in general. In any case, for a more exhaustive review of the current state of research on the effects on the environment and human health of pesticides in Mexico, one can consult the work of García Hernández et al. (2018). They highlight the effects of pesticides on agricultural workers (genetic alterations, decreased semen quality, altered hormonal profile, increased risk of anencephaly, etc.), as well as effects on the environment (DDT concentrations in hawksbill turtle eggs, etc.). The study concludes that there is sufficient evidence to determine that the use of pesticides, both historical and current, is associated with the deterioration of ecosystems and the health of Mexico's population.

Alternatives to the Industrial Agricultural Model

The challenges posed by the adoption of alternative agricultural techniques and strategies in the study area are being mainly led by *civil associations*: from the promotion of organic agriculture to the establishment of local commercial networks through productive empowerment and environmental awareness.[30] In any case, there is still a long way to go because the representativeness of these initiatives in the territory is still scarce. In Tututepec, ECOSTA[31] and the Local Board of Plant Health are the local entities that work to advance more sustainable agricultural models, such as developing and promoting the use of biological controllers to combat pests in the region. Thus, the main alternative to the industrial agricultural model is based on the promotion of organic (or natural) agriculture, as it represents the opposite side to industrial agriculture with respect to the use of synthetic agrochemicals, without excluding other sustainable agricultural models of the region, such as traditional small farmer agriculture.[32]

Saxton's ethnographic work (2015) shows the invisibility of risks associated with agrochemicals due to the marginalized social position of farmers. Based on theories of political ecology, they consider the organizational strength of social movements as the only viable option to lead to the creation of new alternatives for the agricultural model. However, these new alternatives should include a new human–nature relationship since environmental risks are only associated with the effect of productive performance. In order to perceive environmental risk in association with health risk, it would undoubtedly be necessary to perceive the link with the environment in a more comprehensive way. Understanding agriculture beyond the products that are grown would imply taking into account the ecosystem as a whole and our place within it.

One of the principal handicaps that conditions the Mexican agrifood model is the national market and its operation at the structural level. All agricultural production in Oaxaca, Chiapas, Tabasco, and Veracruz is centralized in Mexico City's *supply center* and from there returns to the different states. The central supply works as a monopsony, with very few buyers and their respective receivers, who set the price at which they will buy the product. For example, all the lemon and papaya produced in the study area are marketed in this way, without the possibility of a local and proximate alternative market that guarantees fairer prices. These macrostructural relationships that govern the operation of the national market determine the socioeconomic situation of the population in the study area.

At the state level, the work of RAPAM[33] is important. It strives to achieve changes in public policies in favor of agroecological pest control, for the protection of the rights to healthy food free of pesticides and Genetically Modified Organisms (GMOs), for food sovereignty, and for a pollutant-free environment (Bejarano et al. 2017). Another organization that is leading initiatives to build alternatives to the current agrifood model is CECCAM,[34] with its studies on GMOs, energy reforms, and the consequences of extractive projects on the livelihoods of the country's Indigenous communities.

DISCUSSION

In Tututepec, social representations in the agricultural field reinforce and justify the adoption of *risky* agricultural practices related to the intensive use of agrochemicals and the lack of individual protection. The *lazy* and *weak* categories stain the relationships between the different social agents, mainly between farmers themselves, and connect us with the construction of a masculine identity that faces danger based on a conception of subjective immunity (Douglas 1996). Although the increase in metabolic diseases in the study area is not directly linked to the high use and presence of agrochemicals, the increasing scientific evidence grants them a relevant role in diseases such as diabetes, obesity, and cancer (Rylander, Rignell-Hydbom and Hagmar 2005; Donato and Zani 2010; Uemura 2012; Ruzzin 2012). This fact could be due to a certain ignorance about occupational diseases on the part of institutions, and the *naturalization* of health problems derived from agricultural work by farmers (Menéndez 1981). In any case, it is clear that measures should be taken to eliminate the impacts of agrochemicals as a matter of public health,[35] be it through the development of organic pesticides, comprehensive integrated pest management, or the transformation of the current agrifood system.

With the exception of the organic farmers interviewed, who associate health risk with food quality and environmental contamination, the rest of the farmers do not conceive of agriculture without a high productive yield to cover the needs of the Mexican market, a fact that conditions the productive activity and ties it to the intensive use of agrochemicals. Change to the microclimate in the study area, becoming warmer in recent decades, coinciding with the high rate of deforestation in the region to favor the introduction of industrial agriculture, has not served as a hook to swell the list of environmental defenders. Neither does the fact that the land loses productivity due to the salinization process by the chemicals used during agricultural activity, or that it changes color, or even that the vultures disappear due to the impact on their calcium production in the formation of eggshells, caused by organophosphate products.

Agrochemicals represent a challenge facing the structures and logics that govern contemporary society and profit-oriented business operations (Saxton 2015). The increase in chronic diseases in today's society also challenges us to take radical measures in the field of environmental pollution, which overcomes a theory of the *maximum limits allowed* and the reductionism of the cost–benefit analysis, and places us in a scenario of the vindication of human rights.

CONCLUSIONS

The present work tries to make visible one of the many layers of environmental suffering that farmers endure, highlighting the social representations of risk around the use and presence of agrochemicals in the workplace and food. The concepts "lazy" and "weak" demonstrate how culture influences the representation of risks and, therefore, the adoption of certain practices and discourses. When agriculture is conceived from the cost–benefit analysis (industrial agriculture), the perception of risk becomes ambivalent, influenced by the lack of training and information related to agrochemicals. On the other hand, if we prioritize the right to quality food and the protection of environmental health, the perception of the risk of agrochemicals can lead to the construction of agroecological and sustainable alternatives, as demonstrated by the initiatives implemented by the civil associations of Tututepec. The contributions of the study demonstrate the need for a change in socio-environmental and agrifood policies, highlighting a public health problem related to agrochemicals and linked to the high incidence of metabolic syndrome in the region.

RECOMMENDATIONS

In the face of the ecological crisis that the planet is suffering, the criticism that has arisen from political ecology has highlighted the inefficiency of modern production systems, which generate high ecological (and health) costs, causing an avalanche of research and publications to emerge (Altieri 2014; Altieri and Toledo 2010; Giraldo and Rosset 2016; Patel 2009; Rosset 2003, 2016) who agree that the *knowledge, technologies, and productive strategies of the peasants or small-holder farmers are ecologically sufficient and that must be taken as a starting point in the construction of the agroecological alternatives* claimed by the social movements of global justice and entities such as La Via Campesina, ETC Group, Grain, and PAN.

Along these lines, targets 3, 4, and 5 of SDG 2 (end hunger, achieve food security, and improved nutrition and promote sustainable agriculture) urge governments to ensure the sustainability of food production systems and apply resilient agricultural practices, to double the agricultural productivity of small producers, and to maintain and use genetic resources and traditional knowledge in a fair and equitable way. These proposals fit in with the promotion of peasant agriculture, which is based on short, decentralized production and consumption circuits, and on a balance between food production, ecosystems, and local societies. Likewise, agroecological practices, which produce healthy food, care for the environment and preserve the heritage and cultural tradition of peoples are appropriate, as well as being a key element in the construction of food sovereignty and the process of repeasantization (Torres Martínez and Rosset 2016).

The FAO and PAHO (2017) consider peasant or family farming to be a key factor in achieving food and nutrition security, reducing poverty (as proposed in SDG 1) and achieving environmental sustainability (SDG 15.3); Rosset and Martínez Torres (2016) consider agroecology as one of the solutions to climate change (SDG 13.1), labeling biofuels, GMOs, carbon markets, and the REDD program as its "false solutions."

Producing healthy food from agroecological and diversified agriculture takes care of our health and guarantees a healthy lifestyle and promotes well-being (SDG 3.9). Agriculture without dangerous chemicals avoids contamination of water (SDG 6.3), air, and soil and reduces the diseases and deaths associated with it. Furthermore, it reduces the risk of exposure to chemical products of agricultural workers and its possible negative effects on health (SDG 8.8). But, as the study shows, there is a gap between the perception of the risk of agrochemicals on the environment and the risk on people's health, without yet understanding the close link between environmental and human health. Environmental awareness is needed to recover the health–environment link but also scientific information and studies on the risks associated with agrochemicals.

All the study informants agree that a change in the production model will only be possible if there are structural changes in the logic of the market that revalue and protect organic agriculture and local marketing circuits. In addition, industrial farmers in the study area find it necessary to have specific training in agroecology and, above all, in comprehensive pest management. A methodology widely used in the ECOSTA training workshops is the so-called Campesino-a-Campesino (CAC), which is based on horizontal communication and the sharing of knowledge between peers, and the use of the plots themselves as classrooms (Rosset and Martínez Torres 2016).

In conclusion, not only is training on the environmental effects of pesticides on the population in general necessary but also structural changes are required within the transaction system established by the different agents involved in the agrifood system, as well as promoting the presence of initiatives in favor of organic agriculture in the study area.

ACKNOWLEDGMENTS

Thank you to Pablo Sanchez from the Hunger Project for translating this chapter from Spanish to English. I thank all ECOSTA members and all project participants for their time, dedication, and patience. I thank Mabel Gracia for accompaniment during development of the project and especially the initial contacts and facilities to carry out my field work in Mexico. I am especially grateful to Jordi Brú for his unconditional support throughout the field work, and finally, I thank my parents for the trust placed in me.

NOTES

1. CIMMYT (https://www.cimmyt.org/) and the Rockefeller Foundation funded genetic research programs to produce high-yield varieties and modernize agriculture in nonindustrialized countries. The first results in Mexico were spectacular, but the increase in production was not enough to alleviate world hunger because it does not alter the scheme of concentration of economic power, access to land or purchasing power (Montagut and Vivas 2009).
2. A technological package includes the improved seeds and all the associated agrochemicals (herbicide, insecticide, fertilizer, etc.) that the farmer will need to produce with the "maximum yield," yield that in the long run becomes stagnated or even decreases production. To this, we must add the effect of pollution and degradation of the ecosystem.
3. Some authors believe that crop yields have been stagnant since the 1980s (GRAIN; Entrepueblos; Veterinarians Without Borders; Xarxa de consum solidari; Observatori del Deute en la Globalització 2009).
4. The FAO calculates that, on average, farmers in industrialized countries spend five times more commercial energy to produce a kilo of cereal than farmers in Africa, understanding commercial energy as the gas and fossil fuel required to produce fertilizers and agrochemicals, and that which is used by agricultural machinery (GRAIN et al, 2009: 10).

5. Acronyms: Food and Agriculture Organization (FAO), Pan American Health Organization (PAHO), World Health Organization (WHO), and International Assessment of Agricultural Knowledge, Science and Technology for Development (IAASTD).
6. In the case of Mexico, the value of the energy availability of food, which has remained stable in the last ten years, is among the highest in the world – 3,145 kcal per person per day – but the deficiencies in access give as a result, a heterogeneous scenario: on the one hand, the presence of chronic child malnutrition and, on the other hand, a high prevalence of overweight and obesity in the entire age range.
7. https://www.oecdregionalwellbeing.org/ME20.html [consulted on 05/20/2018].
8. This index is the weighted average of indicators of social needs: education, health, access to basic services and living spaces. The data are from 2010 and have been extracted from: http://www.microrregiones.gob.mx/catloc/Default.aspx?buscar=1&tipo=nombre&campo=mun&valor=tututepec&varent= [consulted on 05/20/2018].
9. https://www.elsiglodetorreon.com.mx/noticia/1562047.laguneros-afectados-por-uso-de-pesticidas.html [last accessed on 01/31/2020].
10. The WHO has estimated that between 2 and 5 million cases of pesticide poisoning occur per years, generating approximately 40,000 deaths, and despite the evidence of negative impacts on human health and the environment, the use of pesticides is increasing worldwide with a growth rate between 4 and 5.4% per year (IAASTD, 2009).
11. https://www.un.org/sustainabledevelopment/es/objetivos-de-desarrollo-sostenible/ [last accessed on 01/31/2020].
12. NOM-003-STPS-1999 establishes the safety and hygiene conditions to prevent the risks associated with agricultural workers in the storage, transfer, and management of plant protection products, pesticides, plant nutrients, and fertilizers. See: http://asinom.stps.gob.mx:8145/upload/noms/Nom-003.pdf [last accessed on 06/08/2020].
13. In Oaxaca, 80% of the territory is communal or *ejidal* property; that is, land ownership is largely social. The agrarian authority that manages the land is the Commissariat for Communal Goods or the *Ejidal* Commissariat, where appropriate.
14. Ecosta Yutu Cuii, SSS, founded in 2004, is an entity dedicated to environmental awareness and the promotion of local development projects, with special emphasis on promoting organic agriculture.
15. The municipal or communal property representatives are positions taken by political authorities.
16. http://www.fao.org/3/a0247s/a0247s05.htm#bm05.1 See too: http://www.fao.org/fao-who-codexalimentarius/sh-proxy/es/?lnk=1&url=https%253A%252F%252Fworkspace.fao.org%252Fsites%252Fcodex%252FStandards%252FCXG%2B92–2019%252FCXG_092e.pdf [last accessed on 06/04/2020].
17. The separation between nature and culture orders much of the Western worldview and has allowed for the separation, both academic and institutional, between the social and cultural dimension (field of study for anthropologists) and the natural dimension (field for biologists, ecologists, physicians, etc.).
18. Institutions, forms of knowledge, worldviews, rules, norms, technological knowledge, modes of communication and government, and forms of property constitute the intangible character of social metabolism that articulates the specific metabolic processes that refer to the flows of energy and matter (appropriation, transformation, circulation, consumption, excretion) of a particular society over time (Toledo 2013).
19. Slash-and-burn or swidden agriculture (*roza-tumba-quema* (RTQ)), is a shifting cultivation or rotational farming production system. It is based on clearing and burning areas for cultivation, followed by a generous fallow period. This provides a greater diversity of land use on the same farm.
20. A *milpa* or cropping field is a diversified production system mainly composed of corn, squash, beans, and chilis.

21. For more information, see: http://ceccam.org/node/2265; http://ceccam.org/node/403; http://ceccam.org/node/366 [last accessed on 05/18/2018].
22. NOM-003-STPS-1999 is the federal standard that establishes the safety and hygiene conditions to prevent the risks to which agricultural workers are exposed, and requires, among others, both employers and farmers, to use PPE. In practice, the fumigation pumps are in poor condition, leak liquid, and come into contact with the farmer's skin, which is rarely protected by suitable protective equipment.
23. During the interviews, the term *liquid* was used to refer to agrochemicals.
24. They would primarily be diseases related to metabolic syndrome (obesity, diabetes, hypertension) and cancer.
25. https://nyeleni.org/spip.php?article38 [last accessed on 06/19/2020].
26. https://infosen.senado.gob.mx/sgsp/gaceta/64/1/2018-10-25-1/assets/documentos/Inic_Sen.Jara_LGDAySA_251018.pdf [last accessed on 06/19/2020].
27. In this instance I am referring to interviewed medical authorities.
28. Of the 13 pesticides most used by informants, all are banned in other countries and classified by international organizations as highly dangerous, with the exception of tordon and esteron. Gramoxone (paraquat), the herbicide most widely used and perceived by informants as "not very risky," is prohibited in 38 countries and classified according to European regulations in category I-II: acute toxicity or mortality in case of inhalation (European Parliament and Council of the EU 2008).
29. https://www.lajornadamaya.mx/2018-06-26/En-Yucatan-se-regala-cancer--con-apoyos-estatales-de-agroquimicos; http://contrapoderweb.com/2018/02/19/cofirmado-los-peces-mueren-por-envenenamiento-y-no-por-la-temperatura-videos/?fbclid=IwAR0fSFMEZBIZEG2lJN5GtWpxL0qE-X7TYSRhWstMo8zFDDzGsyVum1QsIg0 [last accessed on 01/27/2020].
30. For example, ECOSTA offers families environmental and nutritional training, encourages the cultivation of vegetables for self-consumption, and promotes the care of forests as a resource reserve (water, medicinal plants, firewood, etc.), among many other activities.
31. The most cross-cutting activity of the association would be to advise and train in the field of organic agriculture, promoting marketing channels for chemical-free agricultural products and local producers, such as organic cotton and Creole corn projects.
32. The main characteristics of this type of agriculture are biological diversity, the use of natural resources in the area, polyculture, and the use of one's own, inherited, or exchanged seed.
33. Acronym: Pesticide Action Network and Alternatives in Mexico.
34. http://www.ceccam.org/ [consulted on 01/27/2020].
35. https://www.endocrine.org/search/#q=agrochemicals;https://academic.oup.com/edrv/issue/36/6; https://www.bioecoactual.com/2018/06/15/aumenta-numero-pesticidas-disruptores-endocrinos-alimentos/?fbclid=IwAR0rNIUQbxbNYW5aefxbZoRglDFDt4T9hnbMr2dInxoxhb-ydPYqlTnKmgc [consulted on 27/03/2019].

REFERENCES

Alfie Cohen, M. 2017. Riesgo ambiental: la aportación de Ulrich Beck. *Acta Sociológica*, 73: 171–194. https://doi.org/10.1016/J.ACSO.2017.08.006.

Altieri, M. A. 2014. Agroecología, pequeñas fincas y soberanía alimentaria. *Ecología Política*, 38: 25–35. https://doi.org/10.2307/20743515.

Altieri, M. A., and Toledo, V. 2010. La revolución agroecológica de América Latina: Rescatar la naturaleza, asegurar la soberanía alimentaria y empoderar al campesino. *El Otro Derecho*, 42: 163–202.

Arellano, E., Camarena, L., Glascoe, C. Von, and Daesslé, W. 2009. Percepción del riesgo en salud por exposición a mezclas de contaminantes. *Revista Facultad Nacional de Salud Pública, Universidad de Antioquia Colombia*, 27 (3): 291–301.

A/HRC/34/48. 2017. Informe de la Relatora especial sobre el derecho a la alimentación. Consejo de Derechos Humanos de las Naciones Unidas. Anual reporte de la Oficina del Alto Comisionado. https://documents-dds-ny.un.org/doc/UNDOC/GEN/G17/017/90/PDF/G1701790.pdf?OpenElement.

Bauman, Z. 2001. *La postmodernidad y sus descontentos*. Madrid: Akal.

Beck, U. 1998. *La Sociedad del Riesgo*. Hacia una nueva modernidad. Barcelona: Paidós.

Beck, U. 2002. *La sociedad del riesgo global*. Madrid: Siglo XXI de España Editores, SA.

Begueria, A. 2016. *Un equilibrio imperfecto. Alimentación ecológica, cuerpo y toxicidad*. Barcelona: UOC Editorial.

Bejarano, F., Colín, C., González, I. G., Eugenia, I., Rodríguez, M., Martínez, C., … Kubiak, W. 2017. *Los Plaguicidas Altamente Peligrosos en México*. México: RAPAM.

Busqueta, J., Etxezarreta, M., Iglesias, J., Navarro, F., Presas, O., Puig, A., and Teixidó, J. 2017. Apuntes sobre Marx y Naturaleza. Numero 12. Barcelona: Taifa, Informes de Economía Crítica,

Calderón-Garcidueñas, A. L., Waliszewski, S. M., Ruiz-Ramos, R., and del Carmen Martinez-Valenzuela, M. 2018. Time trend tendency (1988–2014 years) of organochlorine pesticide levels in the adipose tissue of Veracruz inhabitants. *Environmental Monitoring and Assessment*, 190: 206. https://doi.org/10.1007/s10661-018-6581-y.

Calvario Parra, J. E. 2007. Masculinidad, riesgos y padecimientos laborales. Jornaleros agrícolas del poblado Miguel Alemán, Sonora. *Región y sociedad*, 19 (40): 39–72. http://www.scielo.org.mx/scielo.php?script=sci_arttext&pid=S1870-39252007000300002.

Castillo-Castañeda, P. C., Gaxiola-Robles, R., Méndez-Rodríguez, L. C., Labrada-Martagón, V., and Zenteno-Savín, T. 2016. Antioxidantes, especies reactivas de oxígeno y daño oxidativo asociado a la presencia de plaguicidas organoclorados en la leche materna. *Nutrición hospitalaria*, 33 (2): 199–511. https://doi.org/10.20960/nh.127.

CECIPROC and ECOSTA. 2018. Propuesta de política pública en relación con la agenda 2030 de desarrollo sostenible (borrador). Villa de Tututepec de Melchor Ocampo. Proposal submitted to the municipal authorities.

CONEVAL. 2015. Medición de la pobreza a escala municipal 2010-2015. Ciudad de México. https://www.coneval.org.mx/Medicion/Paginas/consulta_pobreza_municipal.aspx.

Díaz-Barriga, F. 1996. Los residuos peligrosos en México. *Salud Pública Mex*, 38: 280–291.

Donato, F. and Zani, C. 2010. Chronic exposure to organochlorine compounds and health effects in adults: diabetes and thyroid diseases. *Annali di igiene: medicina preventiva e di comunita*, 22: 185–198.

Douglas, M. 1996. *La aceptabilidad del riesgo según las ciencias sociales*. Barcelona: Paidós.

Douglas, M., and Wildavsky, A. 1983. *Risk and culture. An essay on the Selection of Technological and Environmental Dangers*. Berkeley and Los Angeles: University of California Press.

European Parliament and Council of the EU. 2008. Reglamento (CE) n 1272/2008 de 16 de diciembre de 2008 sobre clasificación, etiquetado y envasado de sustancias y mezclas, y por el que se modifican y derogan las Directivas 67/548/CEE y 1999/45/CE y se modifica el Reglamento (CE) n 1907/2006. https://eur-lex.europa.eu/LexUriServ/LexUriServ.do?uri=OJ:L:2008:353:0001:1355:es:PDF.

FAO; FIDA; UNICEF; PMA y OMS. 2018. El estado de la seguridad alimentaria y la nutrición en el mundo. Fomentando la resiliencia climática en aras de la seguridad alimentaria y la nutrición. Rome: Food and Agriculture Organization. http://www.fao.org/3/I9553ES/I9553ES.pdf.

FAO and PAHO. 2017. Panorama de la seguridad alimentaria y nutricional en América Latina y el Caribe. Santiago, Chile: Food and Agricultre Organization. http://www.fao.org/3/a-i7914s.pdf.

Fénichel, P., and Chevalier, N. 2017. Environmental endocrine disruptors: new diabetogens? *Comptes Rendus Biologies*, 340: 446–452. https://www.sciencedirect.com/science/article/pii/S1631069117301245?via%3Dihub.

García Hernández, J., Leyva Morales, J. B., Martínez Rodríguez, I. E., Hernández Ochoa, M. I., Aldana Madrid, M. L., Rojas García, A. E., and Perera Rios, J. H. 2018. Estado actual de la investigación sobre plaguicidas en México. *Revista Internacional de Contaminación Ambiental*, 34: 29–60. https://www.revistascca.unam.mx/rica/index.php/rica/article/view/RICA.2018.34.esp01.03/46727.

General Directorate of Epidemiology. 2013. Panorama histórico de morbilidad y mortalidad por intoxicación por plaguicidas en México 1995-2012. *Boletín Epidemiológico*, 34 (3): Semana 34. https://www.gob.mx/cms/uploads/attachment/file/12839/sem34.pdf.

Giddens, A. 1994. *Les conséquences de la modernité*. París: L'Harmattan.

Giraldo, O. F., and Rosset, P. 2016. La agroecología en una encrucijada: entre la institucionalidad y los movimientos sociales. *Guaju*, 2 (1), 14. https://doi.org/10.5380/guaju.v2i1.48521.

Giulivo, M., Lopez de Alda, M., Capri, E., and Barceló, D. 2016. Human exposure to endocrine disrupting compounds: their role in reproductive systems, metabolic syndrome and breast cancer. A review. *Environmental Research*, 151: 251–264.

González Mille, D. J. 2010. Aplicación de una metodología de evaluación de riesgo ecológico en fauna acuática de Coatzacoalcos, Veracruz. Doctoral thesis. Universidad Autónoma de San Luis Potosí. http://ninive.uaslp.mx/jspui/bitstream/i/3584/1/DJGM-Tesis Doctorado.pdf.

Gracia Arnaiz, M. 2002. Somos lo que comemos. Estudios de alimentación y cultura en España. Barcelona: Editorial Ariel, SA.

Gracia Arnaiz, M. 2004. Pensando sobre el riesgo alimentario y su aceptabilidad: el caso de los alimentos transgénicos. *Revista de Nutrição*, 17: 125–149.

GRAIN; Entrepueblos; Veterinarios sin fronteras; Xarxa de consum solidari; Observatori del Deute en la Globalització. 2009. *Cocinando el planeta. Hechos, cifras y propuestas sobre cambio climático y sistema alimentario global*. Barcelona: Agència Catalana de Cooperació al Desenvolupament.

GRAIN. 2011. Alimentos y cambio climático: el eslabón olvidado. https://www.grain.org/es/article/entries/4364-alimentos-y-cambio-climatico-el-eslabon-olvidado.

IAASTD. 2009. Global Report. Agriculture at a Crossroads. https://www.globalagriculture.org/fileadmin/files/weltagrarbericht/IAASTDBerichte/GlobalReport.pdf.

INEGI. 2015. México en cifras. http://www.beta.inegi.org.mx/app/areasgeograficas/?ag=20#.

Karam, M. Á., Ramírez, G., Montes, L. P. B., Galván, J. M., Karam, M. Á., Ramírez, G., … Manuel, J. (2004). Plaguicidas y salud de la población. *Red de revistas Científicas de América latina, el Caribe, España y Portugal*, 11: 246–254. http://cienciaergosum.uaemex.mx/index.php/ergosum/article/view/3748/2800.

Küster, Á. S. 2016. Volver a la tierra. Transiciones agroecológicas de los sistemas agroalimentarios hacia la soberanía alimentaria. Doctoral thesis. Universidad de Valencia. https://dialnet.unirioja.es/servlet/tesis?codigo=79238.

Lara Millán, G., and Reyes Cruz, H. 2010. Maíces criollos de Tututepec: cultura, genes y políticas públicas. México: Ecosta Yutu Cuii.

Larrea Killinger, C., and Martínez Mauri, M. 2012. *Contribuciones antropológicas al estudio del desarrollo*. Barcelona: Editorial UOC.

Loomis, D., Guyton, K., Grosse, Y., El Ghissasi, F., Bouvard, V., Benbrahim-Tallaa, L., … Straif, K. 2015. Carcinogenicity of lindane, DDT, and 2,4-dichlorophenoxyacetic acid. *The Lancet. Oncology*, 16: 891–892. https://doi.org/10.1016/S1470-2045(15)00081-9.

Lupton, D. (ed). 1999. *Risk and sociocultural theory: new directions and perspectives*. Cambridge: Cambridge University Press.

Martínez-Hernáez, Á. 2011. *Antropología Médica: Teorías sobre la cultura, el poder y la enfermedad.* Barcelona: Anthropos Editorial.

Menéndez, E. 1981. *Poder, estratificación y salud: Análisis de las condiciones sociales y económicas de la enfermedad en Yucatán.* México: Ediciones de la Casa Chata.

Menéndez, E. 2009. *De sujetos, saberes y estructuras: introducción al enfoque relacional en el estudio de la salud colectiva.* Buenos Aires: Lugar Editorial.

Montagut, X., and Vivas, E. 2009. *Del campo al plato.* Barcelona: Icaria Editorial.

ODELA. 2018. *Polisemias de la alimentación. Salud, desperdicio, hambre y patrimonio.* Barcelona: Edicions de la Universitat de Barcelona.

Ortega-Ceseña, J., Espinosa-Torres, F., and López-Carrillo, L. 1994. El control de los riesgos para la salud generados por los plaguicidas organofosforados en México: retos ante el Tratado de Libre Comercio. *Salud Pública de México*, 26: 624–632.

Patel, R. 2009. Food sovereignty. *Journal of Peasant Studies*, 36: 663–706 https://doi.org/10.1080/03066150903143079.

Pelallo Martínez, N. A. 2010. Evaluación de riesgo en salud en población infantil expuesta a una mezcla de contaminantes en Coatzacoalcos, Veracruz. Doctoral thesis. Universidad Autónoma San Luis de Potosí. http://ninive.uaslp.mx/jspui/bitstream/i/3738/1/DCA1COA01001.pdf.

Pérez, M. A., Navarro, H., and Miranda, E. 2013. Residuos de plaguicidas en hortalizas: Problemática y riesgo en México. *Revista Internacional de Contaminación Ambiental*, 29: 45–64. https://www.revistascca.unam.mx/rica/index.php/rica/article/viewFile/41423/39321.

Porta, M. 2009. Cuerpos tóxicos. *Culturas La Vanguardia*, 388: 2–5. https://forumdedebats.vicentitats.cat/wp-content/uploads/sites/16/2017/12/2009-11-25-Culturas-388-La-Vanguardia-5p.pdf.

Porta, M. 2017. Contaminants en el cos humà. Els tòxics industrials i agrícoles al nostre cos per terra, mar i aire. Conference. http://forumdedebats.vicentitats.cat/diba_projecte/miquel-porta-contaminants-en-el-cos-huma-els-toxics-industrials-i-agricoles-al-nostre-cos-per-terra-mar-i-aire/.

Porta, M. Gasull, M., Puigdomènech, E., Bosch de Basea, M. 2008. *La influencia de la dieta en las concentraciones corporales de Compuestos Orgánicos Persistentes.* Barcelona: IMIM-Hospital del Mar i UAB.

Porta, M., Kogevinas, M., Zumeta, E., Sunyer, J., and Ribas-Fitó, N.; Grupo de Trabajo sobre Compuestos Tóxicos Persistentes y Salud del IMIM. 2002. Concentraciones de compuestos tóxicos persistentes en la población española: el rompecabezas sin piezas y la protección de la salud pública. *Gaceta Sanitaria*, 16: 257–266. https://doi.org/10.1016/S0213-9111(02)71671-3.

Quintanilla, B. 2017. Exposición a plaguicidas y salud humana. Powerpoint presentation. Simposio Nacional de Plaguicidas desde una Perspectiva Bioética. Querétaro (México).

R-PLAFEST. 2014. Reglamento en Materia de Registros, Autorizaciones de Importación y Exportación y Certificados de Exportación de Plaguicidas, Nutrientes Vegetales y Sustancias y Materiales Tóxicos o Peligrosos. México: Diario Oficial de la Federación. http://www.diputados.gob.mx/LeyesBiblio/regla/n109.pdf.

Rodríguez Gómez, G. 2007. Imaginar la soberanía alimentaria y las oportunidades para las agriculturas del México globalizado. *Desacatos*, 25: 101–114.

Rosset, P. 2003. Soberanía Alimentaria: Reclamo Mundial del Movimiento Campesino. *Food Sovereignty: Global Rallying Cry of Farmer Movements*, 9: 1–5.

Rosset, P. 2016. La agroecología como resistencia y Transformación. Boletín Nyeleni, 28: 1–6.

Rosset, P., and Martínez-Torres, M. E. 2016. Agroecología, territorio, recampesinización y movimientos sociales. *Estudios Sociales*, 25: 275–299.

Ruzzin, J. 2012. Public health concern behind the exposure to persistent organic pollutants and the risk of metabolic diseases. *BMC Public Health*, 12: 298. https://doi.org/10.1186/1471-2458-12-298.

Rylander, L., Rignell-Hydbom, A., and Hagmar, L. (2005). A cross-sectional study of the association between persistent organochlorine pollutants and diabetes. *Environmental Health*, 4 (1): 28. https://doi.org/10.1186/1476-069X-4-28.

Saxton, D. I. (2015). Ethnographic movement methods : anthropology takes on the pesticide industry. *Journal of Political Ecology*, 22: 368–387.

Schutter, O. De. 2010. Report submitted by the Special Rapporteur on the right to food. https://undocs.org/es/A/HRC/16/49.

Suárez-Jacobo, A., Alcantar-Rosales, V. M., Alonso-Segura, D., Heras-Ramírez, M., Elizarragaz-De La Rosa, D., Lugo-Melchor, O., and Gaspar-Ramirez, O. 2017. Pesticide residues in orange fruit from citrus orchards in Nuevo Leon State, Mexico. *Food Additives & Contaminants: Part B*, 10 (3): 192–199. https://doi.org/10.1080/19393210.2017.1315743.

Toledo, V. M. 2013. El metabolismo social: una nueva teoría socioecológica. *Relaciones. Estudios de historia y sociedad*, 34 (136): 41–71. http://www.scielo.org.mx/scielo.php?script=sci_arttext&pid=S0185-39292013000400004&lng=es&nrm=iso.

Toledo, V. M., Ortiz-Espejel, B. F., Cortés, L., Moguel, P., and Ordoñez, M. de J. 2003. The multiple use of tropical forests by indigenous peoples in Mexico: a case of adaptive management. *Conservation Ecology*, 7 (3): 9. https://doi.org/10.5751/ES-00524-070309.

Torres Martínez, M. E., and Rosset, P. M. 2016. Diálogo De Saberes En La Vía Campesina: Soberanía Alimentaria y Agroecología. *Revista Espacio regional*, 1 (13): 23–36. http://ceccam.org/sites/default/files/Dialogo%20de%20saberes%20en%20la%20via%20campesina-%20soberania%20alimentaria%20y%20agroecologia.pdf.

Uemura, H. 2012. Associations of exposure to dioxins and polychlorinated biphenyls with diabetes: based on epidemiological findings. *Nihon Eiseigaku Zasshi. Japanese Journal of Hygiene*, 67 (3): 363–374. http://www.ncbi.nlm.nih.gov/pubmed/22781010.

Urquía-Fernández, N. 2014. La seguridad alimentaria en México. *Salud Pública de México*, 56: 92–98. http://sitios.dif.gob.mx/cenddif/wp-content/uploads/2017/12/La-seguridad-alimentaria-en-México.pdf.

Vivas, E. 2014. *El negocio de la comida*. Barcelona: Icaria Editorial.

Widger, T. 2014. Pesticides and global health: 'ambivalent objects' in anthropological perspective. Somatosphere. http://somatosphere.net/2014/08/pesticides-and-global-health-ambivalent-objects-in-anthropological-perspective.html.

Xiao, X., Clark, J. M., and Park, Y. 2017. Potential contribution of insecticide exposure and development of obesity and type 2 diabetes. *Food and Chemical Toxicology*, 105: 456–474. https://doi.org/10.1016/j.fct.2017.05.003.

11 Decolonizing Puerto Rico's Foodscape

Adriana Garriga-Lopez and Shir Lerman Ginzburg

CONTENTS

INTRODUCTION

Is it possible to enact food sovereignty within a colony? In what follows, we critically inspect the relationship between food sovereignty and colonialism in the Puerto Rican archipelago. We describe the context in which efforts to build food sovereignty are happening in the so-called Free Associated State of Puerto Rico, which has been a "possession," overseas territory, or plainly a colony of the United States of America since 1898 and before that was a colony of Spain. We consider the connections between food sovereignty and decolonization, and the limitations to food sovereignty and food justice within this context. Finally, we make note of some of the effects of the global pandemic of COVID-19 on the local Puerto Rican foodscape.

Because of its political subjugation to the United States, Puerto Rico is not a sovereign state and has limited decision-making power in its own socio-political processes. However, Puerto Rico was removed from the list of non-self-governing territories in need of decolonization in 1953 at the behest of the United States. As a result, Puerto Rico is not eligible to be an independent member of the United Nations, since it is considered a territory of the United States. Thus, although Puerto Rican representatives were present by special invitation at the World Summit on Sustainable Development in South Africa in 2002 (Soto-Lacourt 2002) and despite the promise of a web portal, to our knowledge, there is no formal process for implementing the United Nations' Sustainable Development Goals in Puerto Rico as of this writing, except as part of the United States. While the United States has not reported federal SDG data, cities, states, universities, NGOs, and businesses have implemented

DOI: 10.1201/9781003014942-11

measures to advance progress made toward achieving SDGs (Pipa and Brown 2019). The Puerto Rican government partnered with several U.S. organizations, including the United States Forest Service and the Environmental Protection Agency, to collect data on the best ways to implement the SDGs in Puerto Rico (Garofalo 2020).

In the context of this book, we wish to highlight how the UN Sustainability Goals articulate or not with the movements for food sovereignty and decolonization that exists in contemporary Puerto Rico, or the group of islands also known by the Indigenous name of *Borikén*. Control over land, water, and other resources needed to secure food production and subsistence farming on the islands is a hotly contested and troublesome issue given widespread corporate capture of natural resources and public utilities under increasing pressure from settler colonial land grabs, disaster capitalist ventures, debt profiteers, and visitor economy-centric government policies. But there is also plenty of support for local farmers, as well as resistance against imperial policies and agro-tech giants like Monsanto and Bayer.

The small farming and agroecology movements have been particularly salient in recent years, as food sovereignty and food justice have increasingly become part of Puerto Rico's struggle for justice and self-determination against an oppressively undemocratic and increasingly dangerous backdrop shaped by compounding disasters, government corruption, and climate disruption. The ability to decide which foodstuffs are in the markets, how much they cost, how they are produced, and the very cuisine that people relate to or identify with are at the core of food sovereignty in Puerto Rico. As the movements for food justice in Puerto Rico show, redefining sovereignty and decolonization in the twenty-first century is impossible without considering the materiality of self-reproduction through farming, food production, ecological repair, and sustainable market economies.

Food is a thoroughly political element of Puerto Rican social life. And since Puerto Rico is politically subjugated to a great degree, it follows that decolonization is necessary in order to create conditions for food justice at the local level and the movement for food sovereignty builds on a long history of anti-colonial resistance and organizing for national sovereignty. In many ways, this framework may not be compatible with the model of development promoted by the United Nations. In what follows, we organize our commentary around particular Sustainable Development Goals (SDGs) and their relevance to the Puerto Rican context.

SDG 2 (End Hunger)

- Ensure that Puerto Rico receives the same federal assistance for food (either direct foodstuffs or economic assistance to stimulate self-sustaining agriculture).
- Eradicate the Cabotage Laws.

POLITICAL ROOTS OF HUNGER AND FOOD INSECURITY

Puerto Rico is a prime example of how food insecurity intersects with economics and politics to aggravate hunger (Pérez, Sánchez, and Ortiz 2013; Soltero and Palacios 2011). In 1917, the United States passed the Jones Merchant Marine Act (colloquially and henceforth, "Cabotage Laws"), which mandates that only ships flying the U.S. flag may dock in Puerto Rico and that all foreign ships must first dock at mainland U.S. ports, even if they are carrying goods intended for Puerto Rico (Lerman 2017; Rodriguez-Soto 2013). Mainland-based fast food restaurants established a permanent foothold on the island in the late 1950s, influencing the types of foods that are economically and geographically available to Puerto Ricans (Ortíz Cuadra 2013; Rodriguez-Soto 2013). As part of the circulatory migration pattern between the U.S. and Puerto Rico, Puerto Ricans also brought highly processed snack foods back to the island, contributing at least in part to changing dietary patterns and food insecurity on the island (Duany 2002; McGreevey 2018). With the federal government heavily subsidizing corn and soy products and the retail prices of fruits and vegetables increasing, processed foods are economically and energetically cheaper than homegrown and home-cooked foods (Ortíz Cuadra 2013) and Puerto Ricans are rapidly transitioning into a population that consumes more and more processed foods (Colón-Ramos 2017, 2013; Colón-López 2013). Puerto Ricans are required to pay additional taxes to compensate for the transportation of those goods, which account for at least 85% of all of consumer goods (including imported foodstuffs) and which contribute to supermarket food prices being 21% higher than on the U.S. mainland (Beyer 2015; Lerman 2019).

Despite high food prices and Puerto Rico's history as a sugar-producing hub, Puerto Ricans were not eligible for food stamps until 1974, when Section 19 of the Food Stamps Act was expanded to include U.S. colonies (Keith-Jennings and Wolkomir 2020). By 1977, food stamps were heavily utilized on the island: 56% of Puerto Ricans participated, accounting for 8% of total national beneficiaries (Ibid). Due to the expense, Puerto Rico was eliminated from the Food Stamp Act in 1981, and in 1982, the U.S. Department of Agriculture introduced PAN (Programa de Asistencia Nutricional; NAP in English) to provide nutritional assistance to low-income Puerto Rican families via an annual capped block grant of $825 million for the Puerto Rican government to distribute to eligible individuals. Eligibility is determined by the household income level (a family of three can make up to $7,188/month), and participants can have up to $2,000 in the bank, although the maximum monthly benefit through PAN is $200 less than SNAP benefits for a family of three in the United States (Bread For The World 2019; Méndez-Méndez and Fernández 2015).

PAN can only be used for unprocessed foods at supermarkets and grocery stores (Méndez-Méndez and Fernández 2015). Due to the agricultural and economic devastation that Hurricane María left behind, Puerto Ricans were seven times more likely than U.S. residents to be food insecure, and the additional applications for PAN funding strained the overburdened program (Bread For The World 2019). In December 2018, the PROMESA Oversight Board wrote to the Puerto Rico Family Department Secretary, Glorimar Andújar Matos, to recommend that a work requirement of 80 hours/month be attached to PAN in order to stimulate the Puerto Rican economy and labor market and to decrease the reliance on long-term financial aid that the government could not sustain (Carrión and Biggs 2018). This request was not approved due to severely limited job opportunities and to an already-migrating workforce cohort, resulting in an aging, retired population that relies on PAN for assistance.

Although 1.4 million Puerto Ricans receive PAN benefits, the bill for an additional $600 million stalled in Congress in March 2019, leaving PAN participants scrambling for financial assistance. While Congress ultimately approved funding for PAN in June 2019 (González-Colón 2019), the bill's delay in Congress and the subsequent lag before funding was dispersed, caused considerable anxiety among low-income Puerto Ricans and highlighted the hotly-debated role of Puerto Rico's relationship with the United States, both in Puerto Rico and in the United States. The delay in providing food stamps for Puerto Rico until 1974 also underlines a concern that many Puerto Ricans have over the relationship with the United States, that since the United States assumed complete power over Puerto Rico, it should have also accepted responsibility for the island's economic situation, including providing financial assistance for low-income Puerto Ricans to purchase food (Méndez-Méndez and Fernández 2015). Given the high price of food in Puerto Rico, PAN essentially provides its participants with access to the cheapest (and sometimes less nutritious) items to create basic meals, further emphasizing the inequalities in access to food resources in Puerto Rico (Ortíz Cuadra 2013). In 2017, for example, the maximum monthly PAN benefit for a family of five was $499, compared to $771 for a family of five using SNAP, despite grocery prices in San Juan being comparable (or higher) to those in most major mainland cities (Wolkomir 2017).

Puerto Rico's ongoing struggles with bankruptcy and unemployment do not create conditions that favor the creation of new jobs, which would leave un- or underemployed PAN participants even more food insecure. Alejandro García Padilla (the Puerto Rican governor until 2017) declined to follow this recommendation, citing PAN as a social safety net for a food-insecure community, as well as the concern that cutting funding for food would encourage more Puerto Ricans to move to the United States (González-Colón 2019).

Hunger among a great many of the island's population, especially children, is the cost of inaction and governmental neglect in Puerto Rico. The pandemic of COVID-19 exacerbated an already dire situation.

SDG 3 (Ensure Healthy Lives ...)

- Extend Obamacare provisions to Puerto Rico and the other U.S. territories.
- Put more money into health insurance plans so that
  - Doctors will remain on the island.
  - People will get the health services they need.
- Improve hospitals?

Mark Nichter (2008) observed that foods and diets are culturally imbued with meaning, particularly with regard to illness causation. In Puerto Rico, illness causation is politically charged, particularly as it relates to food and the influence of colonialism on local diets.

High poverty rates, a poor economy, and a long-term politically unstable environment contribute to high rates of food insecurity and overall negative health outcomes (Laborde and Sáez-Santiago 2013; Lerman 2017; Mattei et al. 2018; Pérez et al. 2013). High rates of poverty and the cheapness of processed unhealthy foods combine and contribute to an inability to maintain a healthy diet, which in turn are connected to increased risk of food insecurity, which is prevalent in Puerto Rico, affecting 85% of the population (Morales 2019). While this is also true for mainland Americans living in poverty (Duany 2017; McGreevey 2018), it's particularly visceral for Puerto Ricans who need to buy produce instead of growing it as they have in the near past, particularly as Puerto Rico began as an agricultural economy with many people growing their own food in lieu of going out to unaffordable restaurants (Laborde and Sáez-Santiago 2013; Morales 2019). Unhealthy food and life conditions and an increased reliance on cars have created an environment in which Puerto Ricans on the island now live surrounded by poor air quality, little opportunities for physical activity, and little time to spend on their health as many are working several jobs to pay the bills (Acosta-Pérez et al. 2012; Dhokarh et al. 2018).

In Puerto Rico, the plethora of fast food options, the stark dearth of healthy and accessible food options, and the lack of Puerto Ricans' access to their own economic decision-making with regard to food prices and agricultural outputs has led to illness causation and decreased overall health outcomes. For example, Shir Lerman (2019) and Glorisa Canino et al. (2019) independently found that the exorbitant prices of produce and fresh meat, combined with high rates of poverty and unemployment and lack of hope for economic improvement, were associated with elevated levels of diabetes (15.4%), major depression (9.7%), and generalized anxiety (5.2%), all three of which are levels higher than in the general U.S. population.

Furthermore, the tenuous congressional support for PAN also highlights the highly political nature of food insecurity in Puerto Rico, due to the island's reliance on the United States for economic and nutritional support. After Hurricane María, supermarkets were shuttered, farmland, food, and water became polluted, and the food relief boxes that Puerto Ricans received were stuffed with candy, chips, sweetened fruit cups, and canned veggies that exceeded USDA-recommended sodium levels (Herzog 2018; Watson 2018). María also shuttered hospitals and pharmacies and contaminated existing stores of food and water, leading to multiple and deteriorating health problems, such as almost nonexistent access to essential medications and aggravated suicide ideation from stress and lack of resources (Lerman 2019; Michaud and Kates 2017; Rodríguez-Díaz 2018). The spoiled produce and the negligence of the USDA reinforce stark malnutrition in Puerto Rico.

In particular, the ongoing COVID-19 pandemic has deleteriously impacted food insecurity in Puerto Rico. Hurricane María and the January 2020 earthquakes had already worsened an already-fragile food network in Puerto Rico, making people skip meals or eat smaller portions to make food last longer, and even before the pandemic, a 2015 study found that 22% of adults skipped meals because they couldn't afford food (Piser 2020). Once the pandemic hit, food insecurity worsened dramatically. In a 2020 survey of 1,400 households conducted by Dr. Uriyoán Colón-Ramos, 62% of Puerto Ricans stated that they had used a nutrition assistance program in June 2020 alone, an increase of 18% from before the pandemic, while 40% of respondents reported experiencing food insecurity, an increase of 38% pre-pandemic. Coupled with a steep 46% poverty rate and an 8.4% unemployment rate as a result of the pandemic, the reliance on PAN increased from 1.3 million people in February 2020 to more than 1.5 million people in August 2020 and added extra benefits to PAN through July 2020 to match SNAP benefits in the United States (Keith-Jennings 2020). However, when the extra benefits ran out, the average household's benefits dropped sharply from $323 per month in July 2020 to $188 per month in October 2020, highlighting the horrifying lack of resources available to Puerto Ricans for food access (Ibid). Puerto Rico was also left out of the Pandemic-Electronic Benefits Transfer (EBT) Bill, which was introduced in March 2020 and transferred funds for school meals onto debit cards for families: since the funds were tied to SNAP eligibility and Puerto Rico is ineligible for the SNAP program, Puerto Ricans were excluded from necessary financial assistance (Coto 2020; Piser 2020). While Puerto Ricans will benefit from the 2020–2021 bill, the funds were not approved for dispersal until January 14, 2021, ten months after the start of the pandemic; no funds were provided for the summer of 2020, although the funding included the summer of 2021 (Urban Institute 2021). Furthermore, with schools shuttering in March 2020, the vast majority of school cafeterias were closed well into the summer, leaving thousands of children unable to access at least free one meal a day (Coto 2020; Piser 2020).

SDG 8 (Promote Sustained, Inclusive, and Sustainable Economic Growth)

- Improve infrastructure beyond Viejo San Juan?
- Stimulate job development.

Currently, Puerto Rico's economy is heavily invested in the tourism industry, with the tourism-dominated neighborhoods of Viejo San Juan, Condado, (some areas of) Santurce, and Isla Verde (all in San Juan) more economically and infrastructurally well-maintained than the rest of the city or some other parts of Puerto Rico. For example, buses in San Juan run on an irregular schedule and are frequently on strike due to austerity policies that cut funding to public transportation. There is no regular bus system that connects San Juan to the rest of Puerto Rico and the ferry system that connects Vieques and Culebra municipalities to the main island is notoriously unreliable and insufficient.

In general, Puerto Rico is heavily car-dependent except in the tourist-heavy neighborhoods, which are better maintained to encourage tourist foot traffic. When President Barack Obama visited Puerto Rico in June 2011, he stayed for merely five hours, giving a speech at Luis Muñoz Marín International Airport and visiting La Fortaleza, the official San Juan residence of the Governor of Puerto Rico (McGreevey 2018; Morales 2019). Obama's visit was seen by many as merely a ploy for his 2012 reelection campaign, particularly as the only parts of the city that were improved, were those along his route from the airport to La Fortaleza (Klein 2018). Improving the infrastructure throughout Puerto Rico could create more jobs, encourage tourism and facilitate commutes outside of the San Juan metropolitan area, all of which would stimulate the economy. At the same time, tourism has also proven to be destructive to Puerto Rico's natural resources as the tourist demand for coastal resorts, luxury urban development, and tours through Puerto Rico's fragile rainforests and reefs grows despite objections from Puerto Ricans (Hernández-Delgado et al. 2012; Méndez-Lázaro et al. 2014). This highly destructive and extractive form of tourism has been particularly dangerous during the COVID-19 pandemic, when many U.S. tourists patently ignored the curfew and disregarded mask mandates (Acevedo 2021). Additionally, local or internal tourism by island residents and forms of eco-tourism are important markets for small businesses and these are often tied to farming. Local coffee plantations, for example, are a popular destination.

Overall, stimulating Puerto Rico's local economy in ways that support local farmers and business owners will make it easier for Puerto Ricans to consistently afford food and maintain independent decision-making over their own harvests and cuisine. The difficulties of consistent healthy food access, ready availability of unhealthy but heavily advertised food options, and diminishing patterns of exercise, are evident throughout Puerto Rico due to underlying economic, political, and structural barriers. For example, blackberries, which aren't considered native to Puerto Rico, were often prohibitively expensive, at $7.67 for a 6-ounce box ($3.99 at Stop & Shop in the northeastern United States) (Figure 11.1).

As earlier discussed, soaring food prices bear a direct relationship to federal laws regulating shipping to and from Puerto Rico. Removing these imperialist laws would be one way to reduce food costs in Puerto Rico, but it would not necessarily by itself create the conditions for food justice, nor would it create conditions of sustainability for the local food economy and agricultural production. For that to happen, much more is needed.

Food sovereignty can be part of economic growth and stabilization, but it requires an emphasis on local production and consumption of locally grown and processed foods. This kind of emphasis on local food sources is connected to the agroecology movement in Puerto Rico, which itself is part of a broader social movement toward autonomy and self-sustainability that can be thought of as part of the process of decolonization. The tensions that exist between economic development as part of colonial governance and economic activity that is part of locally sustainable and ecologically conscious growth are representative of a global confrontation between our collective survival and a capitalist world order that has literally set the globe on fire.

SDG 13 (End Climate Change)

- End or amend industrial food systems

Puerto Rico is in the midst of the privatization of the Puerto Rico Electric Power Authority (PREPA), a process that is set to capture its substantial energy market in service of U.S. fossil fuel companies. This represents a facet of austerity-driven colonial extraction in Puerto Rico that cuts across the landscapes and societies of both humans and non-human beings in the archipelago. It also constitutes an enormous and missed opportunity to enact the transformation of the Puerto Rican energy grid into a sustainable and ecologically responsible one (De Onís, 2021). Instead of pivoting off the crisis wrought by Hurricane María to lead an energy transition that is necessary to sustain life on Earth, the United States has seen in Puerto Rico's territorial status another opportunity to glut the coffers of a prolific succession of continental-based energy companies with no previous ties to Puerto Rico, nor knowledge of its energy system, and no demonstrated capacity to repair it, much less transform it into an eco-friendly or green infrastructure. While the United States withdrew from the

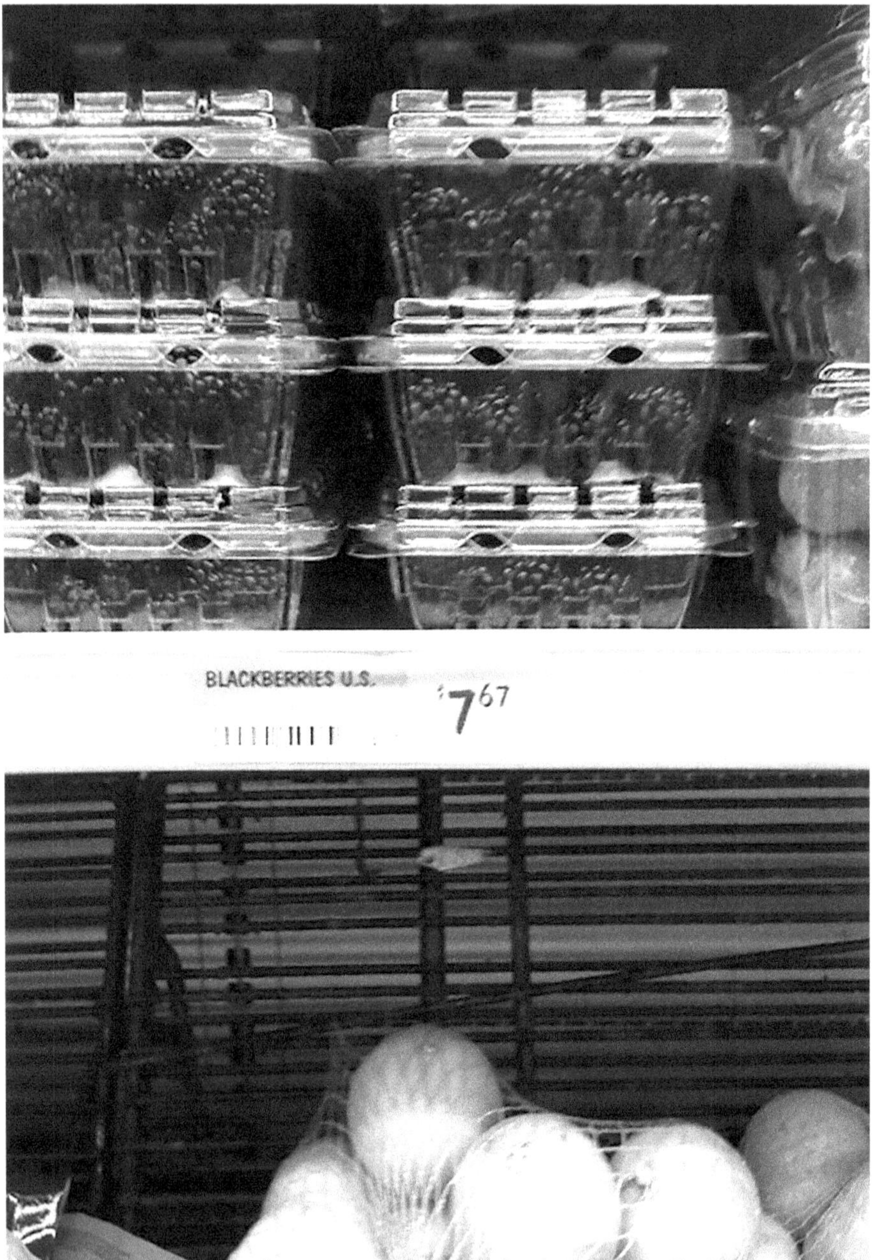

FIGURE 11.1 Price of blackberries in SumerMax, a supermarket in the San Juan neighborhood of Condado, March 2014.

Paris Accord in 2019 and only rejoined it in 2021, Puerto Ricans have consistently demanded, imagined, and worked toward a just energy transition and even called for an "energy insurrection" (Massol Deyá 2018). The privatization of PREPA will not lead to policies that address climate change and to date no federal legislation has emerged to limit or direct energy service provision in an environmentally responsible and socially equitable way.

Clean, renewable energy sources are an important part of food sovereignty and climate justice because they help to sustain the environment and maintain "livable worlds" within Puerto Rico (Lloréns 2021). Making equitable food and energy systems a reality and decolonization are interconnected tasks, and ending industrialized mass food production as we know it will go a long way toward diminishing climate disruption and mitigating the effects of climate change.

SDG 16 (Promote Peace and Inclusive Societies for Sustainable Development)

- End U.S. colonialism in Puerto Rico.
- Assistance to improve structural factors (poverty, unemployment, etc.).

Due to Puerto Rico's political status as a colony, the U.S. exercises political and economic control over the island, including over currency, taxes, and political processes. In this context, the aim of promoting peace and inclusion for sustainable development in Puerto Rico (SDG 16) seems far out of reach, largely due to the absence of political will to resolve Puerto Rico's territorial subjection and the lack of sovereign state power required to enter into and enforce international cooperation agreements, whether that be with the United States or with any other state.

The 2008 recession severely affected Puerto Rico, contributing to an 8.1% unemployment rate (vs. 5.8% nationally) and 45.4% poverty level, compared to 15% nationally. Puerto Rico is over $72 billion in debt, and in May 2017, Puerto Rico entered proceedings to claim Title III relief in federal court under PROMESA (the Puerto Rico Oversight, Management, and Economic Stability Act), which permitted the island to declare its debts as total losses, but also slashed federal Medicare funding and government workers' pensions, and left numerous public health projects unfunded (Orr et al. 2017). Despite the economic crisis in Puerto Rico, the United States government continues to refuse investments needed to improve living conditions, thus affording the United States the economic benefits of exercising control over an overseas territory, without assuming responsibility for a poverty-stricken island.

The most significant step that could be taken to improve structural factors such as poverty and unemployment would be to end U.S. colonialism in Puerto Rico through a process of decolonization and self-determination for Puerto Ricans. Calls for such a process have intensified on the island and from within the United Nations' own Decolonization Committee since 1976, with the latest international declaration calling for self-determination and political independence for Puerto Rico signed in June 2021 (United Nations General Assembly 2021).

CONCLUSIONS

SDGs do not exist in a vacuum. They exist in an interacting set of social, economic, and political contexts that prevent the SDGs from thriving, even in a supposedly developed nation like the United States. The shift from an agrarian economy to a post-industrial economy under U.S. colonialism produced stark food insecurity in Puerto Rico, where at least 85% of commercially available food products are imported from the continental United States. Most residents of these islands can no longer consistently afford to feed themselves and their extended families well and have difficulty accessing local food. The resulting nutritional deficiencies in turn contribute to increased rates of multiple chronic and interlocking diseases such as diabetes, high blood pressure, and depression. These difficulties have only been exacerbated by the COVID-19-related lockdown measures implemented starting in March 2020, which have created significant additional barriers to nutrition for a large percentage of the population as people were unable to leave their house to purchase food, and grocery stores rapidly ran out of sufficient supplies. This has been especially the case for children, who have not been able to receive breakfast and lunch at cafeterias due to school closures. The hurricane season, which ran from June 1st to November 30th, caused additional anxiety as shelters had to maintain physical distancing and had to cap the number of people they could accept, and stores had to limit the amount of supplies that people could purchase in order to ensure sufficient supplies. At the same time, social movements and mutual aid organizations have rapidly generated nutritional support efforts that have become a political flashpoint.

We encourage reform in Puerto Rico, using the SDGs as guidelines for specific recommendations. For SDG 2 (Zero Hunger), we want to ensure that Puerto Rico receives the same federal assistance for food (either direct foodstuffs or economic assistance to stimulate self-sustaining agriculture), particularly by eradicating the Cabotage Laws. For SDG 3 (Ensuring Health Lives), we recommend extending Obamacare provisions to Puerto Rico and other U.S. territories, and putting more money into health insurance plans so that health care providers will remain on the island and people will receive the health services they need. For SDG 8 (Promote Sustained, Inclusive, and Sustainable Economic Growth), we call for improved infrastructure beyond the touristy Viejo San Juan and stimulating job development throughout Puerto Rico. For SDG 13 (Ending Climate Change), we recommend ending or amending industrial food systems in which efficiency is maximized over environmental impact (such as pesticides and untreated animal waste) and which externalizes staggering costs that are transferable to taxpayers. For SDG 16 (Promote Peace and Inclusive Societies for Sustainable Development), we call for an end to U.S. colonialism in Puerto Rico and assistance in improving structural factors, such as poverty and unemployment. In particular, PROMESA needs to be either radically reformed or abolished outright due to its defunding of critical public health measures and depletion of pensions.

REFERENCES

Acevedo, Nicole. (2021). 'Chaotic Situation': Puerto Ricans Indignant at Tourists Breaking COVID Mandates. *NBC News*. https://www.nbcnews.com/news/latino/chaotic-situation-puerto-ricans-indignant-tourists-breaking-covid-mandates-n1261588.

Acosta-Pérez, Edna, Glorisa Canino, Rafael Ramírez, Michael Prelip, Molly Martin, and Alexander N. Ortega. (2012). Do Puerto Rican Youth with Asthma and Obesity Have Higher Odds for Mental Health Disorders? *Psychosomatics, 53*(2): 162–171.

Beyer, Scott. (2015). Puerto Rico, At 11.5%, Has America's Highest Sales Tax. *Forbes Magazine*. https://www.forbes.com/sites/scottbeyer/2015/08/17/puerto-rico-at-11-5-has-americas-highest-sales-tax/.

Bread for the World. (2019). Hunger and Poverty in Puerto Rico. https://www.bread.org/sites/default/files/hunger-poverty-puerto-rico-march-2019.pdf.

Canino, Glorisa, Patrick E. Shrout, Amanda NeMoyer, Doryliz Vila, Katyana M. Santiago, Pedro Garcia, Amarilis Quiñones, Vilmary Cruz, and Margarita Alegría. (2019). A Comparison of the Prevalence of Psychiatric Disorders in Puerto Rico with the United States and the Puerto Rican Population of the United States. *Social Psychiatry and Psychiatric Epidemiology, 54*: 369–378.

Carrión, José B. and Andrew G. Biggs. (2018). "Don't Blame Puerto Rico's Poor Economy on Hurricanes". *Washington Post*. https://www.washingtonpost.com/opinions/dont-blame-puerto-ricos-poor-economy-on-hurricanes/2018/12/17/206a5734-f181-11e8-9240-e8028a62c722_story.html.

Colón-López, Vivian, Geetanjoli Banerjee, Alida María Gertz, Ana Patricia Ortiz, William Calo, Lila J. Finney-Rutten, Uriyoán Colón-Ramos, Bradford W. Hesse, and Guillermo Tortolero. (2013). Behavioral Correlates of Fruit and Vegetable Intake in Puerto Rico: Results from the Health Information National Trends Survey. *Puerto Rican Health Sciences Journal, 32*(4): 194–199.

Colón-Ramos, Uriyoán, Cynthia M. Pérez-Cardona, and Rafael Monge-Rojas. (2013). Socio-Demographic, Behavioral and Health Correlates of Nutrition Transition Dietary Indicators in San Juan, Puerto Rico. *Revista Panamericana de Salud Pública, 34*(5): 330–335.

Colón-Ramos, Uriyoán, Idania Rodríguez-Ayuso, Hirut T. Gebrekistos, Amira Roess, Cynthia M. Pérez, and Lone Simonsen. (2017). Transnational Mortality Comparisons between Archipelago and Mainland Puerto Ricans. *Journal of Immigrant and Minority Health, 19*(5): 1009–1017.

Coto, Dánica. (2020). Puerto Rico to Spend $2B to Fight COVID-19 as Concerns Grow over Allocation. *PBS News*. https://www.pbs.org/newshour/economy/puerto-rico-to-spend-2b-to-fight-covid-19-as-concerns-grow-over-allocation.

De Onís, Catalina M. (2021). *Energy Islands: Metaphors of Power, Extractivism, and Justice in Puerto Rico*. Berkeley, CA: University of California Press.

Dhokarh, Rajanigandha, David A. Himmelgreen, Yu-Kuei Peng, Sofia Segura-Pérez, Amber Hromi-Fiedler, and Rafael Pérez-Escamilla. (2018). Food Insecurity Is Associated with Acculturation and Social Networks in Puerto Rican Households. *Journal of Nutrition Education and Behavior, 43*(4): 288–294.

Duany, Jorge. (2017). *Puerto Rico: What Everyone Needs to Know*. New York: Oxford University Press.

Duany, Jorge. (2002). *The Puerto Rican Nation on the Move: Identities on the Island and in the United States*. Chapel Hill, NC: University of North Carolina Press.

Garofalo, Giovanna. (2020). Puerto Rico Aims to Achieve UN's 2030 Sustainable Development Goals. *Weekly Journal*. https://www.theweeklyjournal.com/politics/puerto-rico-aims-to-achieve-un-s-2030-sustainable-development-goals/article_b1f6417e-e9fe-11e9-83e8-73abb2cb6472.html.

González-Colón, Jennifer. (2019). House Approves $600 Million for the Nutrition Assistance Program (PAN) for Puerto Rico. https://gonzalez-colon.house.gov/media/press-releases/house-approves-600-million-nutrition-assistance-program-pan-puerto-rico.

Hernández-Delgado, Edwin A., Carlos E. Ramos-Scharrón, Carmen R. Guerrero-Pérez, Mary Ann Lucking, Ricardo Laureano, Pablo A. Méndez-Lázaro, and Joel O. Meléndez-Díaz. (2012). Long-Term Impacts of Non-Sustainable Tourism and Urban Development in Small Tropical Islands Coastal Habitats in a Changing Climate: Lessons Learned from Puerto Rico. In *Visions from Global Tourism Industry-Creating and Sustaining Competitive Strategies*. M. Kasimoglu, ed. Pp. 357–398.

Herzog, Hayley. (2018). 10 Facts about Hunger in Puerto Rico. *The Borgen Project*. https://borgenproject.org/facts-hunger-in-puerto-rico/.

Keith-Jennings, Brynne. (2020). Puerto Rico Nutrition Benefit Cuts Risk Food Insecurity, Show Block Grant's Limits. Washington, DC: Center on Budget and Policy Priorities. https://www.cbpp.org/blog/puerto-rico-nutrition-benefit-cuts-risk-food-insecurity-show-block-grants-limits.

Keith-Jennings, Brynne and Elizabeth Wolkomir. (2020). How Does Household Food Assistance in Puerto Rico Compare to the Rest of the United States? Washington, DC: Center on Budget and Policy Priorities. https://www.cbpp.org/research/food-assistance/how-does-household-food-assistance-in-puerto-rico-compare-to-the-rest-of.

Klein, Naomi. (2018). *The Battle for Paradise: Puerto Rico Takes on the Disaster Capitalists*. Chicago, IL: Haymarket Books.

Laborde, Jorge E. and Emily Sáez-Santiago. (2013). Association between Obesity and Symptoms of Depression of Adults in Puerto Rico. *Puerto Rico Health Sciences Journal, 3*, 132–137.

Lerman, Shir. (2017). Disordered Minds and Disordered Bodies: Stigma, Depression, and Obesity in Puerto Rico. In *Foundations of BioSocial Health: Stigma and Illness Interactions*. Lerman, Shir, Bayla Ostrach, and Merrill Singer, eds. Pp. 47–82. Lanham, MD: Lexington Books.

Lerman, Shir. (2019). ¿Qué Sistema de Salud? Broken Health Care in Puerto Rico. *Medical Anthropology: Cross-Cultural Studies in Health and Illness, 38*(3), 210–223.

Lloréns, Hilda. (2021). *Making Livable Worlds: Afro-Puerto Rican Women Building Environmental Justice*. Seattle: University of Washington Press.

Massol Deyá, Arturo. De La Autogestión a la Insurgencia Energética: Una Historia De Supervivencia, Resistencia, y Gobernanza Comunitaria. *Revista Juridica, 3*: 648–654.

Mattei, Josiemer, Martha Tamez, Carlos F. Ríos-Bedoya, Rui S. Xiao, Katherine L. Tucker, and José F. Rodríguez-Orengo. (2018). Health Conditions and Lifestyle Risk Factors of Adults Living in Puerto Rico: A Cross-Sectional Study. *BMC Public Health, 491*: 18. DOI: https://10.1186/s12889-018-5359-z.

McGreevey, Robert C. (2018). *Borderline Citizens: The United States, Puerto Rico, and the Politics of Colonial Migration*. Ithaca, NY: Cornell University Press.

Méndez-Lázaro, Pablo, José J. Terrasa-Soler, Christian Torres-Peña, Paula Guzmán-González, Sulaine Rodríguez, Mariangely Alemán, and Tatiana Seguinot. (2014). Tourism and Climate Conditions in San Juan, Puerto Rico, 2000–2010. *Ecology and Society, 19*(2): 11.

Méndez-Méndez, Serafín and Ronald Fernández. (2015). *Puerto Rico, Past and Present: An Encyclopedia*. 2nd Edition. Santa Barbara, CA: Greenwood Press.

Michaud, Josh and Jennifer Kates. (2017). Public Health in Puerto Rico after Hurricane Maria. *Kaiser Family Foundation*. https://www.kff.org/other/issue-brief/public-health-in-puerto-rico-after-hurricane-María/.

Morales, Ed. (2019). *Fantasy Island: Colonialism, Exploitation, and the Betrayal of Puerto Rico*. New York: Bold Type Books.

Nichter, Mark. (2008). *Global Health: Why Cultural Perceptions, Social Representations, and Biopolitics Matter*. Tucson: The University of Arizona Press.

Orr, Emma, Steven Church, and Michelle Kaske (Producer). (2017, May 17). Puerto Rico's Bankruptcy Fight Is about to Plunge into the Unknown. *Bloomberg*. https://www.bloomberg.com/news/articles/2017-05-11/puerto-rico-debt-donnybrook-kicks-off-with-squabble-over-default.

Ortíz Cuadra, Cruz Miguel. (2013). *Eating Puerto Rico: A History of Food, Culture, and Identity*. Chapel Hill: University of North Carolina Press.

Pérez, Cynthia M., Hesmy Sánchez, and Ana P. Ortiz. (2013). Prevalence of Overweight and Obesity and Their Cardiometabolic Comorbidities in Hispanic Adults Living in Puerto Rico. *Journal of Community Health*, *38*(6), 1140–1146.

Pipa, Anthony F. and Kaysie Brown. (2019). American Leadership on the Sustainable Development Goals. *Brookings Institute*. https://www.brookings.edu/blog/up-front/2019/10/14/american-leadership-on-the-sustainable-development-goals/.

Piser, Karina. (2020). In Puerto Rico, 40 Percent Suffer Food Insecurity with No End in Sight. *Fern's AG: Insider*. https://thefern.org/ag_insider/in-puerto-rico-40-percent-suffer-food-insecurity-with-no-end-in-sight/.

Rodríguez-Díaz, Carlos. (2018). Maria in Puerto Rico: Natural Disaster in a Colonial Archipelago. *American Journal of Public Health*, *108*(1): 30–32.

Rodriguez-Soto, Isa. (2013). *Intergenerational Variation in Cultural Models of Body Size in Puerto Rico*. (Doctor of Philosophy), *Arizona State University*. (3560159).

Soltero, Sandra M. and Cristina Palacios. (2011). Association between Dietary Patterns and Body Composition in a Group or Puerto Rican Obese Adults: A Pilot Study. *Puerto Rican Health Studies Journal*, *30*(1): 22–27.

Soto-Lacourt, Miguel. (2002). Statement by: Estado Libre de Puerto Rico. Presented at the World Summit on Sustainable Development. Johannesburg, South Africa: 30 August 2002. https://sustainabledevelopment.un.org/index.php?page=view&type=255&nr=19753.

United Nations General Assembly. (2021). "Special Committee on Decolonization Approves Text Calling upon United States to Promote Puerto Rico's Self-Determination, Eventual Independence". *Special Committee on Decolonization*. 18 June 2021. https://www.un.org/press/en/2021/gacol3346.doc.htm.

Urban Institute. (2021). State-by-State Guide to the 2020–21 Pandemic EBT Program. https://www.urban.org/state-guide-pandemic-ebt.

Watson, Sara Kiley. (2018). Food Aid to Puerto Rico Is Salty, Sugary, and Unbalanced, Researcher Says. NPR*: Eating and Health*. https://www.npr.org/sections/thesalt/2018/06/22/621036893/food-aid-to-puerto-rico-is-salty-sugary-and-unbalanced-researcher-says.

Wolkomir, Elizabeth. (2017). How Is Food Assistance Difference in Puerto Rico than in the Rest of the United States? Washington, DC: Center on Budget and Policy Priorities. https://www.cbpp.org/research/food-assistance/how-is-food-assistance-different-in-puerto-rico-than-in-the-rest-of-the.

12 Rooftop Farming
A Sustainable Food Production Initiative in Cairo, Egypt

Mahmoud Shaltout, Martina Jaskolski, and Kara Hoving

CONTENTS

INTRODUCTION

Fighting poverty and hunger, eradicating food security, and granting Africans equal access to resources and nutrition are development issues most African nations share. Fast population growth across much of the African continent will lead to vastly increased food and water demands in the near future (van Ittersum et al. 2016). African nations are united in their quest to realize the Sustainable Development Goals (SDGs). Ending Poverty (SDG 1), Zero Hunger (SDG 2), Good Health and Well-being (SDG 3), Economic Equality, and Sustainable Cities and Communities (SDG 11) are among these goals. A United Nations (2019) report on the progress of implementing the SDGs from 2019 shows that the world is currently not on track in regards to reducing the percentage of people living in poverty to less than 3% by 2030, and while poverty is expected to remain above 6% at current projections, hunger was on the rise globally in 2019. A total of 821 million people were undernourished in 2017 (up from 784 million in 2015), with Africa being the continent suffering the highest levels of undernourishment. In 2017, 770 million people faced severe food insecurity (UN 2019). Following a definition developed at the World Food Summit in 1996, the Food and Agriculture Organization of the United Nations

DOI: 10.1201/9781003014942-12

FAO (2006) defines food security as achieved "when all people, at all times, have physical and economic access to sufficient, safe and nutritious food that meets their dietary needs and food preferences for an active and healthy life." Marginalized groups, women, and children are particularly vulnerable to food insecurity. In 2018, one in five children under the age of five years worldwide was stunted in 2018 (UN 2019). Realizing the SDGs means ensuring food security and access to healthy nutrition for all citizens in urban and rural communities across Africa and the world, as well as catering for increasingly urbanized populations. By 2050, almost 70% of the world's population is expected to live in cities (World Bank 2018); African cities are projected to house over 300 million incoming people within the next 25 years (Shirisa and Matamanda 2016). Additionally, Sub-Saharan Africa is the third highest region in terms of urban slum dwellers in the developing world (Jelili 2012). The fact that large segments of Africa's urban populations are lower-income households makes the provision of equal access to affordable as well as healthy, nutritious food supply challenging.

This chapter focuses particularly on urban agriculture and rooftop gardening as a way of growing food in the proximity of consumers in Greater Cairo. Based on iterations by Goldstein (2011) and Hendrickson and Porth (2012), Game and Primus (2015) define urban and peri-urban agriculture as "the growing, processing, and distribution of food and other products through plant cultivation and seldom raising livestock in and around cities for feeding local populations." Urban agriculture has been explicitly linked to the achievement of the SDGs (Game and Primus 2015), as shown in Table 12.1.

Global challenges such as water scarcity and climate change increase both pressure and limitations in the world's struggle to attain the SDGs by 2030. Climate change, water scarcity, and the loss of agricultural land affect particularly arid parts of Africa and require more water and climate-efficient practices in the continent's quest to pave a more sustainable future. SDG 6 specifically targets water-use efficiency across all sectors and a reduction in the number of people worldwide who suffer from water scarcity (UN 2016). In the arid countries of the MENA region, where large segments of the agricultural production sector rely on irrigation, retaining water efficiency while boosting production is particularly important. Integrated water resources management that strengthens local community participation in water management planning and decision-making (SDG 6.5 and 6.B) that should inform efforts to promote urban farming (UN 2016). Climate change and water scarcity are intrinsically linked, as a warmer climate is expected to raise evapotranspiration in agriculture (Abtew and Melesse 2013) and make water-efficient irrigation even more necessary. SDG 13 addresses the aim of tackling climate change and its adverse impacts by promoting resilience (SDG 13.1), awareness and education on mitigating its effects (SDG 13.3) and ultimately incorporating measures into public strategies (SDG 13.2). These measures involve innovative agricultural and food systems, including integrated farming, hydroponic, aquaponics, and aeroponics systems, which increase food productivity while reducing resource use – a much-needed outcome in countries with limited/diminishing fertile land such as Egypt. These innovative systems also address SDG 15, which aims to promote sustainable utilization of terrestrial ecosystems to ultimately decrease desertification and reverse

TABLE 12.1
SDGs Linked to Urban Agriculture

Sustainable Development Goals Linked to Urban Agriculture				
Name of Goal	**Name of TTarget (Shortened), to Be Achieved by 2030**			
Goal 1: End poverty in all its forms everywhere	**1.1** Eradicate extreme poverty for all people everywhere (under 1.25 USD /day)	**1.3** Implement nationally appropriate social protection systems … achieve substantial coverage of the poor and vulnerable	**1.4** Ensure that all men and women, in particular the poor and the vulnerable, have equal rights to economic resources, as well as access to basic services …	**1.5** Build the resilience of the poor and those in vulnerable situations … economic, social, and environmental shocks and disasters
Goal 2: End hunger, achieve food security and improved nutrition and promote sustainable agriculture	**2.1** End hunger and ensure access by all people…to safe, nutritious, and sufficient food all year round	**2.3** Double the productivity and the incomes of small-scale food producers, particularly women…., including through secure and equal access to land, other productive resources and inputs	**2.4** Ensure sustainable food production systems and implement resilient agricultural practices that help increase productivity and production, that help maintain ecosystems.	**2.C** Adopt measures to ensure the proper functioning of food commodity markets … in order to help limit extreme food price volatility.
Goal 3: Ensure healthy lives and promote well-being for all at all ages	**3.4** Reduce by one-third premature mortality from non-communicable diseases through prevention and treatment and promote mental health and well-being			
Goal 6: Ensure availability and sustainable management of water and sanitation for all	**6.4** Substantially increase water-use efficiency across all sectors and ensure sustainable withdrawals and supply of freshwater to address water scarcity and substantially reduce the number of people suffering from water scarcity	**6.5** Implement integrated water resources management at all levels, including through transboundary cooperation as appropriate	**6.b** Support and strengthen the participation of local communities in improving water and sanitation management	

(Continued)

TABLE 12.1 (*Continued*)
SDGs Linked to Urban Agriculture

Name of Goal	Sustainable Development Goals Linked to Urban Agriculture: Name of Target (Shortened), to Be Achieved by 2030						
Goal 7: Ensure access to affordable, reliable, sustainable, and modern energy for all	**7.3** Double the global rate of improvement in energy efficiency						
Goal 11: Make cities and human settlements inclusive, safe, resilient, and sustainable	**11.7** Provide universal access to safe, inclusive, and accessible, green and public spaces, in particular for women and children, older persons, and persons with disabilities.						
Goal 12: Ensure sustainable production and consumption patterns	**12.1** Implement the Ten-Year Framework of Programs on Sustainable Consumption and Production Patterns, all countries taking action, with developed countries taking the lead, taking into account the development and capabilities of developing countries	**12.2** Achieve the sustainable management and efficient use of natural resources	**12.3** Halve per capita global food waste at the retail and consumer levels and reduce food losses along production and supply chains, including post-harvest losses	**12.4** Achieve the environmentally sound management of chemicals and all wastes throughout their life cycle, in accordance with agreed international frameworks, and significantly reduce their release to air, water, and soil…	**12.5** Substantially reduce waste generation through prevention, reduction, recycling, and reuse	**12.7** Promote public procurement practices that are sustainable, in accordance with national policies and priorities	**12.8** Ensure that people everywhere have the relevant information and awareness for sustainable development and lifestyles

(*Continued*)

TABLE 12.1 (*Continued*)
SDGs Linked to Urban Agriculture

Sustainable Development Goals Linked to Urban Agriculture			
Name of Goal	**Name of Target (Shortened), to Be Achieved by 2030**		
Goal 13: Take urgent action to combat climate change and its impacts	**13.1** Strengthen resilience and adaptive capacity to climate-related hazards and natural disasters in all countries	**13.2** Integrate climate change measures into national policies, strategies, and planning	**13.3** Improve education, awareness-raising, and human and institutional capacity on climate change mitigation, adaptation, impact reduction, and early warning
Goal 15: Protect, restore, and promote sustainable use of terrestrial ecosystems, sustainably manage forests, combat desertification, and halt and reverse land degradation and halt biodiversity loss	**15.9** Integrate ecosystem and biodiversity values into national and local planning, development processes, poverty reduction strategies, and accounts		

Source: From (UN 2016).

land degradation (UN 2016). These new technologies may help toward improving nutrition and food security in Africa within the continent's resource boundaries.

In Egypt, the above-mentioned challenges are exacerbated by the country's geography and arid climate. Egypt's landmass – roughly one million square kilometers (km^2) – is mainly desert, and despite government efforts to reclaim desert land for settlements, the majority of Egypt's 98 million strong population live on the thin fertile stretch of Nile and the fertile Nile Delta region (only 5% of Egypt's landmass and includes the two most populous cities, Cairo and Alexandria) (UNICEF Egypt 2019). The Greater Cairo Metropolitan area – the capital of Egypt – lies at the base of the Nile Delta, flanking both sides of the Nile River. The second half of the twentieth century saw a massive expansion of the Greater Cairo area in terms of both population and spatial area (Sims, Sejoume and El Shorbagi 2003). Cairo is now the most populous city in Africa, housing around 20 million people (Central Agency for Public Mobilization and Statistics 2020) with a population density of 19.376 people per square kilometer, the thirty-seventh highest in the world (World Population Review 2019). Egypt is currently classified as a lower middle-income country, the majority of the population living under the poverty line of $3.20 a day (US dollars) (World Bank 2019). The lives of the poor have been worsened by the devaluation of the Egyptian pound in 2016, as well as the removal of subsidies, which has led to a sharp rise in prices of commodities, goods, and services (El Baradei 2019). Additionally, the state-owned Central Agency for Public Mobilization and Statistics (CAPMAS) reported that the percentage of Egyptians living in extreme poverty (under $1.3 daily) rose from 27.8% in 2015 to 32.5% in 2018 (Egypt Today 2019).

Cairo (as well as other urban centers in the Nile Delta) continues to expand, resulting in loss of arable agricultural lands. Analysis of maps shows that over a 24-year period (1991–2015), Egypt has lost 74,600 hectares of fertile agricultural land in the Nile Delta due to urban expansion, and given a business as usual scenario, will lose 87,000 hectares to urban expansion by 2030 (Radwan et al. 2019). This poses a food security problem to a country as populous as Egypt, which since the 1980s has relied on importing foods to sustain its ever-growing population, as relying on local production does not suffice (Galal 2002; Hassan-Wassef 2004). This rapid land loss also endangers the livelihoods of 60% of the population, whose main source of income is the agricultural sector (Radwan et al. 2019). Egypt's food security is not only threatened by land loss, but also by water scarcity and climate change. Egypt solely depends on the Nile for its water supply, and 85% of Egypt's freshwater is used for irrigation purposes (Amer, Abd El Hafez and Abd El Ghany 2017). Egypt's share of the Nile has been 55 billion cubic meters per year since 1959 and is now classified as a water-scarce country as the per capita share of renewable water sources has dropped to below 1,000 m^3/capita/year (about 700 m^3/capita/year) in 2015 (Amer, Abd El Hafez and Abd El Ghany 2017). The country is fast heading into extreme water scarcity, which is expected to hit the country by 2025 (Ministry of Water Resources and Irrigation, Egypt 2014). Additionally, the construction of the Aswan Dam in the late 1960s prevented nutrients and sediments from reaching the Nile Delta, and the outer edges of the Delta are eroding at around 100 m per year (Khedr 2019). On another front, climate change and the subsequent sea level rise (SLR) threaten to submerge 4,500 km of the fertile Delta (UN Environmental Program 2005) and could subsequently lead to a loss of 205–374 billion Egyptian pounds (12–23 billion USD) worth of agricultural GDP by 2060 (Smith et al. 2013).

With a fast-growing population and dwindling natural resources, Egypt faces the challenge of having to significantly boost its food production, while also using much less resources in the process. Currently, Egypt imports approximately 40% of its food supply, while 16% of the population have poor access to food (Sarant 2017). The country was given a ‘moderate’ food security status in 2018 (Global Food Security Index 2018). In fact, Egypt has gone from being the breadbasket of the Roman Empire to the largest wheat importer in the world (Food and Agriculture Organization 2017), importing about 60% of the wheat consumed in the country. Egypt’s population of currently 99.9 million (Central Agency for Public Mobilization and Statistics 2020) grows by a million every 6 months – a growth rate that puts the country into a serious dilemma; having to produce more food each year with diminishing water resources (Jaskolski 2016). The rapid urbanization of Cairo and increasing distances traveled by food from agricultural areas to urban centers begs for an immediate solution to use urban spaces for agriculture to decrease food insecurity.

Almost half of Egypt’s population currently lives in urban areas. This is already higher than the African average of 40% (World Bank 2018). Greater Cairo accommodates over 40% of Egypt’s urban population, currently around 20 million, and is expected to have over 30 million inhabitants by 2050 (General Organization for Physical Planning Egypt 2009). Cairo’s urban structure is characterized mainly by tightly packed multistory buildings, as well as a limited number of green spaces – an average of 0.85 m^2 per citizen in 2015 (Ministry of Planning, Monitoring and Administrative Reform 2018). One result of the expansion of Cairo was the development of informal shantytowns or urban pocket slums – both within the city and on the periphery – to house the huge influx of rural workers unable to afford costly rents in the main urban center (Sims, Sejoume and El Shorbagi 2003; Denis 2006).

Currently, at least 60% of Cairo’s buildings are classified as informal housing; either the owners do not own the land on which they have built, or the building itself was erected where residential housing is not permitted and without following the Egyptian building code (Bayat and Denis 2000). Although the majority of these areas are a result of the post WWII expansion, some have been developed as early as the late nineteenth century. These informal settlements are usually densely packed and populated, and have no green spaces for activity or socializing, and have a high UHIE, similar to disadvantaged urban neighborhoods worldwide (Aboulnaga and Mostafa 2019). These characteristics together create a host of issues, including financial setbacks to an already struggling socio-economic group (higher electric bills through AC/energy usage), exposure to pollutants, as well as less physical activity. Tight urban construction with a lack of urban green space, which in Cairo’s informal areas can be as low as 0.33 m^2 per person (Attia and Amer 2009), coupled with rapid urbanization and greater vehicle use, results in a barrier to physical activity among Cairo’s residents. The urban form living situation in many of Cairo’s informal areas poses a serious challenge to the implementation of SDG 11.7, which demands the provision of universal access to safe, inclusive, and accessible, green and public spaces, in particular for women and children, older persons and persons with disabilities.

Although limited research has examined physical activity levels in urban Egypt, a 1990s WHO study revealed that 73% of urban adults from low socio-economic status (SES) groups and 89% of urban adults from high SES groups had mainly sedentary lifestyles, and demonstrated a positive correlation between sedentary lifestyles and obesity rates (37% and 49%, respectively) (Galal 2002). Over the last few decades, numerous reports and studies have revealed that Egypt is 'the fattest nation in Africa', and among the Middle Eastern countries with the highest prevalence of obesity; one-third of Egyptian adults are classified as obese (Alebshehy et al. 2016; World Health Organization – Eastern Mediterranean Regional Office 2020). SDG 3.4 specifically addresses the percentage of the population that is overweight and obese, targeting to reduce by one-third premature mortality from non-communicable diseases (NCDs) through prevention and treatment, and promote health and well-being (UN 2016). Obesity notably affects twice as many Egyptian women as men (Alebshehy et al. 2016), due to a combination of limited opportunities for physical activity as well as the cultural perception and shaping of women's roles. A substantial number of families within low/middle SES households in Cairo, as in other parts of the country, follow a patriarchal system where men work and women are restricted to the household, often taking care of children and of household chores.

Women are a vulnerable group in society due to their limited access to and ownership of resources, lack of full participation in the labor market and decision-making and lower incomes for the same jobs (Ivers and Cullen 2011; Bishu and AlKadry 2017). Given these inequalities, women are expected to be disproportionately affected by water scarcity, climate change, and food insecurity. In Egypt, the patriarchal system influences women's roles in neighborhoods, families, workplace, as well as their access to the public realm. Patriarchy has a long history in the region, experiencing a revival in the 1970s and 80s under the influence of debates on gender segregation, female modesty, and female involvement in public life – a revival sparked by religious organizations and the media (Moghadam 2004; Rock-Singer 2016). Patriarchy involves the structuring of families under the authority of a senior male head, male-domination over family access to land and resources, as well as decision-making in the household (Moghadam 2004; Yount et al. 2016). Media and public discourses produce men in families as breadwinners, protectors of women's social respectability, and representatives of the family in the public realm. This discursive production can lead men to control female behavior, dress codes, and mobility (Moghadam 2004; Yount et al. 2016). Body politics, the constitution of bodies in a nexus of power and discourse (Foucault 1990) and the performativity of gender roles reinforce the embodiment of such discursive projections of gender roles in everyday life (Butler 1990). Modesty in clothing – covering with a headscarf and traditional clothing – and the avoidance of mixing with men in public are constructed as a reflection of a woman's respectability, and, by extension, her entire family (Walseth and Fasting 2003; Rock-Singer 2016).

Patriarchal norms and lawns have a real impact on women's lives and threaten the achievement of SDG 4, gender equality. In Egypt, only 2% of women own agricultural land, while 5% of women between 15 and 49 who have ever been married own a house (UNICEF 2014). Male-based control and patriarchal structures in Egypt's family organization vary among different geographical parts of Egypt as well as among groups of Egyptian society (Toth 1991) and are dynamic and changing. Patriarchy needs to be examined in the context of complex processes such as the economic system, property and income structures (Moghadam 2004), social class and gender division of labor (Toth 1991), laws, education, family planning, women's agency (Yount et al. 2016), state discourses and the feminist movement (Rock-Singer 2016), as well as youth and feminist activism (Moghadam 2004). While the influx of Western lifestyles, education, and gender concepts shape the life realities of the wealthy families of Cairo, poorer parts of the population financially rely on women's labor for survival. Oftentimes, the middle class holds up the most conservative attitudes toward women's involvement in the formal labor market, gender segregation, and modest, submissive behavior of female family members (Toth 1991). Limited social interaction with others, particularly men, restrict women (particularly from conservative families) in many of Cairo's neighborhoods to the confines of the household for much of their daily lives (Walseth and Fasting 2003). These social norms influence women's access to labor markets, income, green spaces, physical activity, and social contact every day. They display the intricate interconnections between SDG 4, gender equality, SDG 8, decent work, SDG 11.7, access to green and public space and SDG 3, good health and well-being.

Besides gender, social strata, and economic position, geographical location within city space also determines access to green space, mobility, health, and well-being. Densely built urban neighborhoods with a shortage of greenspaces, as well as some types of suburban sprawl, are more prone to effects of the Urban Heat Island (UHI) effect than rural areas (Debbage and Marshall Shepherd 2015), especially during the summer months in a hot and arid climate such as Egypt's. UHI are areas of elevated average air and surface temperatures in cities relative to their surrounding areas (Hamada et al. 2013, Solecki et al. 2005). Causes of UHI include anthropogenic heat release, air pollution, and the replacement of natural surfaces such as soil and vegetation known as green topography with artificial surfaces, such as concrete and asphalt. Such artificial surfaces absorb and retain heat, which, in the context of global urbanization, exacerbates the UHI effect in conglomerations around the world (Hamada et al. 2013; Oke 2011; Voogt and Oke 2003). "Building materials often have thermal properties with a greater capacity to store heat, which is difficult to release. Furthermore, anthropogenic heat from buildings and road traffic also affect the energy balance in an area" (Hamada et al. 2013, 433). UHI can become particularly relevant at nighttime, when urban areas cool down much slower than suburban and rural areas (Solecki et al. 2005). Reducing the UHI effect is thus necessary for addressing SDG 7, which entails access to affordable and sustainable energy for all, particularly SDG 7.3, improving global energy efficiency by 2030 (UN 2016).

In Cairo, the UHI effect ranges from 3.11 to 5.7°C (Aboulnaga and Mostafa 2019), which, as in other cities around the world, can substantially increase energy needs for indoor air conditioning (Hamada et al. 2013; Solecki et al. 2005). Further aggravating the issue is air pollution; traffic, industry, dust, and biomass burning have deteriorated Cairo's air quality for decades. In Cairo, the Nile channels cooler and fresher air through the city, but not all suburbs equally benefit from this cooling effect, and weather conditions such as temperature inversion and dust storms can add high pollution levels to heat. The spatial injustice in the distribution of green areas, with leafy high-end downtown suburbs and compounds on the outskirts of Cairo benefiting from a much higher abundance of trees than informal neighborhoods, characterized by a dense, urban form and multistory buildings divided by narrow alleyways, creates further social and environmental justice in respect to exposure to air pollution. SDG 11.3, which considers access to green space, is thus closely connected with SDG 11.6, which demands a reduction of the per capita environmental impact of cities, with a special focus on air pollution.

Air pollution, associated with numerous adverse health effects including heat stress, lung cancer, asthma, chronic bronchitis, cardiovascular mortality and disability, and premature death (Khafaie et al. 2016; Orru, Ebi and Fosberg 2017; Rajagopalan, Al-Kindi and Brook 2018), will particularly affect the more vulnerable populations (the very old, very young, and the poor) together with urban heat (Solecki et al. 2005). Adaptation measures to heat such as indoor air conditioning is a financial investment not all parts of Cairo's population can afford, placing particularly informal areas at a disadvantage again. A recent study by the Egyptian Meteorological Authority investigated measurements taken by pollution stations across the Greater Cairo area and has shown that emission patterns for several pollutants (sulfur dioxide, nitrogen dioxide, carbon monoxide, ozone and particulate matter) greatly exceed the Egyptian legal exposure limits (Mostafa et al. 2018). Air pollution has also been shown to be strongly associated with an increased risk of obesity and cardiometabolic disease (Jerrett, McConnell and Wolch 2014; Kim et al. 2019). The combination of extreme heat (particularly in summers), lack of green space, air pollution, and cultural factors thus promote a sedentary lifestyle for many Cairenes, placing them at a health disadvantage.

As Kleerekoper et al. (2012, 30) put it, "[t]he relationship between climate and city is reciprocal; the climate influences the ways in which the city space is being used and the climatic performance and needs of buildings. In its turn, the city influences its climate." This reciprocal relationship between cities and their dwellers can work toward improving health and lifestyle in cities, while also helping to mitigate climate change. As many studies have shown, UHI can be mitigated by increasing green spaces, parks, and the number of trees in urban areas (Davies et al. 2008; Hamada et al. 2013; Kleerekoper et al. 2012; Solecki et al. 2005). The bright side to Cairo's urban form is that the majority of Cairo's buildings are buildings of between three and ten-floor height with flat roofs that are accessible for people to walk on. Residents use these roofs to raise poultry, for satellite dishes, for storage, or simply for disposal of debris and garbage (Attia and Amer 2009). Cairo's roofs also function as makeshift housing solutions for the poor. However, the majority of roof space in Cairo is currently unused space. This space provides Egyptians with massive potential to develop green spaces, notably rooftop gardens (RTGs).

ROOFTOP GARDENING AS AN INNOVATIVE FORM OF URBAN FOOD PRODUCTION

Green roofs provide a host of benefits for neighborhoods and communities, specifically for vulnerable groups. Research reveals that urban vegetation reduces temperatures and saves power costs for their respective buildings (Jaffal, Ouldboukhitine and Belarbi 2012; Tsilini et al. 2014; Sharma et al. 2018; Aboulnaga and Mostafa 2019). Green roofs also increase urban biodiversity (Kratschmer, Kriechbaum and Pachinger 2018), sequester CO_2 and remove pollutants from the air. Improved urban environmental conditions and lower health hazards mean lesser health costs to economically vulnerable residents (Peng and Jim 2015). Green roofs may also tackle both food insecurity and income inequality in one single step; produce from these roofs can alleviate food costs and insecurity, promote healthy eating as well as generating income for residents (Whittinghill and Rowe 2012), with specific potential for women and youth. Research also shows that rooftop gardening helps in building communities, as well as promoting social ties in an urban setting (Svendsen et al. 2012; Sonti and Svendsen 2018). Physical and mental health, including greater environmental fitness (less exposure to pollutants, removal of harmful substances from water by soil), less stress (thus reducing incidences of stroke, CVD, and other harmful outcomes) and improved mental health (particularly among women through physical activity), have been associated with green urban spaces (Robbins and Alicia 2015; United States Department of Agriculture 2018). These health benefits are particularly important for women in Cairo's informal neighborhoods who are mainly from traditional families who restrict movement due to cultural factors and household duties.

Cairo is thus clearly in need of urban green spaces, such as green roofs. This need has been acknowledged by the Egyptian Ministry of the Environment, who in cooperation with the German Society for International Cooperation is developing a green roof initiative across the country (Rashed 2019). According to Cairo's current governor, this is part of the sustainable plan to meet Egypt's 2030 vision (Egyptian Streets 2019). These plans are mainly aimed at the city's more affluent neighborhoods on the outskirts of Cairo, as well as the New Administrative Capital city, which lies 40 km east of Cairo. However, Cairo's current economic climate makes it necessary to approach and develop urban green spaces using an affordable model – one that could easily be implemented and maintained, especially in disadvantaged areas. This has been one of the goals of The American University in Cairo (AUC), who has installed, developed, and researched urban green roof systems particularly in Cairo's informal neighborhoods since 2013. The garden was designed and installed with assistance from the US Forest Service's International Programs section, which provides technical assistance on urban green spaces and farming in many countries around the world.

Urban agriculture and rooftop farming as a development solution for the African continent has received scholarly attention as early as the 1990s (Mougeot 1996). Urban farming in African countries such as Uganda or Senegal continues to be studied as a solution to growing urban congestion, degrading living conditions, and poverty (Adigbli 2012; Dubbeling 2011; Orsini et al. 2015; New York Food Policy Center 2019). Highly productive urban farms might also be one way to modernize Africa's farming systems, which researchers have recommended as a way to combat hunger (Harsch 2003). Urban farming is also a solution for improving food security and access to healthy food in the light of water scarcity and population growth – challenges that many African countries face. Bluegreen architecture and the increase of greenspace and planted areas in cities have become strategies for mediating climate change and its adverse effects, as urban plants absorb CO_2, increase shading, absorb pollution, and improve air quality (Depietri and McPhearson 2017; ClimateCentral 2018 [based on data from US Forest Service]).

In Egypt, universities, government research centers, NGOs, as well as foreign and local donors are driving rooftop-farming initiatives. Grants and corporate social responsibility initiatives have greatly assisted with spreading the idea of rooftop gardening and farming across Cairo. A growing number of rooftop-farming initiatives in the city applies a multitude of growing techniques, including media-based planting in barrels and planters and hydroponics and aquaponics systems. Media replacement mixes, usually on a peat and perlite base, are used as lightweight soil replacement in rooftop gardening solutions. Hydroponic systems are soilless growing systems where plant roots sit in water (there are various different systems, for example, deep water and nutrient film technique systems). Aquaponics systems are cyclic solutions in which water is used in a closed cycle for fish and crop farming. While all systems have been trialed on Cairo's roofs, most implemented pilot projects remain disconnected from each other. Recent announcement by Cairo's Governor to make rooftop farming a key strategy for achieving the SDGs, and the opening of a rooftop gardening unit within Egypt's Central Laboratory for Agricultural Climate (CLAC), may give rooftop farming in the city a further political push. In order to ensure that models and initiatives can become a widespread phenomenon across the city, solutions need to be replicable, affordable, sustainable, and easy to implement and operate. Some initiatives focus on creating rooftop farms as small businesses that give their operators an additional income. AUC's efforts, in turn, seek to establish community-based models that encourage residents of informal areas to grow their own food. This chapter analyzes these two approaches, comparing and contrasting their impact, feasibility, and sustainability.

Methodology

This chapter is based on data collection that took place between 2013 and 2019. Informal conversations with rooftop owners in Cairo's informal areas, numerous field trips and assessments to the neighborhoods of Matareya, El Khalifa, Geziret El Dahab, Stabl Antar, and Saft El Laban, meetings with local partner entities and roof owners, as well as the implementation process of 10 rooftop gardens in Cairo form the backdrop of this study. In 2018 and 2019, AUC researchers and students carried out additional sustainability assessments at three sites, as well as a comparative socio-economic study of two sites. This study included conducting a total of over 20 semi-structured, informal key informant interviews and multiple site assessment trips. In 2018, commercial rooftop gardening initiatives, including Schaduf and Urban Greens, were studied and visited. In 2019, researchers held two focus group events in the context of forming a network of rooftop garden actors in Cairo. At the network meetings, roof owners, representatives of NGOs, owners of rooftop-farming businesses, researchers, educators, and students discussed the challenges and opportunities of different rooftop gardening approaches in Cairo.

THE "URBAN COMMERCIAL FARM" MODEL – TURNING ROOFTOPS INTO PROFITABLE PRODUCTION SITES

Commercial farming on rooftops is a model that is being pursued in cities around the world, especially in the global north (Buehler and Jung 2016). This model emphasizes a high level of production for profit, with less attention given to participation or green space provision. Commercial farms are typically large-scale, or the result of a conglomeration of small farms, and tend to be more technologically sophisticated. The high cost of technology and the additional expenses involved with transporting inputs and products onto and off a roof can lead to high production cost, despite the fact that it can be more productive than conventional farming (informal conversation, Brooklyn Grange 2019). As a result, commercial rooftop farms often produce items for the high-end market, driven by the demand of customers who value specialized varieties or organic products, as well as that of restaurants and hotels. Some operators of commercial rooftop farms thus claim that current models of rooftop farming are not yet profitable on their own. Some enterprises choose to marry their food production efforts with other services, for example, the renting out of a rooftop event venue (informal conversation, Brooklyn Grange 2019).

In Cairo, there is no single large-scale rooftop food production initiative yet, but some companies have turned to producing leafy greens in greenhouse-based hydroponics systems. Schaduf, a landscape architecture and urban agriculture start-up founded in Egypt in 2011, is the first company to embark on a project of producing leafy greens on hundreds of rooftops across Cairo, marketed by one centralized entity. The company has since spread to numerous countries throughout the Middle East. Their stated vision is "to provide inspired green solutions that elevate the quality of life through social and environmental change" (Schaduf 2019). Schaduf's 500 Farm Project, launched in 2018, is funded through a grant from a Swiss foundation and aims at significantly boosting rooftop farming in Cairo, following an "urban commercial farm" model. Supplied with infrastructure and training by Schaduf, families across Cairo become part of a food production network that supplies Schaduf with produce, which Schaduf then markets to high-end consumers. Thus far, Schaduf has installed about 200 rooftop farm units in Helwan, a city on the southern edge of Greater Cairo. The project planned to have installed a further 300 units by the end of 2019.

For the 500 Farm Project, Schaduf has designed a simple NFT hydroponics system consisting of a 4×3 m table shaded by a canopy of shade cloth. The start-up partners with local NGOs to recruit families to participate in the project. The recruitment process includes site visits to ensure the structural integrity of the roof as well as the commitment of the household to managing and maintaining the system. Schaduf then holds a four-day training for potential beneficiaries, including training on how to operate the unit, how to conduct organic pest control, and crop-specific care methods, concluding with a practical planting session. About two-thirds of trainee families end up having a unit installed on their roof. Once the units have been installed, Schaduf determines which crops each household should grow based on seasonal variations and market demands. Crops include leafy vegetables such as lettuce, rocket (arugula), basil, and spinach. Each farm receives at least one extension visit per week from among the 10 project engineers and 20 supervisors who provide seeds and fertilizers and to ensure the rooftop systems are working properly. Schaduf has established contracts with main production marketing units, to which the families directly sell their produce. Part of the revenue goes toward paying for the engineers and supervisors and for inputs such as fertilizers and seeds, with the family pocketing about 800 EGP per table per month, equivalent to about 48 USD. Thus, each rooftop farm is designed to cover its own costs and generate revenue, theoretically ensuring long-term sustainability of the project, as extension specialists will still be providing support once the grant runs out.

According to a Schaduf representative, the biggest determinants of farm success under this model are discipline and commitment on the part of the growers. If a farm fails, it is usually because the household would not or could not devote enough time to its upkeep. To ensure that participating households develop a sense of ownership, families are required to pay Schaduf 200 EGP (12 USD) upfront for their unit and another 200 EGP (12 USD) out of their sales revenue, for a total of 400 EGP (about 24 US Dollars). The initiative encourages multiple members of a household, or even whole families, to participate in training events so that management of the farm is a shared effort. Thus far, the program has experienced a failure rate of about 5–10%. Schaduf seeks to continue to introduce new elements to the hydroponics systems, such as automatically timed irrigation pumps, to make the system easier to maintain. One of the challenges identified by Schaduf involves tying the family growers to the market. The volume of crop output from the rooftop farmers is highly variable and still very small, which makes buyers unwilling to enter into contracts. Production marketing units have to agree to a range of crop volume to expect, rather than a specific number.

Although successful in spreading the idea of rooftop food production across Cairo, the urban farm commercial production model means that food producers are removed from their own produce, which is consumed in other suburbs of Cairo. The final destination of the produce from the roofs is the high-end market, including large supermarket chains and specialty grocery stores, which cater to expatriates and the rich top tier of Egyptian society, in which there is a small but growing market segment for fresh and healthy food. The produce is sold at prices ranging from four to 40 times that of conventionally grown produce. At these prices, the produce is unattainable for most of the population, including the rooftop farmers themselves. Even if a growing number of rooftop units brings about economies of scale, Schaduf representatives themselves admit that this will not bring the price down to an affordable level. Thus, this model does little to contribute directly to improved food security or better diets among Cairo's vulnerable populations. Furthermore, the limited size of the upscale market, which the authors estimate to comprise about 2–5% of the total market, means that the potential for this model to expand is very limited. This niche market will be saturated before the full social and environmental benefits of urban farming can be realized.

However, one should not discount the positive effects of the 500 Farm Project's main goal; revenue generation for households in informal areas. The monthly profits from selling produce can be quite significant for families living in areas where the average salary may be less than 1,000 EGP (60 USD) per month (Gawad 2014).

Additionally, the program has given participating families the opportunity to learn about healthy diets, which Schaduf representatives report has motivated the beneficiaries to buy more leafy greens and vegetables for their own consumption using their new source of income. The company emphasizes the educational benefits provided by the program and the provision of new green gathering spaces on formerly derelict rooftops. In the longer run, it remains to be seen how Schaduf is able to ensure a sustainable business model that can financially carry itself once the 500 donor-funded rooftop farms have been put in place. This also concerns the marketing process, which in the current model relies entirely on Schaduf being present as a centralized marketing agency. The small farms are not designed to be stand-alone businesses and are thus relying on a functional overarching entity for their very survival and sustainability.

Another small but upcoming business initiative for rooftop gardening in Cairo that uses hydroponic growing systems is Urban Greens. Urban Greens is a local start-up founded in 2016 by two young men who have studied sustainability and rooftop gardening at university level, and apply their advanced technical knowledge in their respective careers. Their self-funded initiative has resulted in the construction of three rooftop farms located on the roofs of houses owned by a network of family and friends (Figure 12.1). The farms focus on soilless agriculture and are equipped with self-built hydroponic systems in which Urban Greens produce lettuce and other leafy greens, as well as cherry tomatoes and different types of herbs. The friends and business partners also conduct applied research at their facilities, testing the effect of different nutrient solutions, degrees of shading, pipe shapes, and crop varieties for productivity on rooftop farms in a hot, arid environment such as Cairo.

The founders of Urban Greens express a hope that their leading by good example may help to create a new food movement in Cairo that encourages pesticide-free,

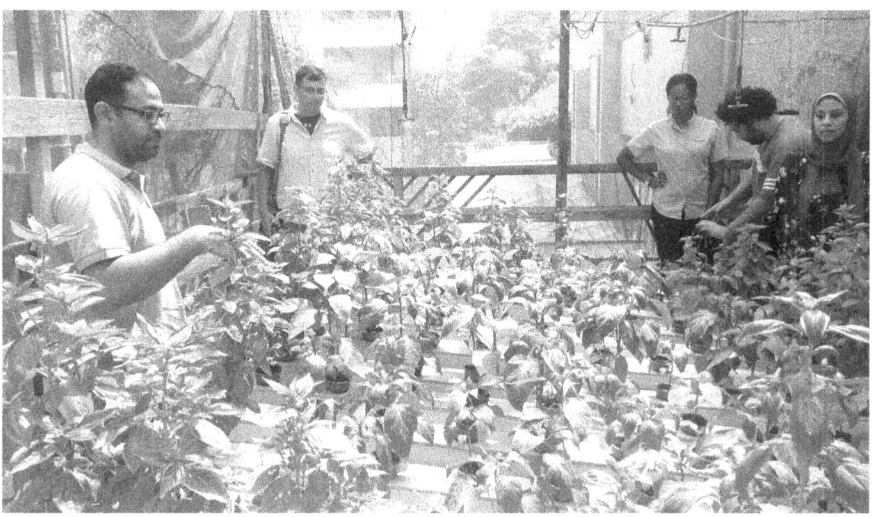

FIGURE 12.1 Urban Greens hydroponics farm in Heliopolis, Cairo.

clean, fresh, and local produce that is affordable to the public and sustainable to the environment. Having created a small model business without the input of donors, the partners want to demonstrate that, with relatively small financial input, it is possible to generate smart agriculture job opportunities in cities. Their systems do not depend on highly specialized and costly technology; rather, they are home-built systems that are tailored to local growing conditions and based as much as possible on locally sourced sustainable materials, such as reused PVC pipes. Besides selling their produce at farmers' markets and select supermarkets, Urban Greens offer tailor-made hydroponic system designs for those who are interested in starting their own rooftop farm. The company owners provide hydroponics consultancies and help interested individuals and companies develop their own business solutions. Believing in the importance of education and awareness, the company provides educational services in the form of theoretical and practical sessions, training courses, workshops, and site visits to their existing urban farms. They also partner with different stakeholders including community-based organizations to develop and implement socially responsible projects focusing on smart and sustainable soilless agriculture techniques. Through their presence at farmers' markets, exhibitions, and fairs, a regular presence in TV shows and documentaries, as well as through the implementation of gardens on the rooftops of company offices and international schools, Urban Greens help spread awareness about the concept of hydroponic rooftop farming in Cairo. Both Schaduf and Urban Greens are model initiatives for running rooftop farms as small commercial businesses by using intensive hydroponic growing systems. The second approach we assess here is one that does not specifically aim at providing rooftop owners with income, but that works to encourage entire urban communities to grow their own food.

COMMUNITY-BASED, NONCOMMERCIAL URBAN FARMING

Another model for urban gardening is household- or organizational-level rooftop farms that produce fresh food for personal consumption, or for sharing within the community. This model's goal is not to generate profit, but to encourage normal citizens, organizations, and other entities to start growing food on their roofs. Besides food production areas, such community-based farms can also include gathering spaces and aesthetic elements that add social and health benefits to food production. As there is no expected revenue stream in this approach, it is important that communities can afford the equipment and gardening inputs – both initially and in the longer run. At AUC, the Research Institute for a Sustainable Environment (later renamed Center for Applied Research on the Environment and Sustainability or CARES) carried out a research project on rooftop farming with technical and financial assistance from the US Forest Service between 2013 and 2019. The joint approach specifically aimed at developing and testing rooftop growing systems and processes that are affordable, easy to implement, operate and maintain, replicable, and scalable within the Egyptian context. The working model and research facility established on AUC's own roof showcased a variety of growing techniques, including an extensive green roof without drainage, several wooden tables, aquaponics and hydroponics system, a vertical farm, as well as barrels, pipes, and planters made from

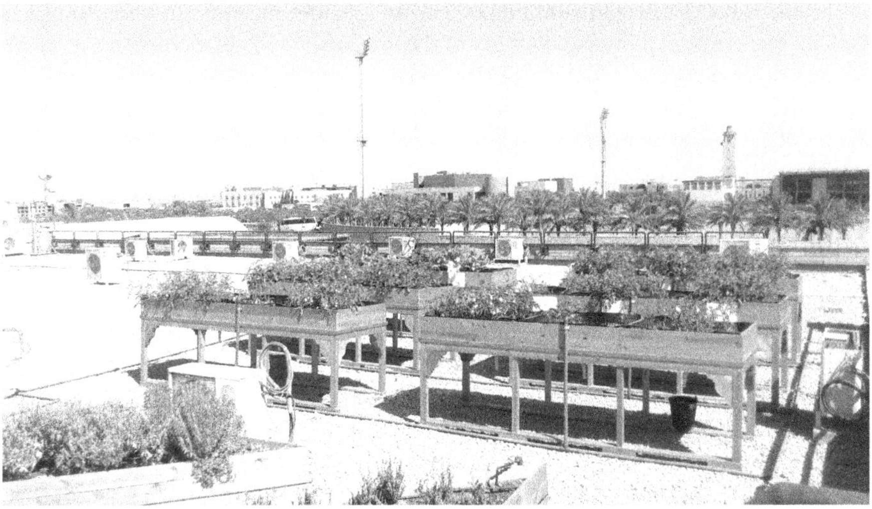

FIGURE 12.2 Rooftop garden and research facility at the American University in Cairo.

reused materials (Figure 12.2). The roof farm also served as a facility for applied research on shading techniques and the use of different fertilizers and growing media in order to fit the systems to the local conditions of climate and resource availability. AUC has also been able to generate funding to build 22 rooftop gardens in urban areas of Cairo, Fayoum, and Marsa Alam as part of development projects funded by corporate donors as part of CSR initiatives, development organizations, and foreign governments.

The projects implemented in different parts of Cairo include rooftop farms implemented on the roofs of schools, orphanages, an NGO that offers after school education programs, a library, an NGO that focuses on cultural heritage conservation, as well as on the roofs of citizens who are seen as local leaders and whose roofs are frequently accessed by neighbors. All of these projects were funded through grant projects and established as models aiming to incentivize replication by neighbors. All rooftop farms were built with materials that were chosen to be cost-effective and available in local neighborhoods. The projects included the implementation of simple wooden raised bed planters, halved plastic barrels with stands built from irrigation pipes, vertical pipe system as well as simple hydroponic systems that used either nutrient film technique (NFT) or deep water systems. Most systems are equipped with drip irrigation facilities. The materials were financed by the projects' budgets, while the community partners were responsible for preparing the roof (which sometimes included adding to the roof wall, improving staircases, or tiling the roof), contributing existing materials as well as labor. Most projects employed a participatory design, whereas some roofs were built using a Design Thinking Methodology process driven by AUC students. In all cases, the community partners and roof owners were heavily involved in the design and implementation of the roof farms. AUC, partly through the engagement of graduate students, has carried out initial research on the socio-economic and community impact of these projects. In order to assess the long-term impact and sustainability of the systems, more comprehensive research is required on how much rooftop garden construction might cost a family, how long the actual, real-life payback times are, what quantities of produce a rooftop garden can produce, and what benefits other than financial benefits can be measured.

The rooftop garden systems implemented as community models cost between 500 and 5,000 USD in total, depending on the size of the roof and the complexity and variety of the installed systems. Besides the planters, community members will have to invest in growing media that replaces heavy soil in rooftop planters. For this media, most commonly coco peat and perlite are used. These are imported materials available in Egypt, but comparatively costly. AUC has conducted research on replacing these inputs with locally available materials. Replacing drip irrigation systems with manual irrigation can further bring down the implementation costs. The running costs of roof farming systems are a challenge for rooftop garden owners in informal neighborhoods, as the yearly upkeep for a garden is estimated to cost between 50 and around 600 USD per year, depending on the type of system and garden size. However, recent research in the form of interviews with rooftop owners has shown that some gardens are able to provide local families with a significant portion of the family's need for fresh vegetables and herbs. As food prices in Cairo are rising, and fresh food is sometimes hard to come by in informal areas, families can save both money and effort by growing their own fresh food on their roofs. Beyond access to fresh food, however, these rooftop gardening owners have also expressed their joy of planting and seeing the plants grow, of being able to consume crops that they have grown themselves, and the pleasure of spending time among the greenery of their roof. Due to the lack of open, green spaces in informal neighborhoods, a seating area placed on a rooftop garden can feel like a small oasis in the midst of a concrete jungle. Our respondents have described the experience as breezy, quiet, relaxing, and soothing. Moreover, the improved rooftops serve as a new gathering space for families, neighbors, and friends. As one roof garden owner put it, the roof had become an equivalent to a living room, and guests of the family now headed straight to the roof instead of to the guest room inside the apartment. On the roofs of schools and educational NGOs, the gardens and farming systems serve as educational spaces where lessons are being carried out, where students spend their lunch breaks, and where individual children can adopt planters for a season, thus learning how to grow and look after plants. The gardens are thus not only spaces for hands-on learning but can also help develop stewardship for plants and green spaces in urban areas. In one informal neighborhood located on the outskirts of Cairo that was swallowed by the city's growth and that went from an agricultural area to a densely built jungle of multistory concrete and brick houses within a matter of ten years, the roof owners used to be farmers. Watching the vegetables grow on the roof of their eight-story building, the owners have expressed a feeling of having reclaimed lost green space for themselves and having restored at least some degree of a farming lifestyle in a brutally urbanized environment (Figure 12.3).

A rooftop gardening network recently founded by AUC project partners that involves several rooftop gardening entities, NGOs, companies, initiatives, and garden owners from Cairo, has identified the access to equipment, materials, input, and

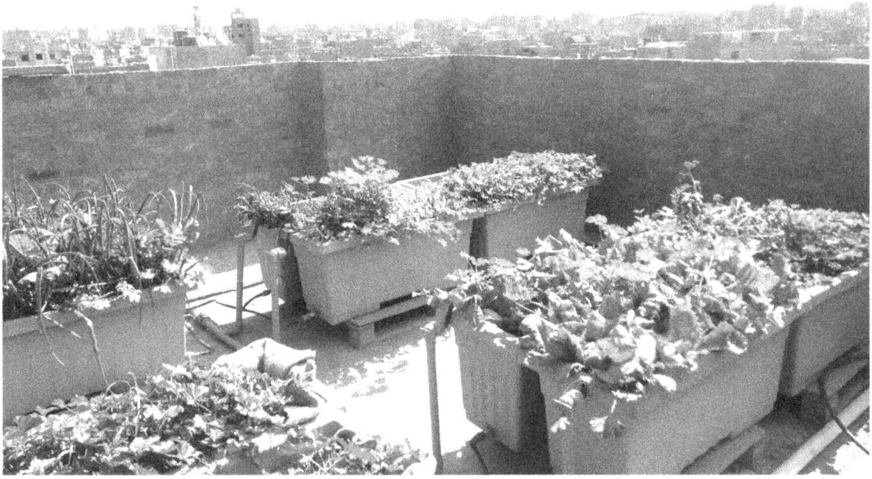

FIGURE 12.3 Rooftop garden at Mish Madrasa, an educational NGO in Saft El Laban, Cairo.

knowledge as one of the major challenges in making rooftop farming a mainstream activity in Cairo. As rooftop gardening in Cairo is not yet as common as it is in other countries, there are no shops as yet that are selling specialized rooftop gardening equipment – let alone in the informal and economically underprivileged neighborhoods of Cairo. One activity the newly formed rooftop gardening network is working on is a series of workshops and competitions (or "buildathons"), that will teach residents of informal areas to turn scrap material frequently found on rooftops into planters. Such knowledge will help residents of informal areas create rooftop farms at negligible costs, which will only leave the relatively low running costs of operation. Savings in purchasing vegetables for families will hopefully make up for the relatively low running costs the rooftop owners will have to bear.

Interviews conducted with garden owners and project partners have shown that, in order to upscale the systems that have been implemented in four different informal neighborhoods of Cairo, it is necessary to build up certain rooftops as gardening hubs. Such local hubs would work to spread rooftop-farming techniques across the neighborhood. It is necessary that there is at least one local champion or leader who ensures that there are informal training sessions, that neighbors learn from each other, and that the knowledge is spread across the neighborhood. In the case of one garden implemented in an informal neighborhood close to Cairo's historic Islamic quarter, the local champion has emerged to be a rapper who sings about the history of his informal neighborhood. Having become locally famous through a number of rap videos posted on his YouTube Channel, the young man has vouched to fight for his vision of greening and improving his neighborhood, while also improving urban access to fresh food (Figure 12.4). Through his YouTube Channel, he plans to release a new rap song about rooftop gardening, and thus hopes to spread the knowledge and awareness about urban farming far beyond the borders of his own neighborhood. In

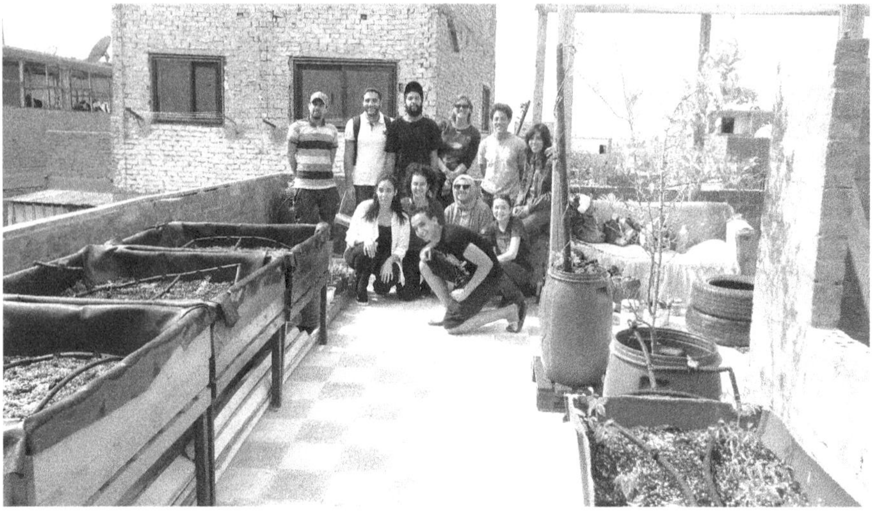

FIGURE 12.4 The local rapper "Khalifa" (center) on his rooftop garden designed in partnership with AUC students (rest of group), implemented with funding from the US Forest Service.

the case of the schools and educational NGOs, the hope is that the future champions will be all the children who are now taking their biology lessons on a roof farm, and who learn how to treasure and cultivate food in an urban space.

DISCUSSION AND CONCLUSIONS

As sustainability initiatives target food security in a context of climate change, water change, population growth, and urbanization in Africa, urban farming projects offer significant advantages. Unused urban spaces, for example, flat rooftops, can be utilized as farms that produce food for urban dwellers, either in the form of a business or for home consumption. Urban farming systems can be highly productive and water efficient, especially where drip irrigation, hydroponic and aquaponics systems are being implemented. One of the current challenges for turning urban farming into a widespread, mainstream practice in cities across Egypt and Africa, is to develop replicable, affordable models that can serve different purposes. We have presented case studies of two different approaches taken in Cairo, Egypt. One approach aims at providing dwellers of economically disadvantaged neighborhoods with an opportunity to use their roofs as small income-generating businesses. This is particularly interesting for female residents of informal areas, who are often culturally bound to the household and do not pursue formal employment. The fact that rooftop gardens are in easy reach for women based mainly at their homes, and that tending to a garden can be combined with other household chores, makes this farming solution particularly suitable for female entrepreneurs in Egypt. The additional monthly income can work as an incentive to promote the model, to facilitate the necessary initial investment and to cover longer-term costs. The relatively high success rate of the model presented shows that there is significant merit in the business approach, which also results in increasing the amount of locally produced food in urban areas.

While the farmers in this model are often not the food consumers, community-based approaches are seeking to turn city dwellers into producers of their own food. By building community hubs and movements of rooftop gardeners and farmers, this model aims at reducing household food expenditures while improving access to fresh food and health. In order to be successful, urban residents of lower-income neighborhoods have to be able to have access to knowledge and materials, as well as to afford both the initial materials as well as the longer-term inputs. Problematically, in all current approaches, inputs are still being covered largely by grants. Enabling rooftop owners to be able to build their own planters, or to learn how to turn unwanted materials into rooftop farms is a challenge that Cairo has yet to overcome. The models introduced here show that rooftop farming is more than a food production activity, as dwellers of densely packed neighborhoods that lack green spaces enjoy the greenery and mental health a rooftop garden can bring. Beyond producing food, we should not forget the social and educational functions, as well as the environmental and health benefits of rooftop gardens, as Cairo is embarking on a citywide initiative to green its roofs.

RECOMMENDATIONS

To date, there are currently no FAO guidelines specifically tailored to urban farming in an Egyptian context. International guidelines on urban agriculture aimed at developing countries urge local governments to promote urban agriculture through policy and tax incentives. Governments should incorporate these initiatives into their efforts to alleviate poverty and food security issues. Moreover, the guidelines stress building linkages between production and markets in order to create self-sufficient systems. Since commercializing this activity may lead to it becoming a more masculine domain, recommendations stress the importance of allowing women greater access to the market aspect of urban agriculture (FAO 2001).

Promoting food security through the creation of self-sufficient urban agriculture systems could not come at a more crucial time. They are of utmost importance given the recent COVID-19 pandemic, which threatens to negatively impact food security. A recent article in the leading Egyptian state newspaper, Al-Ahram, written in April 2020, states that Egypt is food secure for four months, but the pandemic threatens to increase food prices and cause shortages due to shipping difficulties – between rural and urban Egypt, as well as halted imports from other countries (Mounir 2020). Both food shortages and rising prices will take their toll on Egyptians, particularly on vulnerable lower-income urban populations. As lockdowns and physical distancing rules and practices have been binding people to their homes all over the world, people have been valuing the possibility to grow fresh food at home. In Cairo, the confinement to the small apartments in crowded neighborhoods has further limited daily contact with greenery and nature for many of the city's residents. Having access to greenery during the COVID-19 global pandemic has served as a mental outlet for rooftop garden owners, decreasing feelings of anxiety and providing a small space of freedom and normality during a time that has turned many of our urban habits and lifestyles upside down. Correspondence with rooftop garden owners in Cairo who have kept to their homes during the curfew periods revealed that their gardens have also encouraged them to follow healthier diets, while farming and maintenance tasks provided them with a daily sense of accomplishment.

The experience of going through a global pandemic such as COVID-19 shows us that transformations of our urban spaces can lead to overall healthier and more sustainable lives. Increasing green spaces and fostering rooftop gardening in Cairo may improve the city's future resilience to global challenges including pandemics and climate change. Based on FAO's guidelines and the author's own research and project experience, the following list presents recommendations that may help urban rooftop projects thrive within Cairo:

- Rooftop gardening programs should be integrated into Cairo's city strategy for meeting the SDGs. While the current focus is on constructing new developments away from the city center, goals to increase the per capita availability of green space across the city should be an integral part of future city planning strategies. This would not only count as a measure of climate change mitigation but would also increase shading, help prevent flooding and improve air quality and public health.
- There is a lack of awareness in Cairo about the potential benefits of rooftop gardening. Urban farming technologies and implementation should form part of teaching and learning at secondary and tertiary levels of education. Professional training courses for rooftop gardening could help establish a business landscape around rooftop gardening in Cairo.
- In order for rooftop gardening to become a widespread practice of urban farming in Cairo, it is necessary to spread the word about tested and successful cost-efficient, easy-to-build, and easy-to-maintain rooftop-farming systems. Current efforts of the Cairo Rooftop Gardening Alliance to support the uptake of the practice could be replicated and multiplied with the help of grants (for example through CSR), as well as similar volunteering initiatives.
- Small grants and tax incentives could provide motivation for residents of informal areas to invest in rooftop gardening technology. Special grants for youth and female entrepreneurs could help engage young people and women in urban food production.
- Business incubators and grant incentives could encourage entrepreneurs to start producing urban farming and rooftop gardening equipment in Egypt. The local production of simple sets and tool kits could help develop a widespread availability of rooftop gardening infrastructure across Cairo and other parts of Egypt. This plan should also incorporate and stress the role of women in the process, and allow them access to market elements.
- More research is needed regarding the quantitative impact of rooftop gardening in regard to socio-economic as well as environmental gains in Cairo. The availability of solid data for Cairo could help drive the necessary policies.

REFERENCES

Aboulnaga, M., and M. Mostafa. 2019. "Mitigating Heat Islands Effect in Mega Cities through Districts' Prioritisation for Urban Green Coverage Applications: Cairo – Egypt as a Case Study." *Renewable Energy and Environmental Sustainability 4* 5.

Abtew W., and A. Melesse. 2013. "Climate Change and Evapotranspiration." In *Evaporation and Evapotranspiration*, by W. Abtew and A. Melesseeds (eds), 197–202. Springer, Dordrecht.

Adigbli, K.E. 2012. "*Developing Senegal's Urban Agriculture*." *Inter Press Service*. http://www.ipsnews.net/2012/11/developing-senegals-urban-agriculture/.

aldinger

Alebshehy, R., N.M. Shuaib, J.D. Mbako, D. Barffo, and R.K. Nuotol. 2016. "Determinant Analysis of Obesity among Adult Females in Egypt." *Egyptian Journal of Hospital Medicine 65* 662–669.

Amer, M.H., S.A. Abd El Hafez, and M.B. Abd El Ghany. 2017. "Water Saving In Irrigated Agriculture in Egypt." *International Commission on Irrigation and Drainage (ICID)*. https://www.icid.org/WatsrSaving_Egypt.pdf.

Attia, S., and A. Amer, 2009. "Green Roofs in Cairo; A Holistic Approach for Healthy Production Cities." Procedures of the Annual Greening Rooftops for Sustainable Communities Conference, Atlanta, GA.

Bayat, A., and E. Denis. 2000. "Who Is Afraid of Ashwaiyyat? Urban Change and Politics in Egypt." *Environment and Urbanization 12*(2) 185–199.

Bishu, S.G., and M.G. Alkadry. 2017. A Systematic Review of the Gender Pay Gap and Factors That Predict It. *Administration and Society 49*(1): 65–109.

Brooklyn Grange. 2019. Informal Conversation with the Owner during a Tour of the Facility. New York City. https://www.brooklyngrangefarm.com.

Buehler, D., and R. Jung. 2016. "Global Trends and Current Status of Commercial Urban Rooftop Farming." *Sustainability 8* 1108–1124.

Butler, J. 1990. *Gender Trouble*. Routledge, New York/Oxon.

Central Agency for Public Mobilization and Statistics. 2020. *Central Agency for Public Mobilization and Statistics*. https://www.capmas.gov.eg/HomePage.aspx?lang=2.

ClimateCentral. 2018. "The Power of Trees." Tools Developed with Data from the US Forest Service. www.climatecentral.org.

Davies, R.G., O. Barbosa, R.A. Fuller, J. Tratalos, N, Burke, D. Lewis, P.H. Warren, and K.J. Gaston. 2008. "City-Wide Relationships between Green Spaces, Urban Land Use and Topography." *Urban Ecosystems 11* 269–287.

Debbage, N., and J. Marshall Shepherd. 2015. "The Urban Heat Island Effect and City Contiguity." *Computers, Environment and Urban Systems 54* 181–194.

Denis, E. 2006. "Cairo as Neo-Liberal Capital? From Walled City to Gated Communities." In *Cairo Cosmopolitan: Politics, Culture, and Urban Space in the New Globalized Middle East*, by D. Singerman, and P. Amar (eds), 44–72. American University in Cairo Press, Cairo.

Depietri, Y., and T. McPhearson. 2017. "Integrating the Grey, Green, and Blue in Cities; Nature-Based Solutions for Climate Change Adaptation and Risk Reduction." In *Nature-Based Solutions to Climate Change Adaptation in Urban Areas. Theory and Practice of Urban Sustainability Transitions*, by N. Kabisch, H. Korn, J. Stadler, and A. Bonn, 91–110. Springer, Cham.

Dubbeling, M. 2011. "Integrating Urban Agriculture in the Urban Landscape." *Urban Agriculture Magazine 25* 43–46.

Egypt Today. 2019. 32.5% of Egyptians Live in Extreme Poverty; CAPMAS. August 1. https://www.egypttoday.com/Article/1/73437/32-5-of-Egyptians-live-in-extreme-poverty-CAPMAS.

Egyptian Streets. 2019. Cairo to Begin Planting Gardens on Rooftops. July 15. https://egyptianstreets.com/2019/07/15/cairo-to-begin-planting-gardens-on-rooftops/.

El Baradei, L. 2019. "Egypt's Currency Devaluation & Impact on the Most Vulnerable." *International Relations and Diplomacy* 7(07) 303–316.

Food and Agriculture Organization of the United Nations (FAO). 2001. *Urban and Peri-Urban Agriculture: A Briefing Guide for the Successful Implementation of Urban and Peri-Urban Agriculture in Developing Countries and Countries of Transition*. http://www.fao.org/fileadmin/templates/FCIT/PDF/briefing_guide.pdf.

Food and Agriculture Organization of the United Nations (FAO). 2006. Food Security. Policy Brief June 2006 Issue 2.

Foucault, M. 1990. *The History of Sexuality, Volume 1*. Vintage Books, New York.

Galal, O. 2002. "The Nutrition Transition in Egypt: Obesity, Undernutrition and the Food Consumption Context." *Public Health Nutrition 5(1A)* 141–148.

Game, I., and R. Primus. 2015. *Urban Agriculture*. GSDR 2015 Brief published by the United Nations. 1–13.

Gawad, I.O. 2014. "The Rise of Rooftop Gardens in Informally Developed Areas in Egypt; Exploring the Abilities and Boundaries." *ArchCairo 6th International Conference Proceedings* 208–223. ARCHCAIRO 2014, Cairo.

General Organization for Physical Planning (GOPP) Egypt. 2009. Vision of Cairo 2050: Within a National Vision of Egypt. https://cairofrombelow.files.wordpress.com/2011/08/cairo-2050-vision-v-2009-gopp-12-mb.pdf.

Global Food Security Index. 2018. *International Food Security Map*. http://foodsecurityindex.eiu.com/.

Goldstein, M. 2011. *Urban Agriculture: A Sixteen City Survey of Urban Agriculture Practices across the Country*. Page 4. Retrieved from http://www.georgiaorganics.org/Advocacy/urbanagreport.pdf.

Hamada, S., T. Tanaka and T. Ohta. 2013. "Impacts of Land Use and Topography on the Cooling Effect of Green Areas on Surrounding Urban Areas." *Urban Forestry & Urban Greening 12* 426–434.

Harsch, E. 2003. "Senegal: To Fight Hunger, Modernize Farming." *Africa Recovery 17*(1) 14.

Hassan-Wassef, H. 2004. "Food Habits of the Egyptians: Newly Emerging Trends." *East Mediterr Health Journal 10*(6) 898–915.

Hendrickson, M.K. and M. Porth. 2012. *"Urban Agriculture — Best Practices and Possibilities. University Of Missouri Division of Applied Social Sciences*." http://extension.missouri.edu/foodsystems/urbanagriculture.aspx.

Ivers, L.C., and Cullen, K.A. 2011. "Food Insecurity: Special Considerations for Women." *American Journal of Clinical Nutrition 94*(6) 1740S–1744S.

Jaffal, I., S.-E. Ouldboukhitine, and R. Belarbi. 2012. "A Comprehensive Study of the Impact of Green Roofs on Building Energy Performance." *Renewable Energy 43* 157–164.

Jaskolski, M. 2016. "Managing Egypt's Limited Supply of Fresh Water – Challenges of Sustainability, Water Scarcity and Food Security." *German Science Monitor* 3–8. December.

Jelili, O. 2012. "Urbanisation and Future of Cities in Africa: The Emerging Facts and Challenges to Planners." *Global Journal of Human Social Science 12*(7) 6–12.

Jerrett, M., J. McConnell, and L. Wolch. 2014. "Traffic-Related Air Pollution and Obesity Formation in Children: A Longitudinal, Multilevel Analysis." *Environmental Health 13* 49.

Khafaie, M.A., Yajnik, C.S., Salvi, S.S., and Ojha, A., 2016. "Critical Review of Air Pollution Health Effects with Special Concern on Respiratory Health." *Journal of Air Pollution and Health 1*(2) 123–136.

Khedr, M. 2019. "Challenges and Issues in Water, Climate Change, and Food Security in Egypt." In *Conventional Water Resources and Agriculture in Egypt*, by A.M. Negm (ed), 229–243. Springer, Cham.

Kim, J.S., Chen, Z., Aldereteb, T.L., Toledo-Corral, C., Lurmann, F., Berhane, K., and Gilliland, F.D. 2019. "Associations of Air Pollution, Obesity and Cardiometabolic Health in Young Adults: The Meta-AIR Study." *Environment International 133* 105180.

Kleerekoper, L., M. van Esch, and T. Baldiri Salcedo. 2012. "How to Make a City Climate-Proof, Addressing the Urban Heat Island Effect." *Resources, Conservation and Recycling 64* 30–38.

Kratschmer, S., M. Kriechbaum, and B. Pachinger. 2018. "Buzzing on Top: Linking Wild Bee Diversity, Abundance and Traits with Green Roof Qualities." *Urban Ecosystems 21* 429–446.

Ministry of Planning, Monitoring and Administrative Reform (MPAR). 2018. "Egypt's Voluntary National Review 2018." Sustainable Development Goals Knowledge Platform. https://sustainabledevelopment.un.org/content/documents/20269EGY_VNR_2018_final_with_Hyperlink_9720185b45d.pdf.

Ministry of Water Resources and Irrigation, Egypt. 2014. *"Water Scarcity in Egypt."* https://drive.google.com/drive/folders/0B3XQwpMpDWiXUVh1ZHBfdW1DZ3c.

Moghadam, V.M. 2004. "Women and the Changing Family in the Middle East." *Journal of Comparative Family Studies 35*(2) 137–163.

Mostafa, A.N., A.S. Zakey, A.S. Monem, and M.M. Abdel Wahab. 2018. "Analysis of the Surface Air Quality Measurements in the Greater Cairo (Egypt) Metropolitan." *Global Journal of Advanced Research 5*(6) 207–214.

Mougeot, L.J.A. 1996. "An Improving Domestic and International Environment for African Urban Agriculture." *African Urban Quarterly 11* 137–153.

Mounir, S. 2020. "Egypt: Is Food Secure?" http://english.ahram.org.eg/NewsContent/50/1202/366809/AlAhram-Weekly/Economy/Egypt-is-food-secure.aspx.

New York Food Policy Center. 2019. "Micro Gardens, Senegal: Urban Food Policy Snapshot." http://www.nycfoodpolicy.org/senegal-microgardens/.

Oke, T.R. 2011. "Urban Heat Islands." In *The Routledge Handbook of Urban Ecology*, by I. Douglas, D. Goode, M. Houck, and R. Wang (eds), 120–131. Routledge, Abingdon, Oxon.

Orsini, F., R. Kahane, R. Non-Womdim, and G. Gianquinto. 2015. "Urban Agriculture in the Developing World: A Review." *Agronomy for Sustainable Development 33*(4) 695–720.

Orru, H., Ebi, K.L. & Forsberg, B. 2017. "The Interplay of Climate Change and Air Pollution on Health." *Current Environmental Health Reports 4* 504–513.

Peng, L.L.H., and C.Y. Jim. 2015. "Economic Evaluation of Green-Roof Environmental Benefits in the Context of Climate Change: The Case of Hong Kong." *Urban Forestry & Urban Greening 14*(3) 554–561.

Radwan, T., G. Blackburn, D. Whyatt, and P. Atkinson. 2019. "Dramatic Loss of Agricultural Land Due to Urban Expansion Threatens Food Security in the Nile Delta, Egypt." *Remote Sensing 11*(3) 332.

Rajagopalan, S., Al-Kindi, S.G., Brook, R.D. 2018. "Air Pollution and Cardiovascular Disease: *JACC* State-of-the-Art Review." *Journal of the American College of Cardiology 72*(17) 2054–2070.

Rashed, M. 2019. *"EGP Government Starts Green-Roofing Initiative and Here's Why You Should Follow."* October 10. https://scoopempire.com/egp-government-starts-green-roofing-initiative-and-heres-why-you-should-follow/.

Robbins, K.L., and S.T. Alicia. 2015. "Metro Nature, Environmental Health, and Economic Value." *Environmental Health Perspectives 123*(5) 390–398.

Rock-Singer, A. 2016. "The Salafi Mystique: The Rise of Gender Segregation in 1970s Egypt." *Islamic Law and Society 23* 279–305.

Sarant, L. 2017. "Egypt: Space to Grow." *Nature 544* S14–S16.

Schaduf. 2019. *About Schaduf.* https://schaduf.com/.

Sharma, A., S. Woodruff, M. Budhathoki, A.F. Hamlet, F. Chen, and H.J.S. Fernando. 2018. "Role of Green Roofs in Reducing Heat Stress in Vulnerable Urban Communities — A Multidisciplinary Approach." *Environmental Research Letters 13*(5) 094011.

Shirisa, I., and A. Matamanda. 2016. “Addressing Urban Poverty in Africa in the Post-2015 Period. Perspectives for Adequate and Sustainable Housing.” *Journal of Settlements and Spatial Planning* 7(1) 79–87.

Sims, S., M. Sejoume and M. El Shorbagi. 2003. *“Understanding Slums: Case Studies for the Global Report on Human Settlements 2003.”* Development Planning Unit Multimedia Projects, London. http://www.ucl.ac.uk/dpu-projects/Global_Report/pdfs/Cairo.pdf.

Smith, J., L. Deck, B. McCarl, P. Kirshen, J. Malley, M. Abd Rabo, and United Nations Development Program. 2013. *Potential Impacts of Climate Change on the Egyptian Economy.* http://www.eeaa.gov.eg/portals/0/eeaaReports/CCRMP/6.%20Potential%20Impact%20of%20Climate%20Change%20on%20the%20Egyptian%20Economy/Potential%20Impact%20of%20CC%20on%20the%20Egyptian%20Economy%20English.pdf.

Solecki, W.D., C. Rosenzweig, L. Parshall, G. Pope, M. Clark, J. Cox, and M. Wiencke. 2005. “Mitigation of the Heat Island Effect in Urban New Jersey.” *Global Environmental Change Part B: Environmental Hazards* 6(1) 39–49.

Sonti, N.G., and E.S. Svendsen. 2018. “Why Garden? Personal and Abiding Motivations for Community Gardening in New York City.” *Society and Natural Resources 31*(10) 1189–1205.

Svendsen, E.S., L.K. Campbell, N. Falxa-Raymond, J. Northridge, E. Stone, and C. Mees. 2012. “Introducing a Longitudinal Study of Community Gardeners and Gardens in New York City.” *Cities and the Environment (CATE) 5*(1) 11.

Toth, J. 1991. “Pride, Purdah and Paychecks: What Maintains the Gender Division of Labor in Rural Egypt?” *International Journal of Middle East Studies 23*(2) 213–236.

Tsilini, V., S. Papantoniou, D.-D. Kolokotsa, and E.-A. Maria. 2014. “Urban Gardens as a Solution to Energy Poverty and Urban Heat Island.” *Sustainable Cities and Society 14* 323–333.

UN Environmental Program. 2005. Potential Impact of Sea Level Rise: Nile Delta. https://www.grida.no/resources/6479.

UNICEF. 2014. Egypt Demographic and Health Survey 2014. www.unicef.org/egypt/reports/egypt-demographic-and-health-survey-2014.

UNICEF Egypt. 2019. Country Background: Egypt. https://www.unicef.org/egypt/country-background#_ftn1.

United Nations. 2016. Final List of Proposed Sustainable Development Goal Indicators. https://sustainabledevelopment.un.org/content/documents/11803Official-List-of-Proposed-SDG-Indicators.pdf.

United Nations. 2019. #Envision2030: 17 Goals to Transform the World for Persons with Disabilities. https://www.un.org/development/desa/disabilities/envision2030.html.

United States Department of Agriculture. 2018. “Urban Nature for Human Health and Well-Being.” https://www.fs.fed.us/sites/default/files/fs_media/fs_document/urbannatureforhumanhealthandwellbeing_508_01_30_18.pdf.

van Ittersum, M.K., L.G.J. van Bussel, J. Wolf, P. Grassini, J. van Wart, N. Guilpart, and L. Claessens. 2016. Can Sub-Saharan Africa Feed Itself? Proceedings of the National Academy of Sciences, Dec 12, 2016. https://www.pnas.org/content/early/2016/12/07/1610359113.

Voogt, J.A., and T.R. Oke. 2003. “Thermal Remote Sensing of Urban Climates.” *Remote Sensing of Environment 86* 370–384.

Walseth, K., and K. Fasting. 2003. “Islam’s View on Physical Activity and Sport Egyptian Women Interpreting Islam.” *International Review for the Sociology of Sport 38*(1) 45–60.

Whittinghill, L.J., and D.B. Rowe. 2012. “The Role of Green Roof Technology in Urban Agriculture.” *Renewable Agriculture and Food Systems 27* 314–322.

World Bank. 2018. Urban Population (% of Total Population). https://data.worldbank.org/indicator/SP.URB.TOTL.IN.ZS.

World Bank. 2019. Poverty & Equity Brief, Arab Republic of Egypt. April. https://databank.worldbank.org/data/download/poverty/33EF03BB-9722-4AE2-ABC7-AA2972D68AFE/Archives-2019/Global_POVEQ_EGY.pdf.

World Bank. 2020. *Urban Development*. https://www.worldbank.org/en/topic/urbandevelopment/overview.

World Health Organization — Eastern Mediterranean Regional Office. 2020. *Obesity*. http://www.emro.who.int/health-topics/obesity/.

World Population Review. 2019. *Cairo Population 2019*. http://worldpopulationreview.com/world-cities/cairo-population/.

Yount K.M., K.E. VanderEnde, S. Dodell, and C. Yuk Fei. 2016. "Measurement of Women's Agency in Egypt." *Social Indicators Research 128* 1171–1192.

13 The Bee City Movement in Canada

Jennifer Marshman

CONTENTS

INTRODUCTION[1]

Crisis in the Anthropocene

We are in the midst of what is being called a mass extinction (Kolbert 2014; Thomas et al. 2004; Wake & Vredenburg 2008). Multiple factors, including a changing climate, are contributing to mass species extinctions and the myriad socio-ecological crises of our time. These crises are not random or passive – they are directly linked to human activity (IPCC 2018; Schultz 2011). As we approach an uncertain future faced with the accelerating impacts of a changing global climate and an unprecedented rate of species extinctions and resource depletion, some of our most vital life support systems are degrading including many of the key elements in healthy and diverse systems of food production. Of particular concern in this new epoch is the decline in health, and in numbers, of many pollinating insects. Human and ecological health is dependent on pollinators in myriad, interconnected ways, from providing food, fiber, and medicine, to supporting the very web of life that sustains living organisms on Earth. In this chapter, we probe the food–people–nature nexus and address the links between people and nature through the food system.

One of the most salient expressions of this nexus is the relationship between people and pollinators, and the human dimensions of pollinator conservation. In particular, we highlight the important contribution of bees to ecosystem health and resilience.

DOI: 10.1201/9781003014942-13

This chapter draws on doctoral research in human geography at Wilfrid Laurier University, Waterloo, Ontario, Canada (Marshman 2019; Marshman, Blay-Palmer, & Landman 2019). In it, we ask if and how municipalities can play a role in pollinator conservation, especially in urban spaces, and we introduce the Bee City movement. Healthy and diverse pollinator populations can help "ensure plant–pollinator phenological synchrony," or the seasonal timing of pollinator emergence in the spring with the flowering of plants that they pollinate (Bartomeus et al. 2013, 331; Memmott et al. 2007). Given the importance of pollinators to diverse and nutrient-dense diets for people and myriad other species, this is of great topical concern.

Evidence indicates that there are significant declines in both insect biomass and on the plant species that are dependent on insect pollination (Biesmeijer et al. 2006; Hallmann et al. 2014; Kopek & Bird 2017). A 2019 review shows that over 40% of insects are at risk of extinction globally over the next few decades (Sanchez-Bayo & Wyckhuys 2019). It is important to understand the human dimensions of human–pollinator interactions, since human activity is responsible for creating the conditions that threaten these populations of pollinating insects, including habitat fragmentation and destruction and anthropogenic climate change. Through the Bee City movement, municipalities can play an important role in drawing attention to pollinator conservation and act as a catalyst for stewardship and action toward climate change mitigation. While Bee Cities have the potential to perpetuate a dysfunctional and unsustainable system of socio-ecological production (including food systems), the positive benefits of creating new forms of production and inclusion can help to dismantle some of these detrimental conditions.

The Bee City Movement

The Bee City movement began in the United States in Asheville, North Carolina in 2012, through the vision of pollinator advocate Phyllis Stiles and members of the Buncombe County Chapter of the North Carolina State Beekeeping Association. In June 2018, Bee City USA joined the Xerces Society for Invertebrate Conservation. This organization protects the natural world through the conservation of invertebrates and their habitats (Bee City USA 2019; Xerces Society 2021). In 2016, environmentalist Shelly Candel championed the movement in the City of Toronto, making Toronto the first Bee City in Canada. The numbers of Bee Cities continue to grow year by year in both Canada and the United States. At the time of writing, there are 48 Bee Cities in Canada, including 32 in Ontario where research interviews took place, and 127 in the United States. In Canada, schools, businesses, and faith groups have also received the Bee City designation, in addition to the municipal affiliates.

Bee Cities sign a resolution to support and protect bees and other pollinators by creating habitat, celebrating achievements, and raising awareness through education. Bee Cities require commitment and action from local officials who work with concerned citizens to establish how these criteria will be enacted. Small-scale, local predictions of climate change are difficult, but municipalities are uniquely situated to understand their local mitigation and adaptation needs. Place-based planning can play a key role in climate adaptation strategies (Marshman, Blay-Palmer, & Landman 2019; Measham et al. 2011).

Bee Cities commit to pollinator education, celebration, and habitat creation, but the ways in which Bee Cities do this is determined at the local level. These conservation strategies help to create the space needed for Bee City affiliates to highlight and maximize their existing policies and programs (Bee City USA 2019), as well as build on and create new measures to support and protect pollinators.

METHODS

This research was done using a multi-site, collective case study of the Bee City movement in Canada. Data collection took place between October 2018 and July 2019 through 41 interviews with Bee City board members, volunteers, and municipal staff, ranging in length from 0.5 to 2 hours. Participant observation, surveys, and document analysis also contribute to overall theme development. Seventeen of the eighteen Bee Cities that were recognized in Ontario during the research period participated in this qualitative study.

Interview participants were asked questions on the following topics: motivations for becoming a Bee City, perspectives on the need for such a program, barriers and facilitators to implementation, details about their working group, project goals and sustainability, champions within their program, and overall Bee City plan. A thematic, interpretivist analysis was undertaken with interview transcripts using NVivo v12. This research was funded by the Social Sciences and Research Council of Canada (SSHRC), with support from Wilfrid Laurier University and the Laurier Centre for Sustainable Food Systems and is approved by the Laurier Research Ethics Board.

WHY THE CONCERN FOR BEES?

There are an estimated 20,000 species of bees on Earth, of which seven are honey bees of the genus Apis (Sen Nag 2018). The European honey bee *Apis mellifera* is the most widely managed pollinator on Earth with an estimated 81 million hives (IPBES 2016) with hives housing up to 100,000 bees (Canadian Honey Council 2018). Commercial hives are mobile and can be physically moved between locations to provide pollination services. Hives are managed similarly to other domesticated animals such as chickens, sheep, or pigs. Globally, pollination has an estimated market value of up to $577 billion USD annually (IPBES 2016).

Mainstream concerns for bees grew in response to colony collapse disorder (CCD), which widely affected beekeepers in the United States in 2006/2007 (Atkins & Atkins 2016; Suryanarayanan & Kleinman 2016). CCD is the name given to the phenomenon when entire managed colonies die off or disappear suddenly (Atkins & Atkins 2016; Kosek 2011; Suryanarayanan & Kleinman 2016). While CCD is less of a burden than it was a decade ago, the overall health of the managed honey bees and seasonal colony losses continue to be concerning for bee keepers around the world. There is concern for bees across continents and generations. From primary schools (Blackawton et al. 2011), to horticultural groups (Ontario Horticultural Association 2010), to mass media campaigns (General Mills 2020), the European honey bee has become something of a charismatic micro-fauna or flagship species (Marshman

2019; Matteson & Langellotto 2010). Flagship species are defined as "popular charismatic species that serve as symbols and rallying points to stimulate conservation awareness and action" (Barua, Gurdak, Ahmed, & Tamuly 2012, 1458).

While tracking and quantifying populations and losses are well established for the European honey bee, data for the health and numbers of North America's 4,000 native bee species are conspicuously lacking (Colla & MacIvor 2017). Overall, there is evidence that wild pollinators are in decline, both in numbers and in distribution (Baldock et al. 2015; Colla 2016; FAO 2018; Godfray et al. 2014; Goulson 2013; OMAFRA 2016; Wojcik et al. 2018). Available data also indicates that more than half of the known ~4,000 native bee species in North America are in decline with nearly one in four at risk of extinction (Kopec & Burd 2017).

For some, there is a direct cognitive pathway between bees and honey. However, of the estimated 20,000 species of bees on Earth, only a few produce honey that is collected by humans. Most bees are ground-nesting bees who tend their own nests without the help of a colony or workers the way honey bees do. In terms of pesticides, honey bees are the only insect model for regulatory pesticide risk assessments (Franklin & Raine 2019); they are favored for their extensive breeding programs and easy mobility in constructed hives. According to formal assessment standards (e.g., the International Union for Conservation of Nature's Red List of Threatened Species, the Canadian Species at Risk), the European honey bee is not at risk of extinction, and yet remains the focus of conservation politics and best management practice interventions (Chan et al. 2019; Colla & MacIvor 2017). Gaps in our understanding of the status of wild, unmanaged, bees resulting from this "surrogacy approach" (Franklin & Raine 2019, 1) further increase the risk to many native bee species through exclusion from marketing, education, policy, and planning considerations.

Along with the ecosystem services provided to people, wild pollinating insects are considered a keystone species (USDA n.d., 2), defined as "the glue that holds a habitat together" (Denchak 2019). Pollinators are needed to help maintain healthy ecosystems and are essential for plant reproduction and plant diversity which can help to mitigate climate shocks. The presence (or absence) of wild pollinators can reflect the health of an ecosystem making them important bioindicators (Naeem et al. 2020). This is important because indicator species can help with strategic conservation as well as help with biodiversity monitoring (Ibid), One Bee City volunteer said, "people know about bees, and the peril of bees, because of honey bees." In this way, bees are uniquely situated to inspire their own rallying call – to act as a gateway to (re)connect people with the rest of nature, through their charismatic presence and importance in ecosystems.

CLIMATE CHANGE, POLLINATORS, AND FOOD

Climate change negatively affects availability, access, utilization, and stability of food security (Mbow et al. 2019) and negative impacts on global crop production are already apparent (Ray et al. 2019). In the coming decades, food systems will face increasing demand from a growing global population as well as increasing environmental pressures from climate change which will impact the quality and quantity of food (Myers et al. 2017). The consumption of resource intensive food, such as meat and dairy, is rising in emerging economies (Ranganathan et al. 2016). Along with the additional contributions to atmospheric greenhouse gasses, these changes are likely to create new landscapes of food production including deforestation through subsistence activities and large-scale commercial agricultural activities which further reduces habitat and forage for pollinating insects. Conversely, awareness of the foraging needs of pollinating insects can help to draw attention to mitigative ecosystem management (Table 13.1).

A changing climate is also concerning due to disruptions to seasonal timing of pollinator emergence and the flowering of plants (Memmott et al. 2007). In North America and Europe, bumble bee species are not moving northward with the warming trend in addition to losing their southern range limits. This timing disruption results in a decoupling of plants and pollinators which impacts plant fertility (Hegland et al. 2009; Kearns, Inouye, and Waser 1998). An overreliance on managed bees as a monocultural pollination system, could further exacerbate the risks associated with a loss of biodiversity and Millenia of plant–pollinator coevolution.

Pollinator-dependent crops contribute an estimated 35% of global crop volume, including the foods that provide people with many vitamins and nutrients that lead to a healthful diet (Eilers et al. 2011) (Table 13.1). Micronutrient deficiencies, also known as hidden hunger, can prevent people from thriving and cause irreversible health effects. There are currently an estimated 2 billion people suffering from hidden hunger globally. Pollinators provide important ecosystem services through pollination

TABLE 13.1
Select Contributions of Pollinating Insects to Achievement of the Sustainable Development Goals

Sustainable Development Goals: Goal 1
SDG 1 is concerned with ending poverty in all forms. Pollinators contribute positively in both direct and indirect ways. Directly, beekeeping can provide a source of income in urban and rural settings. Indirectly, many smallholder farmers can benefit from education around the important contributions of both wild and managed bees to sustainable crop production.
Sustainable Development Goals: Goal 2
SDG 2 is concerned with improved nutrition and promoting sustainable agriculture. Given the significant contribution of pollinating insects to crop success, any discussion about nutritious and healthful diets necessarily includes pollinator health.
Sustainable Development Goals: Goal 13
SDG 13 is concerned with action to combat climate change. Awareness of the foraging needs of pollinating insects can help to draw attention to mitigative ecosystem management.
Sustainable Development Goals: Goal 15
SDG 15 is concerned with protecting, restoring, and promoting sustainable use of terrestrial ecosystems. Pollinators contribute significantly to the diversity of flowering plants providing food and resources for people and other animals.

that contributes more than 90% of the vitamin C, 100% of Lycopene and the majority of the antioxidants β-cryptoxanthin and β-tocopherol, lipids, vitamin A and related carotenoids, calcium and fluoride, and a large portion of folic acid in healthful diets (Eilers et al. 2011, e21363). These numbers make it clear that declines in pollinator populations could result in further increases in non-communicable diseases, especially in existing at-risk populations (Marshman, Blay-Palmer, & Landman 2019).

Significant financial implications are also projected with pollinator declines. The loss of pollinators could result in a loss of between US$235 billion and US$577 billion in annual global crop output (IPBES 2016). A lack of wild pollinators in large-scale monocropping systems creates an overreliance on managed honey bees and associated risks and costs. For example, an estimated 75% of all commercial hives in the United States are employed for the California almond bloom (Bond, Plattner, & Kevin 2014), and gross revenue from pollination services by managed honey bees was an estimated $655.6 million in 2012 (Ibid). A loss of bees who account for an estimated 70% of pollination could lead to an increasing pollination problem requiring supplemental hand pollination which is already happening in places like China, Brazil, and Uganda. In addition, hand pollination has been shown to be unsustainable due to both time constraints and the extremely high cost of human labor (Partap & Ya 2012).

In North America, we do not know the true impacts of a need to manually pollinate plants beyond human food crops, such as those needed to provide the food and resources for other animals. An increase in the cost of food production puts not only farmer livelihoods at risk, but also creates the potential for a new form of food elitism where only people who can afford the increased costs of food can afford to eat those foods (Marshman, Blay-Palmer, & Landman 2019). This would only serve to exacerbate an already significant barrier to maintaining nutritious and sufficient diets for the ¾ billion people living in extreme poverty globally.

IMPORTANT ECOLOGICAL LANDSCAPES

Urban spaces can provide important habitat for pollinating insects (Baldock et al. 2015; Hall et al. 2017). For example, urban spaces can present a greater diversity of flowering plants than conventional agriculture composed of a monoculture of commodity crops. This point should not be trivialized. As cities are the sites of the highest consumption and therefore a significant driver of a changing global climate, providing a variety of foci for urban greening is optimal. Urban agriculture is one such opportunity and can provide food for people and habitat for pollinating insects who contribute important ecosystem services resulting in enhanced quality of life (Jim 2013).

There is a substantial body of literature on the benefits of urban agriculture, including mitigating food insecurity, global climate change, the urban heat island effect, and the various forms of malnutrition, as well as the creation of more sustainable and resilient communities through reskilling (De Zeeuw & Drechsel 2015). Urban agriculture is not new – for as long as there have been cities, people have been growing food and raising animals within city limits. There are more than 800 million people practicing urban agriculture globally, much of which is subsistence production in developing countries, as well as a growing number in North American cities (Blecha & Leitner 2014; Blum 2017; Wolch & Emel 1998). Along with pollinating an estimated 90% of the flowering plants on Earth which provide food and resources for myriad species, pollinators are a key ingredient for productive agricultural activities globally including food grown in urban and peri-urban agriculture.

Urban agriculture provides an additional benefit in that it provides a proximal source of fresh food. While urban agriculture is not a substitute for parks and other greenspace, it does provide a complimentary growing-space (Contesse, van Vliet, & Lenhart 2018). Promoting urban agricultural activities is an opportunity for Bee Cities that is not currently being optimized by the majority of affiliates; however, the potential is there. Instead, most Bee Cities are currently emphasizing education and citizen engagement, and less so on habitat restoration on private and municipal property.

Foregrounding the needs of bees through enhanced urban environments helps to increase community resilience in direct and indirect ways. Growing food in residential yards, community gardens, and other urban venues provides a source of fresh foods and an alternative to resource intensive turf grass that is effectively a 'food desert' for pollinating insects. Among other benefits, urban food growing can enhance physical activity and reduce overall stress in gardeners (Baldock et al. 2015). Beyond the many positive health impacts, improved pollination has the potential to boost crop yields by 25% (FAO 2018). An increase in plant diversity is a key feature of urban agriculture which can support a diverse assemblage of pollinating insects. The contribution of many of the non-Apis species to pollination services is less well understood than for honey bees, but there is a growing literature indicating that a diversity of pollinators (i.e. not a monoculture of honey bees) enhances pollination success and provides more stable and productive ecosystem services (City of Toronto 2018; Lowenstein et al. 2015; Pfiffner & Müller 2016; Rogers, Tarpy, & Burrack 2014).

Decisions about how to manage vacant urban land and residential properties can yield large benefits for people and insects alike, including threatened and endangered species (Hall et al. 2017). Pollinator conservation emphasizing healthy ecosystems provides a 'big picture' or systems approach to a healthy environment. One Municipal staff person said, "I think our municipality and the work that [we're] doing, it's more about healthy environments than it is about the bees." This illustrates that activities aimed at improving habitat and forage for bees helps to create an important reciprocity and healthier urban environments for everyone.

STAKEHOLDER PERCEPTIONS OF BENEFITS

Leadership and Education

Two interwoven threads that emerged from this research were leadership and education. For the City of Toronto, becoming the first Bee City in Canada in 2016 was opportune because it occurred during the same time period when the city was launching their Pollinator Protection Strategy (2018) to support diverse pollinator communities, contribute to resilient ecosystems, and enhance urban biodiversity.

Becoming a Bee City was an opportunity to attract a wider audience for the strategy which is an important tool for municipalities who are planning for pollinator-friendly spaces. A former Toronto City Councillor who helped champion becoming a Bee City, along with others including Parks Program Officers, recognized the opportunity to promote the strategy and provide leadership for other communities. She said, "when Toronto does a policy and does something, and leads the way, a lot of the GTA [greater Toronto area] will follow… it's that domino effect."

Much like the City of Toronto, the Environmental Stewardship Coordinator in the Township of King was motivated to become a Bee City to be a leader in the pollinator movement and encourage surrounding municipalities to get involved. The Township of King received their Bee City designation in November 2017.

The City of Niagara Falls also saw Bee City designation as an opportunity. They had just developed their green burial section and they dedicated two acres of their busiest cemetery to pollinator habitat including native plants and educational signage. The Manager of Cemetery Services said that it offered a unique opportunity for community engagement, and was intentional about choosing an urban cemetery for their project where "hundreds of walkers and cyclists and visitors each week … are now taking notice of the green burial section and they're stopping and they're getting out of their cars and they're reading the signs." The City of Niagara Falls received Bee City designation in March 2018.

The City of Guelph has been providing education and an annual pollinator symposium through a pollinator-focused nonprofit called Pollination Guelph. Many organizations turn to this group, along with established researchers from the University of Guelph, for the latest in pollinator research and information (Pollination Guelph 2019). Pollination Guelph was acting primarily within a local context and recognized the need for a national organization to help propel and organize conservation efforts on a larger scale. It was municipal staff, with a representative from Pollination Guelph, that initially applied for the designation. The Program Manager of Trails and Natural Areas Stewardship for the city recognized Bee City designation as a way to "do a better job of leveraging the work that has already been happening in the community." A Community Stewardship Coordinator with the city additionally stated that the community and city have already been "doing a lot of stuff but it also keeps us accountable." A municipal staff person admitted that becoming a Bee City wasn't a motivator for increasing the amount of work being done, but instead it was about creating engagement opportunities and supporting "the underlying work of having communities get engaged in their natural areas … through the lens of pollinators." In these ways, the Bee City designation acts to highlight activities and accomplishments in a novel way, provide an example for other municipalities who are interested in the Bee City designation, and provide a platform for education and engagement. The City of Guelph received Bee City designation in June 2018.

Bee City Canada hosts "Buzz Webinars" as a knowledge sharing platform since December 2018, often presented by Bee City affiliates (Bee City Canada, n.d.). The webinars are hosted live and recorded for future viewing on the Bee City Canada YouTube channel. The webinars present a wide range of topics, from bee-related art, to bee-friendly farming, to specific municipal Bee City programs, and more. There is a breadth of webinar topics, each with an intimate connection to bee health. With so many different modalities of learning, these webinars present an additional option for engaging with issues of pollinator health and conservation. Remote education through webinars became an important engagement strategy during the COVID-19 pandemic that abruptly stopped in-person activities in March 2020 in many Canadian provinces and around the world.

On March 11, 2020, the World Health Organization declared COVID-19 to be a global pandemic. This swiftly altered business as usual in many countries around the world, including Canada. In a few short weeks, Canada saw unprecedented economic and social changes. To contain the spread of the novel virus, borders were closed, schools were closed, businesses ground to a halt. While some sectors were deemed essential (Government of Canada 2020), many people found themselves working remotely from their homes. Online communication became the "new normal" for many, and experts anticipate the shift to online communication to continue beyond the COVID-19 pandemic even after precautions are lifted (Orol 2020).

In Canada, more than 80% of post-secondary institutions offer online courses (Levkoe et al. 2020), but one of the contributing factors to the unprecedented nature of the pandemic was the shift to online communication beyond educational institutions. While some municipal projects have been delayed due to pandemic precautions, organizations like Bee City Canada, who have an established online platform for information sharing, are well situated to continue to provide that information. Making connections in this way allows for ongoing networking and knowledge mobilization, even when individual projects are delayed.

BEYOND LOCAL – CREATING NETWORKS

Bee Cities create a network of interconnected entities that are practically and theoretically joined by the "Bee City" designation (Marshman & Knezevic, forthcoming). Membership in social networks provides benefits and resources not necessarily gained without access to those networks (Eriksson 2011). In September 2018, Bee City Canada held the first Bee City Pollinator Summit for Bee Cities in Ontario, Canada. The summit was attended by over 100 people and provided an opportunity for Bee Cities to share their challenges and successes. Participants agreed that the Summit has been a highlight of the Bee City experience. A staff person from the City of Kitchener said, "We attended the Bee City summit. I would say that was a really good start to start making those connections, and meeting those people, and seeing where staff fits in on their respective Bee City committees." This form of knowledge sharing creates opportunities for municipalities to learn from each other, gauge progress, evaluate successes, and gain insights about their programs by learning about what other Bee City affiliates have accomplished within their respective programs (Marshman & Knezevic, forthcoming).

Many of the Bee City affiliates recognize that there are benefits to being part of a network. Some respondents identified the importance of being part of something bigger, being part of a movement. A Bee City volunteer said being a Bee City is important because it gives people a way to "feel like they're part of something really big." Social movements and networks, or those movements which are interested in social change, can enhance sustainability, resilience, and be a facilitator of wide scale transformation (Blay-Palmer, Sonnino, & Custot 2016). This has important implications including the potential for social movements to merge for mutual support and success. Food system change – moving away from industrialized practices including intensive pesticide use and monoculture cropping – is growing, but still lacking. A movement to protect, conserve, and raise awareness about bees as pollinators is one more avenue for engagement that can contribute to more resilient and ecologically diverse, food systems and practices. One municipal staff person said, "we want to be making sure we're managing our natural assets in ways that are resilient and healthy and sustainable – so the Bee City program will be supportive in that sense."

Implications

Addressing pollinator declines through municipal conservation efforts is an important intervention to ensure a healthy future for people, pollinators, and the planet. True conservation efforts require transdisciplinary approaches from healthy soils, to mitigating urban heat islands, to understanding the impacts of human activities on healthy ecosystems. There are relevant links between the literature on human well-being, contact with nature, and the kinds of urban environments that benefit bees.

It is becoming increasingly clear what contribution pollinating insects such as bees play in helping to achieve the Sustainable Development Goals. New research suggests that bees contribute to the achievement of 15 of 17 SDGs, and at least 30 SDG targets (Patel et al. 2021). The SDGs provide an interesting convergence of priorities and approaches that can help draw attention to the mitigating needs of both wild and managed bee species. In particular, Bee Cities provide an opportunity for social movements to merge for mutual support and success.

Cities can provide important habitat for pollinating insects, and with urban populations expected to be nearly ¾ of the global population by 2050, the importance of recognizing urban spaces as pollinator habitat in conservation planning is clear. There are obvious linkages that can be made between Bee City efforts and underutilized urban spaces. For example, municipalities can use the Bee City designation to legitimize changes to conventional urbanization such as yard, boulevard, roadway, or underutilized green space naturalization.

Since insect pollination is such an integral part of a healthy and productive food systems, opportunities exist for collating existing efforts to promote and enhance food security. Given how Bee Cities at the local level can catalyze collective action, creating a network of unique Bee Cities across the country unites these cities in shared identity and creates integration of awareness that is relevant in the local context. One regional example is The Region of Waterloo in Ontario which consists of three cities and four townships. In the fall of 2019, The Region voted unanimously to become the first Bee Region in Canada. The Regional Chair stated in a news release that becoming a Bee Region "supports [Waterloo Region's] environment and climate action goals, as well as allows all seven local municipalities to work together to promote healthy habitats for bees" (Region of Waterloo 2020, para. 3).

With evidence pointing to global hunger on the rise (FAO 2018), the potential to increase and enhance collaborative efforts in a number of areas is also promising. For example, urban food growing, whether intentional or accessory food growing, also has implications for pollinating insects. Intentional food growing includes activities such as community gardens, urban own-growing, urban food forestry, market gardening, and more. Accessory food growing includes things like the planting of fruit-bearing trees by municipalities along boulevards and in residential neighborhoods. Fruit set on fruit producing trees and shrubs on municipal property can be enhanced by pollination services of bees providing them, and people, with a source of foraged food.

With a growing number of Bee Cities across North America, there is an intentional effort to foreground pollinator health in municipal planning. With active implementation, this has potentially far reaching tendrils from increasing interest and awareness to the creation of pollinator habitat on municipal, private, and residential property with all the associated benefits. In these seminal years of Bee Cities in Canada, pure conservation value has not been measured or evaluated. The links between food security and robust pollinator populations are clear, however, the Bee City movement would benefit from more research to document how Canadian Bee Cities are actively contributing to conservation efforts in their respective cities, and if and how these efforts help to improve and enhance climate mitigation and adaptation strategies.

With that said, important components of conservation efforts such as awareness building, education, and engagement, are all integral to the Bee City movement and apparent in each Bee City program. In addition, Bee Cities report that leadership, recognition, and networking are all important aspects to their respective Bee City programs. The conservation potential, leveraged by municipal will and resources, is significant. The former communications director of Bee City Canada said, "There is a knowledge transfer happening… but I think we are just kind of scratching the surface."

NOTE

1. This chapter contains excerpts from two published, and cited, articles from a doctoral dissertation.

REFERENCES

Atkins, J., & Atkins, B. (2016). *The Business of Bees: An Integrated Approach to Bee Decline and Corporate Responsibility*. Greenleaf Publishing Limited: Sheffield.

Baldock, K. C., Goddard, M. A., Hicks, D. M., Kunin, W. E., Mitschunas, N., Osgathorpe, L. M., … Memmott, J. (2015). Where is the UK's pollinator biodiversity? The importance of urban areas for flower-visiting insects. *Proceedings of the Royal Society B: Biological Sciences*, *282*(1803), 20142849.

Bartomeus, I., Park, M. G., Gibbs, J., Danforth, B. N., Lakso, A. N., & Winfree, R. (2013). Biodiversity ensures plant–pollinator phenological synchrony against climate change. *Ecology Letters*, *16*(11), 1331–1338.

Barua, M., Gurdak, D. J., Ahmed, R. A., & Tamuly, J. (2012). Selecting flagships for invertebrate conservation. *Biodiversity and Conservation*, *21*(6), 1457–1476.

Bee City Canada. (n.d.). Bee City Canada YouTube page [webpage]. Retrieved June 2020 from https://www.youtube.com/channel/UCJcvunxZkieNkEygIJ1HL9A/videos.

Bee City USA. (2019). Website. Accessed Aug 2019 from https://www.beecityusa.org/.
Biesmeijer, J. C., Roberts, S. P., Reemer, M., Ohlemüller, R., Edwards, M., Peeters, T., … Kunin, W. E. (2006). Parallel declines in pollinators and insect-pollinated plants in Britain and the Netherlands. *Science*, *313*, 351–354.
Blackawton, P. S., Airzee, S., Allen, A., Baker, S., Berrow, A., Blair, C., … Lotto, R. B. (2011). Blackawton bees. *Biology Letters*, *7*, 168–172.
Blay-Palmer, A., Sonnino, R., & Custot, J. (2016). A food politics of the possible? Growing sustainable food systems through networks of knowledge. *Agriculture and Human Values*, *33*(1), 27–43.
Blecha, J., & Leitner, H. (2014). Reimagining the food system, the economy, and urban life: new urban chicken-keepers in US cities. *Urban Geography*, *35*(1), 86–108.
Blum, J. (Ed.). (2017). *Urban Horticulture: Ecology, Landscape, and Agriculture.* Boca Raton, FL: CRC Press.
Bond, J., Plattner, K., Hunt, K. (2014). Fruit and Tree Nuts Outlook: Economic Insight. US Pollination-Services Market. USDA Economic Research Service Situation and Outlook FTS-357SA. Retrieved online March 2021 from https://www.ers.usda.gov/publications/pub-details/?pubid=37060.
Canadian Honey Council. (2018). Bee Facts. Retrieved online July 2020 from https://honeycouncil.ca/bee-facts/.
Chan, D. S. W., Prosser, R. S., Rodríguez-Gil, J. L., & Raine, N. E. (2019). Assessment of risk to hoary squash bees (*Peponapis pruinosa*) and other ground-nesting bees from systemic insecticides in agricultural soil. *Scientific Reports*, *9*(1), 1–13.
City of Toronto. (2018). Toronto Pollinator Protection Strategy: Draft Priorities and Actions. Retrieved from https://www.toronto.ca/wp-content/uploads/2017/11/9819-Toronto-Pollinator-Strategy-Booklet-Draft-Priorities-and-Actions-2017.pdf.
Colla, S. R. (2016). Status, threats and conservation recommendations for wild bumble bees (*Bombus* spp.) in Ontario, Canada: a review for policymakers and practitioners. *Natural Areas Journal*, *36*(4), 412–426.
Colla, S. R., & MacIvor, J. S. (2017). Questioning public perception, conservation policy, and recovery actions for honeybees in North America. *Conservation Biology*, *31*(5), 1202–1204.
Contesse, M., van Vliet, B. J., & Lenhart, J. (2018). Is urban agriculture urban green space? A comparison of policy arrangements for urban green space and urban agriculture in Santiago de Chile. *Land Use Policy*, *71*, 566–577.
Denchak, M. (2019). Keystone Species 101 [NRDC Website]. Retrieved online March 2021 from https://www.nrdc.org/stories/keystone-species-101.
de Zeeuw, H., & Drechsel, P. (Eds.). (2015). *Cities and Agriculture: Developing Resilient Urban Food Systems.* Routledge: London.
Eilers, E. J., Kremen, C., Greenleaf, S. S., Garber, A. K., & Klein, A. M. (2011). Contribution of pollinator-mediated crops to nutrients in the human food supply. *PLoS One*, *6*(6), e21363.
Eriksson, M. (2011). Social capital and health – implications for health promotion. *Global Health Action*, *4*(5611), 1–11.
FAO, IFAD, UNICEF, WFP and WHO. (2018). *The State of Food Security and Nutrition in the World 2018. Building Climate Resilience for Food Security and Nutrition*. FAO: Rome. Retrieved online July 2020 from http://www.fao.org/3/i9553en/i9553en.pdf.
Franklin, E. L., & Raine, N. E. (2019). Moving beyond honey bee-centric pesticide risk assessments to protect all pollinators. *Nature Ecology & Evolution*, *3*:1373–1375.
General Mills. (2020). Bring Back the Bees Campaign. [Website]. Accessed July 2020 from https://www.cheerios.ca/bringbackthebees/.
Godfray, H. C. J., Blacquiere, T., Field, L. M., Hails, R. S., Petrokofsky, G., Potts, S. G., … McLean, A. R. (2014). A restatement of the natural science evidence base concerning

neonicotinoid insecticides and insect pollinators. *Proceedings of the Royal Society B: Biological Sciences*, *281*(1786), 20140558.

Goulson, D. (2013). An overview of the environmental risks posed by neonicotinoid insecticides. *Journal of Applied Ecology*, *50*(4), 977–987.

Government of Canada. (2020). Guidance on Essential Services and Functions in Canada During the COVID-19 Pandemic. Retrieved online June 2020 from https://www.publicsafety.gc.ca/cnt/ntnl-scrt/crtcl-nfrstrctr/esf-sfe-en.aspx.

Hall, D. M., Camilo, G. R., Tonietto, R. K., Ollerton, J., Ahrné, K., Arduser, M. … Threlfall, C. G. (2017). The city as a refuge for insect pollinators. *Conservation Biology*, *31*, 24–29.

Hallmann, C. A., Foppen, R. P., van Turnhout, C. A., de Kroon, H., & Jongejans, E. (2014). Declines in insectivorous birds are associated with high neonicotinoid concentrations. *Nature*, *511*(7509), 341–343.

Hegland, S. J., Nielsen, A., Lázaro, A., Bjerknes, A. L., & Totland, Ø. (2009). How does climate warming affect plant-pollinator interactions? *Ecology Letters*, *12*(2), 184–195.

IPBES. (2016). The Assessment Report of the Intergovernmental Science-Policy Platform on Biodiversity and Ecosystem Services on Pollinators, Pollination and Food Production. Retrieved September 2019 from https://www.ipbes.net/assessment-reports/pollinators.

Intergovernmental Panel on Climate Change (IPCC). (2018). Summary for Policymakers. In *Global Warming of 1.5°C*. Pp.1-24. Masson-Delmotte, V., Zhai, P., Pörtner, H.-O., Roberts, D., Skea, J., Shukla, P. R., Pirani, A., Moufouma-Okia, W., Péan, C., Pidcock, R., et al., [Eds.]. World Meteorological Organization: Geneva, Switzerland.

Jim, C. (2013). Sustainable urban greening strategies for compact cities in developing and developed economies. *Urban Ecosystems*, *16*, 741–761. https://doi.org/10.1007/s11252-012-0268-x.

Kearns, C. A., Inouye, D. W., & Waser, N. M. (1998). Endangered mutualisms: the conservation of plant-pollinator interactions. *Annual review of ecology and systematics*, *29*(1), 83–112.

Kolbert, E. (2014). *The Sixth Extinction: An Unnatural History*. A&C Black: London.

Kopec, K. & Burd, L. A. (2017). Pollinators in Peril: A Systematic Status Review of North American and Hawaiian Native Bees. Retrieved from the Center for Biological Diversity https://www.biologicaldiversity.org/campaigns/native_pollinators/index.html.

Kosek, J. (2011). The Natures of the Beast: On the New Uses of the Honeybee. In *Global Political Ecology*. Peet, R., Robbins, P., & Watts, M. [Eds.], (pp. 242–266). Routledge: New York.

Levkoe, C. Z., Knezevic, I., Appavoo, D., Moraes, A., & Scott, S. (2020). Serving up food studies online: teaching about "food from somewhere" from nowhere. *Food, Culture & Society*, *23*(3), 434–453.

Lowenstein, D. M., Matteson, K. C., & Minor, E. S. (2015). Diversity of wild bees supports pollination services in an urbanized landscape. *Oecologia*, *179*(3), 811–821.

Marshman, J. (2019). Communing with bees: a whole-of-community approach to address crisis in the Anthropocene. *Journal of Agriculture, Food Systems, and Community Development*, *9*(A), 87–110.

Marshman, J., Blay-Palmer, A., & Landman, K. (2019). Anthropocene crisis: climate change, pollinators, and food security. *Environments*, *6*(2), 22.

Matteson, K. C., & Langellotto, G. A. (2010). Determinates of inner city butterfly and bee species richness. *Urban Ecosystems*, *13*(3), 333–347.

Mbow, C., Rosenzweig, C., Barioni, L. G., Benton, T. G., Herrero, M., Krishnapillai, M., … Xu, Y. (2019). Food security. 5SM: 1-18. In *Climate Change and Land: an IPCC Special Report on Climate Change, Desertification, Land Degradation, Sustainable Land Management, Food Security, and Greenhouse Gas Fluxes in Terrestrial Ecosystems*. Shukla, P. R., Skea, J., Calvo Buendia, E., Masson-Delmotte, V., Pörtner, H.-O., Roberts, D. C., Zhai, P., Slade, R., Connors, S., van Diemen, R., Ferrat, M., Haughey, E., Luz,

S., Neogi, S., Pathak, M., Petzold, J., Portugal Pereira, J., Vyas, P., Huntley, E., Kissick, K., Belkacemi, M., Malley, J. [Eds.]. Intergovernmental Panel on Climate Change: Washington, DC.

Measham, T. G., Preston, B. L., Smith, T. F., Brooke, C., Gorddard, R., Withycombe, G., & Morrison, C. (2011). Adapting to climate change through local municipal planning: barriers and challenges. *Mitigation and Adaptation Strategies for Global Change*, *16*(8), 889–909.

Memmott, J., Craze, P. G., Waser, N. M., & Price, M. V. (2007). Global warming and the disruption of plant–pollinator interactions. *Ecology Letters*, *10*(8), 710–717.

Myers, S. S., Smith, M. R., Guth, S., Golden, C. D., Vaitla, B., Mueller, N. D., … & Huybers, P. (2017). Climate change and global food systems: potential impacts on food security and undernutrition. *Annual Review of Public Health*, *38*, 259–277.

Naeem, M., Huang, J., Zhang, S., Luo, S., Liu, Y., Zhang, H., … An, J. (2020). Diagnostic indicators of wild pollinators for biodiversity monitoring in long-term conservation. *Science of The Total Environment*, *708*, 135231.

Ontario Horticultural Association. (2010). A Guide to Creating a Pollinator Patch. Retrieved online July 2020 from https://feedthebees.org/wp-content/uploads/2011/07/Roadsides.pdf.

Ontario Ministry of Agriculture Food and Rural Affairs (OMAFRA). (2016). Pollinator Health Action Plan. Retrieved online July 2020 from https://collections.ola.org/mon/30001/333570.pdf.

Orol, R. (2020). After the Pandemic, Teleconferencing and E-learning Could Be the New Normal. Retrieved online July 2020 from https://www.cigionline.org/articles/after-pandemic-teleconferencing-and-e-learning-could-be-new-normal.

Partap, U., & Ya, T. (2012). The human pollinators of fruit crops in Maoxian County, Sichuan, China: a case study of the failure of pollination services and farmers adaptation strategies. *Mountain Research and Development*, *32*(2), 176–186.

Patel, V., Pauli, N., Biggs, E., Barbour, L., & Boruff, B. (2021). Why bees are critical for achieving sustainable development. *Ambio*, *50*(1), 49–59.

Pfiffner, L., & Müller, A. (2016). Wild Bees and Pollination. Research Institute of Organic Agriculture (FiBL).

Pollination Guelph [Website]. (2019). Accessed June 2020 from https://www.pollinationguelph.ca/.

Ranganathan, J., Vennard, D., Waite, R., Dumas, P., Lipinski, B., & Searchinger, T. (2016). Shifting Diets for a Sustainable Food Future. World Resources Institute. Retrieved June 2020 from http://www.indiaenvironmentportal.org.in/files/file/Shifting_Diets_for_a_Sustainable_Food_Future.pdf.

Ray, D. K., West, P. C., Clark, M., Gerber, J. S., Prishchepov, A. V., & Chatterjee, S. (2019). Climate change has likely already affected global food production. *PLoS One*, *14*(5), e0217148. https://doi.org/10.1371/journal.pone.0217148.

Region of Waterloo. (2020). Waterloo Region Becomes the First Bee Region in Canada. Retrieved online July 2020 from https://www.regionofwaterloo.ca/Modules/News/index.aspx?feedId=ab159244-c732-45c7-b4c9-67b38b43eed5&newsId=ed3f7427-658a-47b6-9563-040464aa9548.

Rogers, S. R., Tarpy, D. R., & Burrack, H. J. (2014). Bee species diversity enhances productivity and stability in a perennial crop. *PloS One*, *9*(5), e97307.

Sanchez-Bayo, F., Wyckhuys, K. (2019). Worldwide decline of the entomofauna: a review of its drivers. *Biological Conservation*, *232*, 8–27.

Schultz, P. W. (2011). Conservation means behavior. *Conservation Biology*, *25*(6), 1080–1083.

Sen Nag, Oishimaya. (2018). The Seven Different Types of Honey Bees. Retrieved from https://www.worldatlas.com/articles/the-seven-species-of-honey-bees-living-today.html.

Suryanarayanan, S., Kleinman, D. (2016). *Vanishing Bees: Science, Politics, and Honeybee Health*. Rutgers University Press: New Brunswick, NJ.

Thomas, J. A., Telfer, M. G., Roy, D. B., Preston, C. D., Greenwood, J. J. D., Asher, J., … Lawton, J. H. (2004). Comparative losses of British butterflies, birds, and plants and the global extinction crisis. *Science*, *303*(5665), 1879–1881.

USDA. (n.d.) Attracting Pollinators to Your Garden Using Native Plants. Retrieved online March 2021 from website https://www.fs.fed.us/wildflowers/pollinators/documents/AttractingPollinatorsV5.pdf.

Wake, D. B., & Vredenburg, V. T. (2008). Are we in the midst of the sixth mass extinction? A view from the world of amphibians. *Proceedings of the National Academy of Sciences*, *105*(Supplement 1), 11466–11473.

Wojcik, V. A., Morandin, L. A., Davies Adams, L., & Rourke, K. E. (2018). Floral resource competition between honey bees and wild bees: is there clear evidence and can we guide management and conservation?. *Environmental Entomology*, *47*(4), 822–833.

Wolch, J. R., & Emel, J. (Eds.). (1998). *Animal Geographies: Place, Politics, and Identity in the Nature-Culture Borderlands*. Verso: New York.

Xerces Society for Invertebrate Conservation. (2021). [Website]. Accessed February 2021 from https://www.xerces.org/.

14 Walking the Middle Path of Food Sovereignty, Food Security, Nutrition, and Health in Chiang Mai Province, Thailand

Preety Gadhoke

CONTENTS

INTRODUCTION

The purpose of this study was to engage in fieldwork with farmers across four rural Indigenous and non-Indigenous villages in the Chiang Mai Province of Northeastern Thailand. This study was a result of a partnership with the International Sustainable Development Studies Institute (ISDSI) (ISDSI 2018) to gain access to their network

DOI: 10.1201/9781003014942-14

of farming villages in the Chiang Mai Province. Questions that this study posed to answer include: How are rural Indigenous and non-Indigenous farmers across four villages in Chiang Mai Province adapting to climate change? What are local perceptions and actions on food security, nutrition, and health? What are the implications for strategies that the world can learn from these case studies on increasing food security, climate change resilience, and enhancing access to healthy diets that are local and sustainable? The chapter reveals key themes about food sovereignty, food security, nutrition, and health as they relate with the United Nations Sustainable Development Goals (SDGs) – particularly SDG 1 (Eliminate Poverty), SDG 2 (No Hunger), SDG 3 (Good Health and Well-Being), SDG 10 (Reduce Inequality), SDG 13 (Climate Change Resilience), and SDG 15 (Sustainable Use of Terrestrial Ecosystems) – through fieldwork in four rural Thai highland villages. *Emic* themes include climate change resilience, Buddhist principles of walking the middle path of harmony and balance, Nature as God and animist belief systems, principles of sufficiency economy, environmental justice, organic farming, agency, and sustainable development. Health and nutrition-specific themes, including protecting adults and children from infectious diseases; the importance of stress management through social interactions and support; as well as connecting with Mother Nature, and addressing community health concerns and maintaining harmony and balance in community life.

BACKGROUND AND CONTEXT

Indigenous peoples around the world exhibit "enduring resilience" while experiencing devastation and trauma of the past and present histories. Considered among the most underserved people in the world, Indigenous people globally live with higher rates of communicable and noncommunicable diseases, higher mortality rates, and lower life expectancies than their non-Indigenous counterparts (DESA 2020). The COVID-19 pandemic poses a new threat to their health and survival, but also new opportunities for resilience and coping strategies among Indigenous people. In this chapter, I describe the Hmong and Karen Indigenous people in the context of food and health sovereignty through traditional rituals, sustainable agroforestry, household gardens, and crop fields, and engage in handicrafts and innovative eco-tourist ventures to thrive in today's competitive market economy of the Northeastern highlands of Thailand. Through a "Right to Food" based lens, this chapter describes the role of the Royal Projects for supporting local Indigenous and rural food sovereignty through interviews with organic and nonorganic farmers for climate change resilience and food sovereignty and security to improve equity and reduce social and health disparities. A holistic and integrated local view of harmony in rural life centers upon the forest as a giver, provider, and a teacher for climate change resilience. Key lessons include learning from, being sensitive to the changes in, living off of, and caring for the forest, and transference of local Indigenous, intergenerational knowledge. The ongoing COVID-19 pandemic provides a "wake-up call" for such Indigenous people by revealing the transparent fissures and fractures of inequitable and unequal social structures that are addressed in the 2030 United Nations Sustainable Development Goals (SDGs) (UN SDG COVID-19 2021).

The Kingdom of Thailand's long coastlines, rapidly growing economy, fragile agroforestry system, and susceptibility to weather extremes make it vulnerable to climate change and food insecurity (UNDP 2020; UNDP 2019, 6). With a population of 68.9 million, Thailand is an upper middle-income country that is ranked as the twentieth most populous country with key economic sectors (service, industry, and agriculture). The agriculture sectors, which include crop agriculture, forestry, and fisheries, employ about 31% of Thailand's workforce (2018) and contribute to about 8.1% of the country's Gross Domestic Production (GDP) (2018), key to providing nutrition to rural populations (UNDP 2019, p. 6). Located in Southeast Asia's tropical peninsula in the monsoon region, Thailand covers 513,120 km^2 (UNDP 2019, 6). The country's five regions, North, Northeast, Central, East, and South, are extremely diverse. The North is mountainous and highly fertile. Situated in a monsoon region, Thailand has three seasons: hot, wet, and cool, with mean temperatures between 22 and 32°C. Thailand is susceptible to extreme weather, including droughts, floods, and tropical storms. Moreover, despite banning logging in 1989, Thailand continues to have problems with deforestation, which exacerbates the impacts of fluctuating weather patterns (UNDP 2020).

In the ninth century B.C., the Mon and Khmer people established kingdoms that included large areas of what is now Thailand. Over time, Thailand's culture and identity were influenced greatly by its interactions with South Asia, across religious, social, political, and cultural domains. In 1238, when Sri Intraditya declared independence in the Central region from the Khmer people during the Sukhothai Period (1238–1438 A.D.), with the people taking the name "Thailand" quite literally meaning "free" to distinguish themselves from Tai people still under foreign rule. Hence, the kingdom of Sukhothai was formed with its first king, King Ramkhamhaeng, or Rama the Great (1279–1298) (LOC 2007).

Over the last 30 years, Thailand has observed marked increases in temperatures and rainfall patterns, which has had a drastic effect on food production, specifically rice, which is essential to the country's food security (UNDP 2020). In order to adapt to climate change, the Thai Kingdom has implemented demand-side management and energy conservation programs. Climate change has implications for each of the 17 Sustainable Development Goals (SDGs) with the goal to ultimately achieve Zero Hunger (SDG 2). SDG13 on climate change action highlights adaptation as a key mechanism to combat climate change and its impacts with several targets (UNDP 2019).

Climate change is placing the agriculture sector at risk in Thailand. For instance, Thailand has been described as

> experiencing average growing season maximum temperatures of above 34 degrees Celsius, which is a temperature threshold above which rice yields can be negatively affected unless corrective action is taken. These trends are expected to continue, and the area of the country affected is projected to grow as the climate changes further.
>
> *(UNDP 2019, 6)*

Moreover, "agriculture is the main income basis for poor farmers. Thus climate change has a tremendous impact on poor individual farmers and has aggravated the poverty issue" (UNDP 2019, 6). These plans "identify a need for research and innovative climate change response action to enhance overall resilience of the country" (UNDP 2019). Additionally, another document called the *National Disaster Prevention and Mitigation Plan* (2015) "supports integrated policies on climate change and disaster preparedness initiatives" with Thailand's flagship sufficiency economy philosophy (UNDP 2019, 7). Thailand's highest-level policy document that guides the national climate change response is called the *Climate Change Master Plan* (CCMP 2015–2030). The plan is focused f on seven sectors, including public health, agriculture and food security, and natural resource management (UNDP 2019, 7). On this topic, the UN SDGs applicable are SDG 13.1 (Strengthen resilience and adaptive capacity to climate-related hazards and natural disasters in all countries); SDG 13.2 (Integrate climate change measures into national policies, strategies, and planning); and SDG 13.3 (Improve education, awareness-raising and human and institutional capacity on climate change mitigation, adaptation, impact reduction, and early warning) (SDG 2021).

On the issue of health expenditures, Thailand spends about 4.2% of its Gross Domestic Product (GDP). Life expectancy at birth in Thailand for males and females in 2019 was 74 and 81 years of age, respectively. As a quickly economically rising country, Thailand has drastically reduced the burden of infectious diseases and seen a rapid increase in noncommunicable diseases as well as traffic injuries. Yet, there are health disparities facing a triple burden of infectious diseases, noncommunicable diseases, along with food insecurity and hunger burden. Data from FAO 2020 report indicate existing disparities in terms of child stunting, wasting, as well as food insecurity and hunger across regions in Thailand (FAO 2020).

In terms of infectious diseases, the latest data on the Mekong Malaria Elimination Programme, using July–September 2021 data – including Cambodia, China, Lao People's Democratic Republic, Myanmar, Thailand, and Vietnam – Thailand reported 899 cases, a 32% decrease compared to the same period in 2020. The current COVID-19 statistics, as of January 6, 2022, include a total of 2.245 million confirmed cases and 21,780 confirmed deaths.

METHODS

In July 2019, I worked with ISDSI Executive Director, Mark Ritchie, and his staff to coordinate fieldwork in four of their upland partner villages. ISDSI began as an initiative of the Center for International Programs at Kalamazoo College and is now officially recognized as a nonprofit foundation by the Thai government. It is an experiential learning institute that runs study abroad programs through relationships with local communities on sustainable development and agroforestry with many universities in the United States. ISDSI assisted me in setting up interviews with upland farmers and local community members. Using purposive sampling, I interviewed both organic and nonorganic farmers in the four villages to gain an understanding of the local contexts of food systems, nutrition, health, and well-being. Two out of the four villages are Indigenous, specifically, a Karen and a Hmong community. This study was approved by the St. John's University Institutional Review Board (IRB). All participants provided oral consent of their participation, including audiotaping and photography during interviews. This study was made possible by a

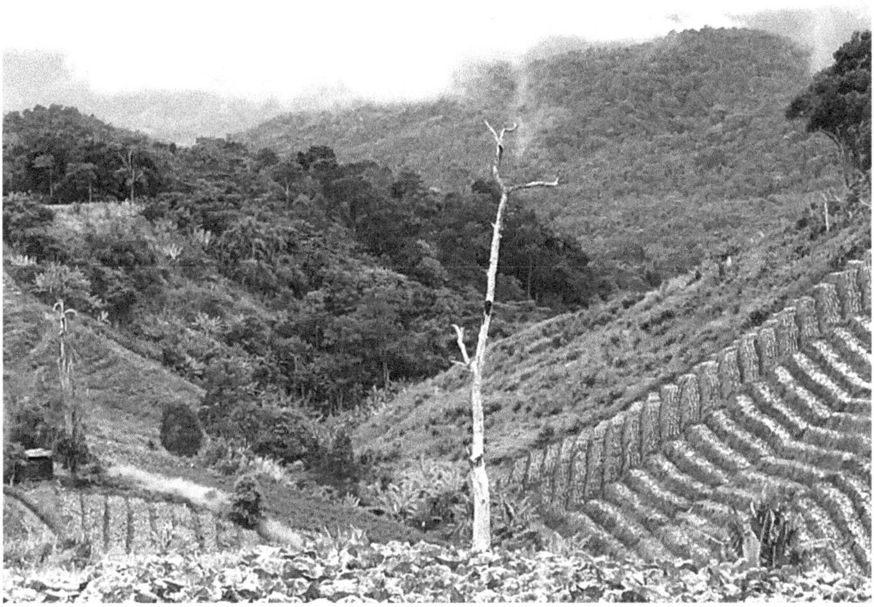

FIGURE 14.1 Hmong cabbage fields at mountain top.

Catholic Relief Services Global Research Grant for the academic year 2019–2020 (Figure 14.1).

FARMING IN THE HIGHLANDS

Our drive into the highlands was a pilgrimage to visit Mother Nature where she co-mingles with the clouds. The silver minivan with curtained windows rolled through winding roads that grew narrower as they zig zagged through thick, lush forests carrying us gently up the mountain. After one stop along the way at a sewing shop at the entrance of Mae Sa Mai village, we piled into a black pickup truck driven by the leader of the Hmong village, Kor Kiat. He took us further up to the Hmong village's farm at the top of the hills. Weaving through narrow winding roads, after a rainfall, we drove through the thicket where the trees enveloped us overhead, carrying us upward. Along the way, we saw smaller farms, until we reached the apex. It was then that the sky burst open, touching the farms with foggy, misty fingers over hundreds of acres of blossomed cabbages over the rolling hills. In 2019, the year before COVID-19 when I traveled to Thailand for my fieldwork, Chiang Mai was experiencing a drought, evident when looking across that foggy mountain top covered by gorgeous cabbage blooms. Standing close to the cabbage plants I could smell the rot. Taking a closer look, I could see the shriveled and burned corners of

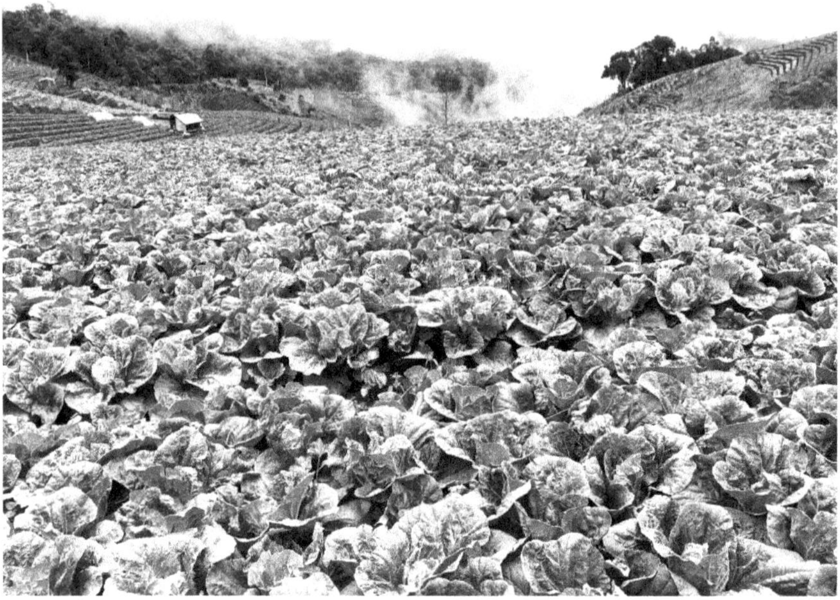

FIGURE 14.2 Cabbage wilted during ongoing drought.

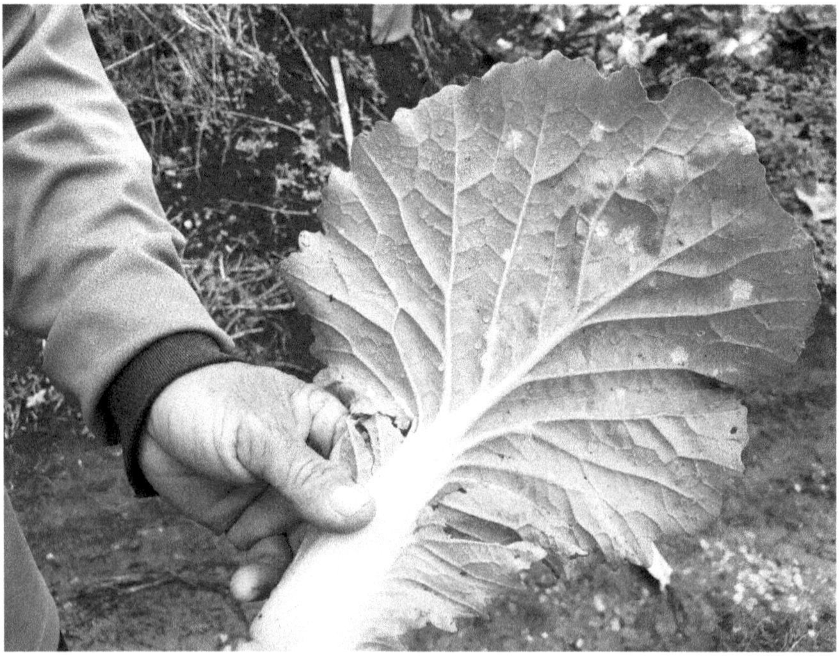

FIGURE 14.3 Wilted cabbage leaf in Hmong farmer's hand.

the cabbage leaves at the edges where the biggest leaves were and also at the very top of the cabbage flower (Figure 14.2).

Kasem, a Hmong village leader, explained me that this would be a costly loss for the village (Figure 14.3).

> This whole area is about 30,000 baht [~U.S. $900.00] worth of vegetables. Crops, when well grown, we can buy [other foods] from the buyers… If not, we eat just vegetables, mostly string beans, cabbage, white cabbage, and tomatoes and the like.

Entering the Mae Sa Mai village, we stopped at the tourist textile shop where we met Kor Kiat outside. The air was cooler and the clouds were gray up here. The front showroom had the most intricate, indigo-dyed jackets, pants, and tops hanging, with a step down into the back sewing room. Women were sewing indigo textiles including Kor Kiat's wife, and a woman with a baby. Kor Kiat pointed to the *Gon Chon* tree that produces hemp that they dry and weave into the delicate and creamy cloth. He showed us the different stages of the plant from a live plant outside the shop to dried stalks, loose fiber, and woven hemp sheets. We piled into Kor Kiat's pickup truck, and he drove us on an unpaved road past the main village to a village farm at the top of the hills (Figure 14.4).

UN SUSTAINABLE DEVELOPMENT GOALS TO REDUCE POVERTY AND HUNGER AND IMPROVE HEALTH

This research project underscored the importance of achieving the United Nations Sustainable Development Goals (SDGs), especially among underserved rural and Indigenous communities for achieving equity and health. Related to the immediate discussions on food, nutrition, and health, this fieldwork underscores the interrelationship between the UN SDGs, especially SDG 1 (End Poverty in All Its Forms Everywhere); SDG 2 (End Hunger, Achieve Food Security and Improved Nutrition, and Promote Sustainable Agriculture); and SDG 3 (Ensure Healthy Lives and Promote Well-Being for All at All Ages) (SDG 2021) for the sustainable development of vulnerable rural Thai communities, both Indigenous and non-Indigenous. In order to address food security, nutrition, and health of these communities, targets and indicators pertaining to eliminating poverty, eliminating hunger and food insecurity, and having access and availability of quality health care locally are necessary for achieving good health and well-being, the implications of which will be described further in this chapter in the Discussion and Conclusions sections (Figure 14.5).

CLIMATE CHANGE RESILIENCE IN INDIGENOUS POPULATIONS

Mae Sai Ma village, sitting at the top of the mountain, represents some of the 240,000 Hmong living, second only to the 300,000 Karen who are also among the highland Indigenous people of Thailand. Since the communist takeover in Laos in 1975, a large diaspora of the Hmong population sought political asylum refugee status in Europe and North America (Culas 2004, 98). Originating in Laos, the Hmong left China in the late 1800s instigated by clashes with the Chinese. The stimulus for the Hmong

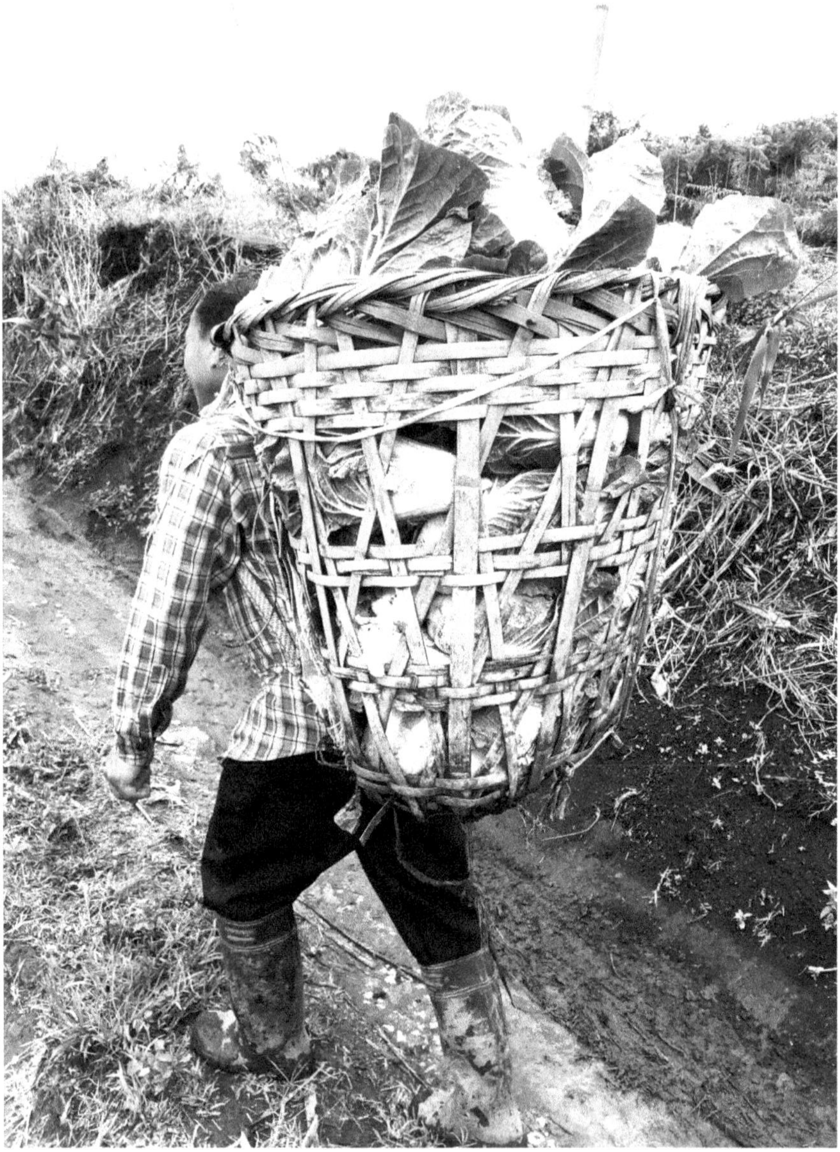

FIGURE 14.4 Cabbage basket on Hmong farmer's back.

migration to largely uninhabited highlands was the search for growing opium poppy, which quickly exhausts the soil, a practice that spread quickly across the Hmong at that time (Culas 2004, 66). With a combination of fertile forest and access to trade routes, the Thai highlands became a place that, as the Royal King and Queen visiting the area observed, became a place where "the hill tribes [grew] opium but were poor," Just as Kor Kiat stated among the cabbage fields at the top of the mountain.

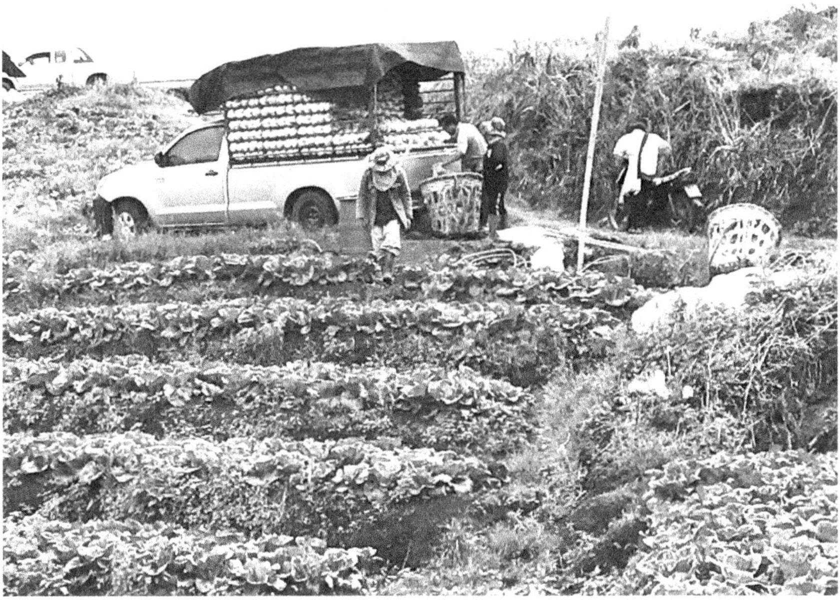

FIGURE 14.5 Cabbage being loaded on truck by Hmong farmers.

In Mae Sa Mai, Kasem had shared that they had not always been growing produce:

> We [The Hmong people of Mae Sa Mai] used to grow opium and rice 30 years ago. We let the land go and let it regenerate. After the Royal Project began, we were funded to stop growing opium and grow vegetables for our livelihood instead.

The traditional belief systems of the Hmong and Karen people in Thailand are similar in their emphasis on the importance of attaining a balance of life in harmony with their natural resources. They use natural resources in every aspect of life from food through farming, hunting, and gathering to housing, clothing, medicine, and performing rituals and ceremonies such as births, weddings, and funerals. Moreover, both Indigenous peoples share the importance of transferring traditional knowledge intergenerationally through teachings, songs, legends, stories, rituals, and daily practices in their homes and also on farms and in agroforestry. Both cultures also share in their animist beliefs of "nature as God" that influences their practices of sustainable development. Yet, there are some key differences between the Hmong (Mae Sa Mai) and the Karen (PhaMon). At Mae Sa Mai, the farmers picked fresh green beans and cabbage to take back to their home to prepare farm-to-table food for us in their home (Figure 14.6).

While the Hmong plant cash crops, the Karen focus on wet rice and swidden cultivation with an emphasis on producing rice, eco-tourism efforts through Homestays and traditional coffee roasting, which I was able to partake in with a group during

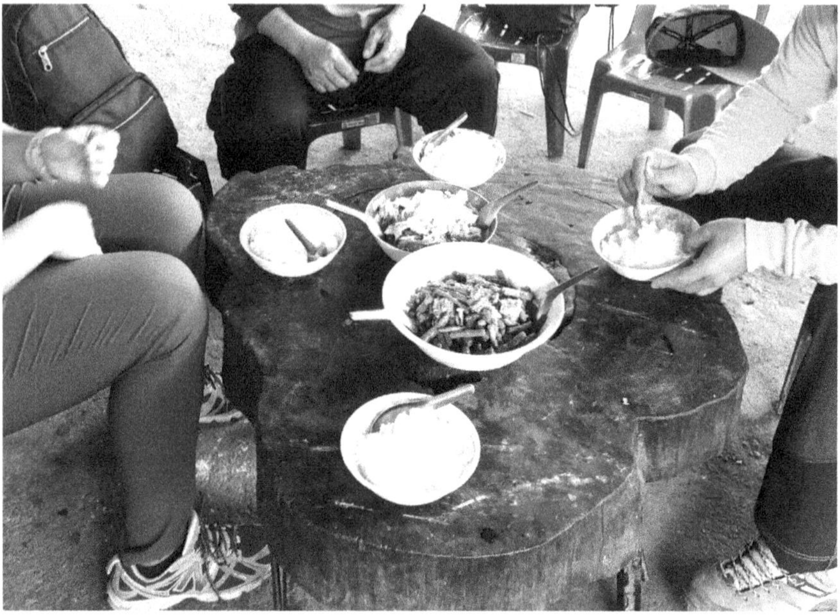

FIGURE 14.6 Farm-to-table meal with Hmong family.

my stay. There were three of us who stood in front of a clay pot placed on a homemade mini earthen stove. We were given handmade stirrers and a cup of green coffee beans to start heating over the mini stove. We stirred the coffee beans on low heat for a while and, when we were happy with the roast, transferred the beans onto a flat sifting plate handmade with straw. We blew air on to the beans to remove any dried particles and transferred the beans into a paper bag. I made a light roast; Khun Sit brought out a coffee grinder, ground some of my beans, and then it was added to hot water in a French press to steep. He repeated this for the others and we sat on the floor on the veranda and sipped the freshest coffee that I have ever had. It had a delicate flavor and a smooth finish (Figure 14.7).

Erosion of social-cultural traditions relates to the degree to which these communities have had to work on commercial economies, religion, and formal education. Moreover, the Thai Constitution, which is deemed the highest law of the land, provides some recognition of customary natural resource management by tribal and Indigenous Peoples does not have all articles put into practice. IMPECT (the Inter-Mountain Peoples Education and Culture in Thailand Association) and FPP (Forest Peoples Programme) have called for certain actions to increase tribal sovereignty, including engaging these communities in participatory action research (such as this fieldwork project), educating the public about tribal and Indigenous Peoples, aiding in cooperative solutions to tribal and Indigenous problems, as well upholding cultural rights and rights of Indigenous communities across Thailand (FPP 2020).

The Royal King then set up the Royal Project in 1969 to "improve the lives and well-being of hilltribes ... reduce opium cultivation [and] restoring forests upstream"

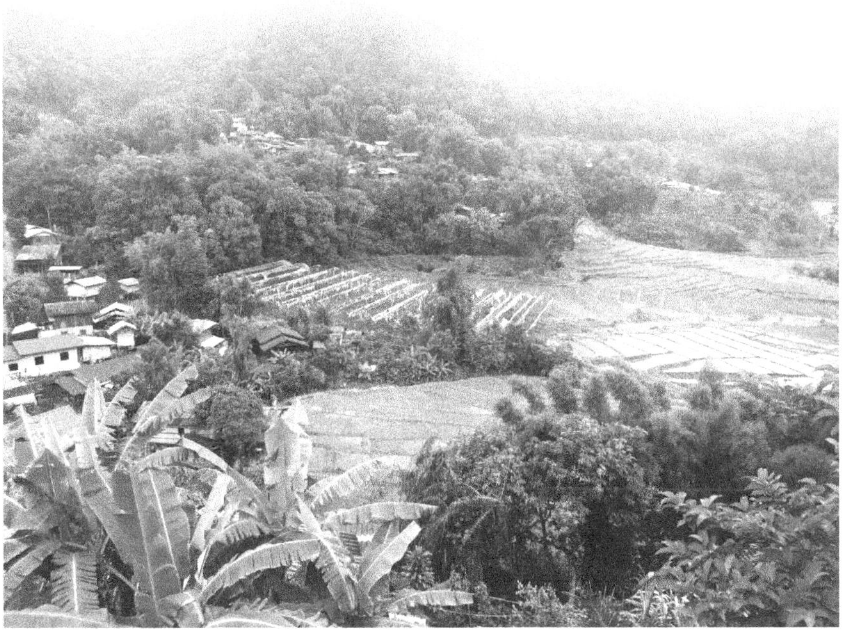

FIGURE 14.7 Panoramic view of Karen Village and rice paddies.

(Royal Project Foundation 2012). The Royal Development Project focuses upon Thai highland communities for integration across land use planning, agroforestry, soil and water conservation, research, processing, transportation, distribution, and marketing. The project emphasizes sustainable development in these highlands of hill tribes for poverty reduction and improved health behaviors such as hygiene and key health outcomes, such as life expectancy (Royal Project Foundation 2012). The Thai government developed a relief program to increase the ability of the highland communities to earn more income through legal means (Royal Project Foundation 2012). Furthermore, UN SDGs focused on improving equality of populations are relevant to this discussion on Indigenous and non-Indigenous community capacity strengthening, specifically, SDG 10.2 (Empower and promote the social, economic, and political inclusion of all, irrespective of age, sex, disability, race, ethnicity, origin, religion, or economic or other status); SDG 10.3 (Ensure equal opportunity and reduce inequalities of outcome, including by eliminating discriminatory laws, policies, and practices and promoting appropriate legislation, policies, and action in this regard); and SDG 10.4 (Adopt Policies, especially Fiscal, Wage, and Social Protection Policies, and Progressively Achieve Greater Equality) (SDG 2021).

On the interlinkages between farming, economic development, and downstream effects on community health, Pi Aun, an organic farmer stated (Figure 14.8):

> This year has been the toughest drought, so it has affected the rice paddies. It's too late to do anything. Because of the drought, there is no water in the rice paddies, and this

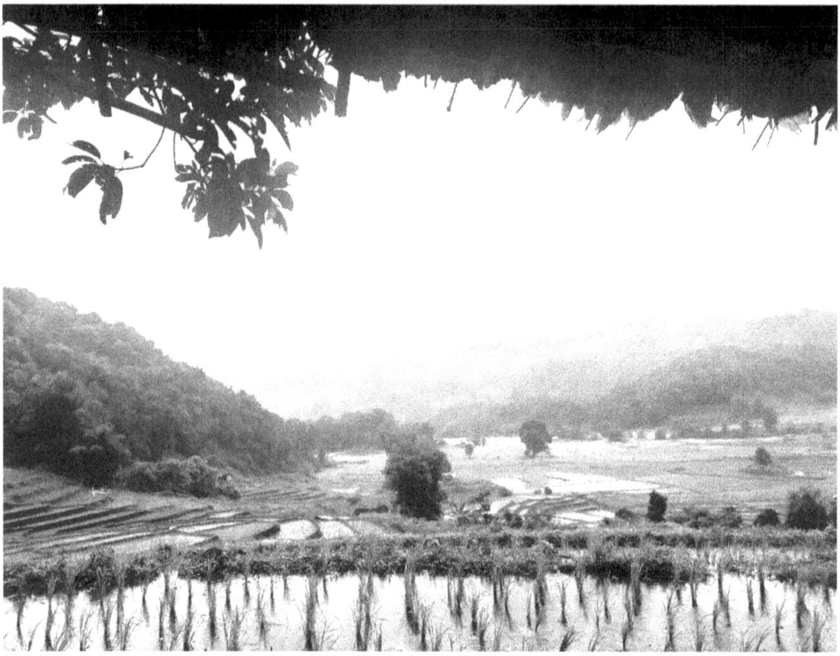

FIGURE 14.8 View of rice paddies from homestay rental in Karen Village.

> has delayed the rice growth. The farmers can adapt by growing baby corn up in the hills in the fall. During this time of year, when rice paddies are wet, cows go up the hill, and they have a bell around their neck to hear them. They have some problem with tigers up in the hills but they rarely would kill a cow...If households each had their own gardens, this would alleviate the problem of food insecurity as well as having a coalition of organic farmers who take care of each other, trade, support each other, and also plan ahead and act out of sovereignty.

COVID-19 IMPACT ON THAILAND'S FOOD SYSTEM, NUTRITION, AND HEALTH

Looking back at 2015, before the pandemic, the countries of the United Nations committed to the 2030 Agenda for Sustainable Development. This agenda recognized the importance of looking beyond hunger toward the goals of ensuring access to safe, nutritious, and sufficient food for all people all year round, and of eradicating all forms of malnutrition (SDG 2 Targets 2.1 and 2.2). Importantly, as the COVID-19 pandemic continues to evolve, the FAO's 2020 State of Food Security and Nutrition in the World report (FAO 2020) attempts to foresee some of the impacts of this global pandemic on food security and nutrition. However, given that the continuing devastation that COVID-19 will cause is still largely unknown, it is important to recognize that any assessment at this stage is subject to a high degree of uncertainty and should be interpreted with caution (FAO 2020).

The most recent estimate for 2019 shows that prior to the COVID-19 pandemic, almost 690 million people, or 8.9% of the global population, were undernourished. Since 2014, the number of hungry people worldwide has been slowly rising. The new estimate for 2019 has revealed that an additional 60 million people have become affected by hunger since 2014. If this trend continues, the number of undernourished people is expected to exceed 840 million by 2030. Hence, the world is not on track to achieve Zero Hunger, even without the negative effects that COVID-19 will likely have on hunger.

Preliminary projections based on the latest available global economic outlooks, also presented in this report, suggest that the COVID-19 pandemic may add an additional 83 to 132 million people to the ranks of the undernourished in 2020 (FAO 2020). Beyond hunger, a growing number of people have had to reduce the quantity and quality of the food they consume. For Thailand, the country placed a ban on international tourists in April 2020 and was able to quickly control the spread of COVID-19 for the rest of 2020. Since December 2020, however, there has been an early rise in the rates of COVID-19 across the country (FPP 2020).

When Thailand's nationwide lockdown was imposed on March 26, 2020, the highland communities were reported as being "less anxious" than city dwellers. IMPECT, an Indigenous organization based in Chiang Mai Province that works closely with Indigenous communities in northern Thailand, shared how the abundance of food in these communities made them self-sufficient, and even with a surplus for sharing. IMPECT helped coordinate food relief drives to share food supplies outside their villages to distribute rice, vegetables, dried foods, and fruits grown on their lands to both urban and rural areas, including Chiang Mai, Chiang Rai, and Bangkok. They reached out to those hardest hit by the lockdown, particularly the Indigenous people who had lost their jobs and/or were unable to return home from the city. IMPECT and the Indigenous Media Network (IMN) also helped monitor the conditions of the elderly across regional communities. Many Indigenous communities also observed rituals and ceremonies to lessen their anxiety and help alleviate their worries about the pandemic. With the help of their community leaders, they were able to set up strict quarantine areas across their communities and practiced strict lockdown measures (FPP 2020). As a result, some have noted potential human rights violations of Indigenous Peoples during COVID-19 that resulted in lack of access to forests risking their food security and livelihoods (Cultural Survival 2020).

Traditional agricultural systems have been devastated by the COVID-19 pandemic. According to the most recent 2020 FAO report, rural communities have continued to face an increase in food insecurity since 2014 (FAO 2020) that was worsened by the pandemic.

Pi Aun spoke about how the farmers were very poor and felt neglected by the Thai government, which underscores the importance of implementing UN SDG 2, particularly, SDG 2.1 (By 2030, end hunger and ensure access by all people, in particular, the poor and people in vulnerable situations, including infants, to safe, nutritious and sufficient food all year round); SDG 2.3 (By 2030, double the

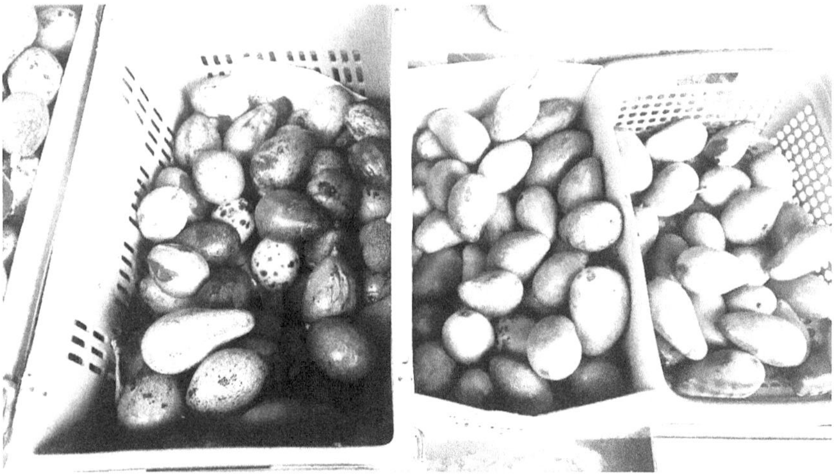

FIGURE 14.9 Fresh produce (avocados and mangoes) at local Karen farm stand.

agricultural productivity and incomes of small-scale food producers); SDG 2.4 (By 2030, ensure sustainable food production systems and implement resilient agricultural practices that increase productivity and production, that help maintain ecosystems, that strengthen capacity for adaptation to climate change, extreme weather, drought, flooding, and other disasters and that progressively improve land and soil quality); and SDG 2.c (Adopt measures to ensure the proper functioning of food commodity markets… in order to limit extreme food price volatility) (SDG 2021) (Figure 14.9).

THE RIGHT TO FOOD AND FOOD SOVEREIGNTY

The Kingdom of Thailand does not explicitly guarantee a right to adequate food (FAO n.d.). Now more than ever, it is necessary to take a rights-based approach to food sovereignty, food security, nutrition, according to the United Nations Food and Agriculture Organization, and health, according to the WHO Alma Ata conference. The "Right to Food" was first established in Article 25 of the 1948 Universal Declaration of Human Rights (UDHR) and was incorporated into Article 11 of the 1966 International Covenant on Economic, Social and Cultural Rights (ICESCR). Starting in the 1990s, interest grew in integrating a human rights approach for population-wide policies to end forms of injustice and oppression, through adequate standards of living including food, clothing, housing, and medical care, and social services. Through this rights-based approach, the UN integrated human rights into the Millennium Development Goals agenda. Without a right to food approach, we cannot guarantee life, dignity, and human rights.

In Mae Sa Mai, Kasem discussed Indigenous sovereignty with me.

He stated that owning his business helps him have a sense of peace and happiness, which he believes is important for sovereignty.

Since the 2008 global food crisis, governments have turned their attention to food policy and support for rural farmers (Field 2016). Both food sovereignty and food security are concepts that emphasize the need to increase food production and productivity to meet future demand. While food security "Food security exists when all people, at all times, have physical and economic access to sufficient, safe and nutritious food to meet their dietary needs and food preferences in order to lead a healthy and active life." In contrast, food sovereignty refers to the political empowerment of small-scale farmers, who are rural and Indigenous (Figure 14.10), by focusing on

> food for the people, valuation of food providers as essential for sustainable livelihoods, locally sustainable food systems, promoting knowledge and skills, and recognizing the upholding the deeply cultural roots of people's relationship with nature and their environment, recognizing the intricate and delicate relationship between ecosystems and human health, wellness, and resilience.
>
> *(Nyeleni 2007, iv–v)*

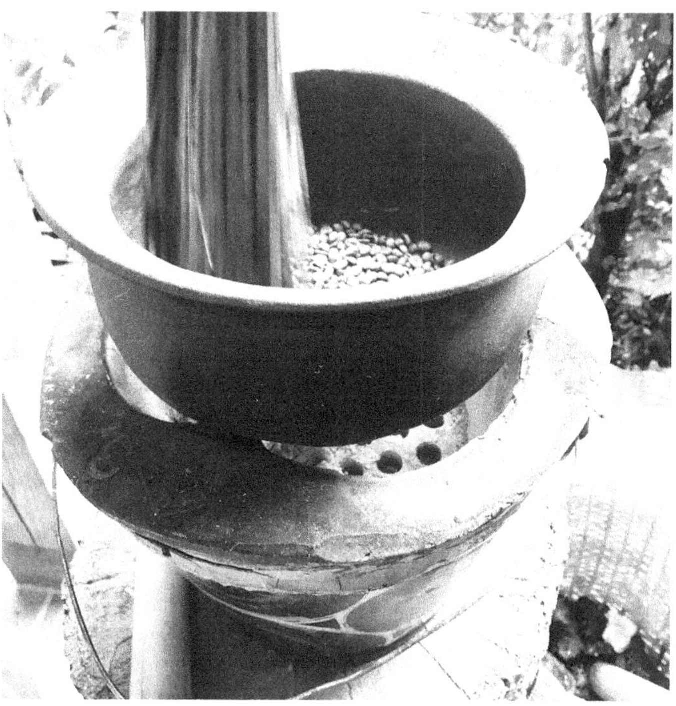

FIGURE 14.10 Roasting coffee beans with eco-tourists.

FOOD SOVEREIGNTY AND INDIGENOUS COMMUNITIES

Food sovereignty holds specific meanings for many Indigenous communities. Defined in 1996 by La Via Campesina, a group of peasant and small-scale farmers wanted to articulate a common response to neoliberalism and the dominant market economy and to defend their rights to land and seeds. The term was defined in 2007 by the Declaration of Nyeleni as "the right of peoples to healthy and culturally appropriate food produced through ecologically sound and sustainable methods, and their right to define their own food and agriculture systems" (Nyeleni 2007). The declaration highlights the importance of placing food producers and consumers, rather than corporations, at the heart of food systems policies; the need to include the next generation in food production, as well as empower food producers and artisans; the importance of environmental, social, and economic sustainability; and the need for transparent trade as well as equality between genders, racial groups, and social classes. Everyone in the food chain is positioned as a potentially powerful actor. The food sovereignty movement is built on the foundation of social justice because a food system must work to correct historical and structural injustices by focusing on the distribution of culturally appropriate foods that must be accomplished while strengthening community, livelihoods, and environmental stability. Food sovereignty connects production and consumption of food in a sustainable way (Nyeleni 2007).

Pi Pui walked me through her seed project area and organic farm. She pointed out the beautiful squash, basil, dragon fruit winding up a tree, pineapple, and other plants. She showed me the shed where she was preparing the seeds and another shed where she was growing shoots that would soon be ready to plant in the next season.

PhaMon, a Karen village, is located on another mountain along windy roads outside Chiang Mai. Unique to PhaMon, they have invested in community-based ecotourism as entrepreneurial ventures, including a pink house overlooking their rice paddies and another homestay opportunity at a private farm house owned by an entrepreneur, Inthanon, an Indigenous Karen who is an advocate for Indigenous sovereignty, as well as has his own eco-tourism venture involving coffee roasting. Inthanon graciously hosted me, along with a German traveler and his partner, and other local Thai travelers. Khun Sit invited us to his parents' home, a hand-built traditional Karen hut. The Karen have an animist belief system, where, as Khun stated: "Nature is God. It is important to share food and preserve and conserve nature" (Figure 14.11).

Food sovereignty is a top priority for non-Indigenous villagers in the Chiang Mai area as well. For instance, a third village where I conducted fieldwork was Mae Tha, where organic farming started years ago by an innovative collective. Pi Aun, a third-generation organic farmer and activist and member of the local organic farming coalition, talked about sovereignty as we walked around the large agroforestry land:

> Before we turned to organic farming, we had to work very hard for monocropping. I stopped monocropping because of the debt that we incurred. So we had to buy a couple cows, then we sold the cows and got rid of our debt from year by year. Every time my wife sold crops, I saved ½ of a piggy bank. I can save money because I am fully reliant on my crop, self-sufficient economy. Now, years later, I have a lot of teak from agroforestry, and grow some fruit. For instance, my house is built off all of the wood from my land.

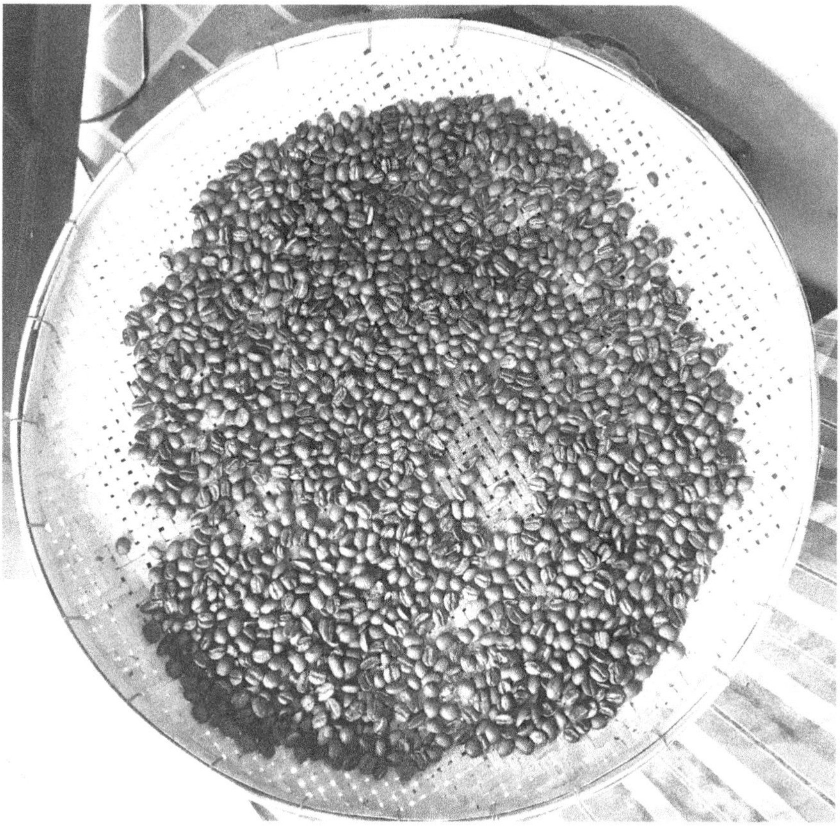

FIGURE 14.11 Roasted coffee beans for eco-tourism.

He additionally spoke about the need for sovereignty:

> We have [many] interests. We work in the community. We have a café. We work with schools and more than 30 groups or organizations, women's groups, men's groups, and a health center. At the end of the year, we have a community report and get plans together for next year now.

Pi Aun met us at the organic arabica cafe early in the morning. He rode in on his motorcycle with a backpack on his back. I met his son at the end of the day along with his wife as we returned to the cafe to have a drink and chat. It was here that he shared some history about organic farmers in the Chiang Mai region. He stated that years ago, they rode horses locally and the Thai government did not recognize them as a people, given that they were not only physically hidden from society in the highlands but were also invisible to them, not recognized nor financially supported by the government. This was the impetus behind their self-sufficiency movement, which involved hiring a nongovernmental organization (NGO) from Germany to help them develop an integrated agroforestry system.

Our vision of sustainable agriculture needs a new generation to join the initiative. I'm a third generation who studied in Bangkok and came back. We are really poor people. The older men didn't go to school beyond grade 4. We have had 11 members return home. We work on resource management and sustainable agriculture, how to plant, and traditional ceremonies for respecting water and trees. In the past, we learned from the outside (Europeans). Now we are learning about our practices. Families gain a lot of debt going to school in Bangkok and farmers are also loaning money. Younger generations are going to the first step, talking to the second generation up a stair, and third generation up another stair. Leaders are first talking and speaking. We got data now, in the past, we didn't know about data.

SOVEREIGNTY, FOOD AND NUTRITION, AND COMMUNITY HEALTH

The farmers all spoke about the interconnectedness between having sovereignty which, in turn, helps to provide good food and nutrition to their communities, and attaining holistic health, in terms of both physical and mental health. In their worldview, the farmers across the four villages shared their strengths-based approaches toward defining their own food security, nutrition, and health status. Again, in their cultural construct informed by sufficiency economy principles, they believe that they make do with what they have as resources and foods that are available. Meat is the most expensive food and, while they may not have access to it, they remain focused on being self-reliant and providing the most balanced meals that they can for their families and living within their means. Upon inquiring about food security and hunger, farmers across all four villages were not aware of any formal governmental, nongovernmental or academic food assessments conducted among their communities, nor was there any perception of food insecurity. Despite having enjoyed accelerated economic growth, Thailand continued to face a burden of food insecurity and hunger as a result of budget cuts on social service programs prior to COVID-19. Food insecurity and nutrition are inextricably linked, as revealed in the farmer interviews across the four villages in Chiang Mai during my fieldwork. Food insecurity can lead to different manifestations of malnutrition. One vital element that explains this connection is the food that people eat, specifically, the quality of their diet. Food insecurity can affect diet quality in different ways, potentially leading to undernutrition as well as overweight and obesity, both spectrums are types of malnutrition. Ensuring access to a healthy diet is a prerequisite for achieving the SDG target of eradicating all forms of malnutrition. For this reason, food security and nutrition-focused agriculture upstream is necessary for the future well-being of societies (Figure 14.12).

Pi Aun and Paw Pat both said that because they practice agroforestry planning ahead for a year, they do not observe food insecurity in their farming group and village. But Paw Pat and Pi Aun did state that having drought does not help, and also that they were not aware of food insecurity in their villages. Food insecurity has not been formally measured in these rural villages, and therefore, the discussion on food security reflects more of their perceptions rather than the state of food security in their villages.

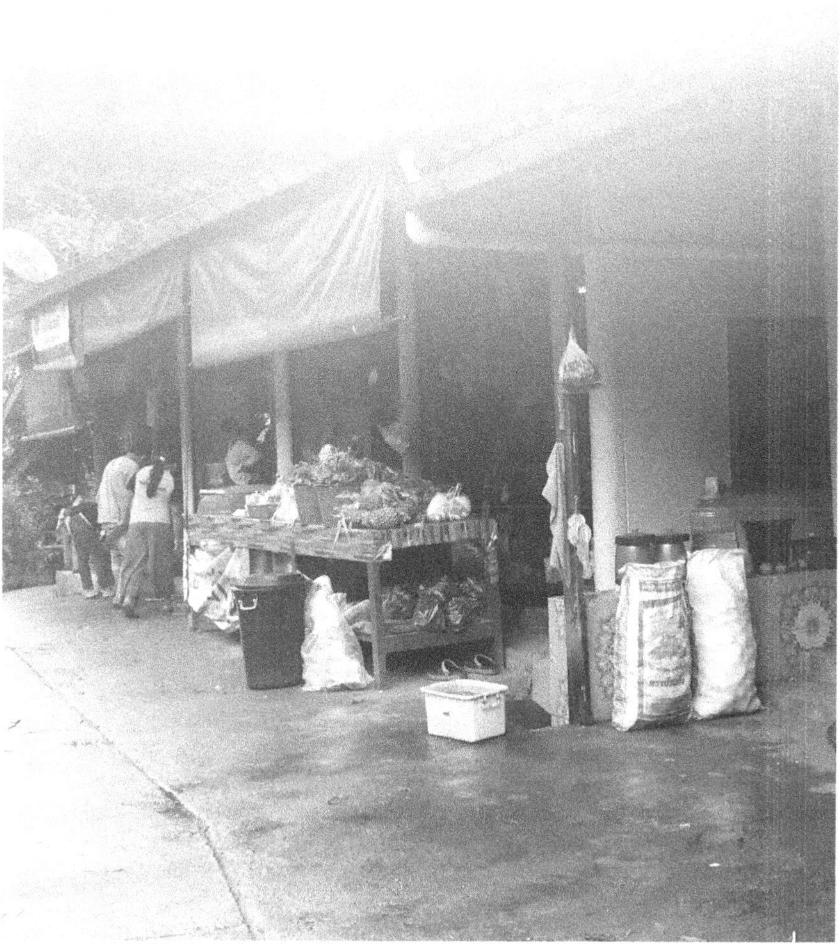

FIGURE 14.12 Karen Village farm stands.

In Don Phon, where the organic farming movement began decades ago, the father or organic farming, Paw Pat sat in the community room cross-legged and talked to us, as we sat around him on the floor:

> Because households each have a garden, we do not have food insecurity. The gardens provide food for each household.

Evidence from published studies reports that food insecurity exists in rural Thailand caused by reduced purchasing power, which leads to reduced consumption of nutritious, balanced meals (Isvilanonda and Bunyasiri 2009). In Mae Sa Mai, Kasem and his colleague that I spoke with did inform me that families do not get nutritious meals when they cannot sell at a competitive price at the downhill market, and cannot afford to buy meat.

Back in Mae Sa Mai village, Kasem discussed community health needs that links sovereignty, food security, and health altogether:

> There are three things that we need. First we need to live in a good atmosphere that is good for health and the body. Second, we need to grow our own food. And third, we need to take care of our own mental health and owning his business helps him have a sense of peace and happiness.

The farmers discussed the importance of stress management. For instance, in Don Jieng, Mae Wines described the interlinkages between stress, health, and the importance of going into nature to reset and calibration of harmony and balance:

> The main problem is heat and stress. Stress causes high blood pressure and diabetes. Lots of villagers have appointments with the local doctor. I go to the farm and listen to music to bring my pressure and stress down.

In Don Jieng, Pi Pui stated the importance of nature as resetting one's mind and alleviating stress:

> I go to the jungle and farm, sit under a tree and it makes me feel less stressed. Older people stay at home, they cannot come out in the extreme weather.

General conceptions of health among the Hmong were described as hard work, living by traditional ways and taking herbal medicines as the first line of therapy, as Kasem stated:

> Hmong people work very hard. Elders work very hard all their life and maybe look healthy because of the hardwork in the fields...In the first few days of being ill, we live by our traditional way through herbal medicines. If we get worse, then we go to the hospital.

Conceptions of being healthy were described by Kasem as being stress-free and achieving life's goals through hard work across Indigenous and non-Indigenous perspectives:

> To be stress free, some people live a long life if they are not educated and not stressed.

Back in Mae Sa Mai, Kasem said:

> The health promotion center is nearby, about 4 kilometers away. Children get fevers once in a while. Otherwise we are healthy." For when they need a hospital for special care or tertiary/emergency care, we go to Nakhon Ping hospital, which is about 20 kilometers away. Access to health care and public health is easier than before. Ever since we got funding from the Royal [Thailand] Projects, it has raised our quality of life and health status.

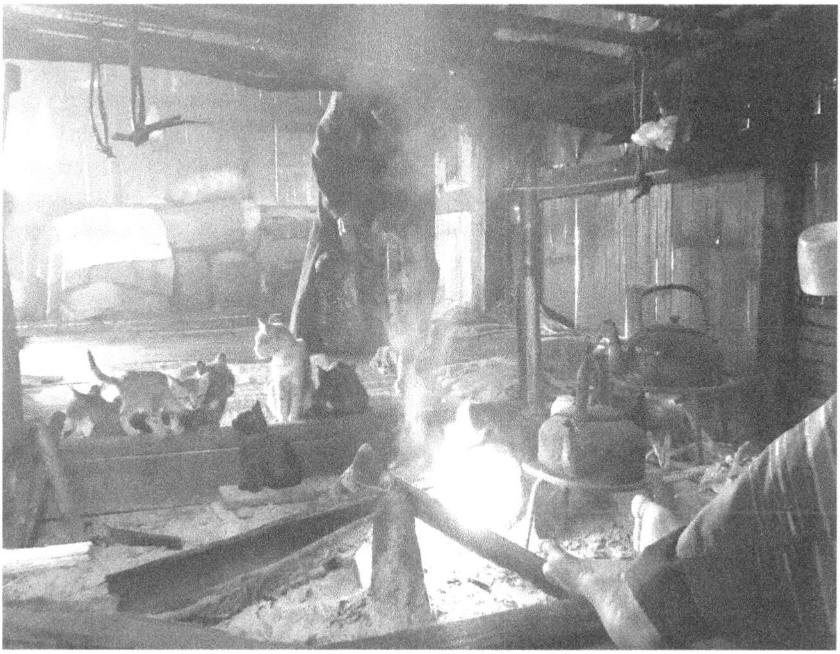

FIGURE 14.13 Hearth inside Karen family home.

Mental health and stress came up as important themes, given the stressors that tribal and Indigenous communities face. Khun Sit stated:

> People decompress with communication and being with relatives. Everybody knows each other in our village. We eat out at each other's homes. That is a way to decompress, such as having four other homes to eat at during the week. It is the job of the host to feed them and it's our culture to feed and take care of each other.

In terms of health risks, Khun Sit mentioned (Figure 14.13):

> on the issue of health risks and the health status of FaMine, dengue fever and malaria are a risk here. But because of climate change, there has been a drought and a delay in the monsoon or wet season. So, dengue and malaria have not started to be a concern yet this year.

In the last three decades, Thailand's health departments have expanded to address community health needs from urban centers to the most remote communities at low to no cost. Majority of Thailand's population falls under universal coverage for preventive and primary care (Chiang Mai City Life 2022). Khun Sit described high rates of malaria and dengue fever in his community and that, because of the drought, they had not yet seen malaria or dengue fever impacting the locals yet. (Monsoon season would start soon after I left Chiang Mai to return home.)

SUFFICIENCY ECONOMY PHILOSOPHY FOR SUSTAINABLE DEVELOPMENT

Sufficiency Economy is the unique, innovative philosophy of sustainable development adopted by the Kingdom of Thailand, and is founded on Buddhist principles of moderation or the "middle path" of life, as well as principles of self-awareness and reasonableness whose meanings are intertwined and interdependent across individual, community, and national levels (PRD Thailand n.d.).

At the individual level, it reflects the philosophy of leading a simple life, one that is based on living on resources necessary, living within one's own means and not taking advantage of others. On a community level, it refers to having solidarity in joint decisions for the benefit of community members and utilizing natural resources sustainably (UN 2020). On the national level, it refers to taking a holistic approach to develop interdependent systems (UN 2020). "Sufficiency" pertains to living in moderation in a way that is sufficient for development and buffering systems against internal and external shocks across individual, community, and national levels. At the same time, this sufficiency economy must be built on moral Buddhist principles of moderation, balance, harmony, patience, perseverance, and diligence (Mongsawad 2010).

According to the Royal Project Foundation, there are five distinct strategies for sufficiency economy centered on building a sufficient economy (which includes having sufficient income and community capacity building, as well as preservation of nature and land): (1) planning for land use; (2) afforestation in appropriate areas; (3) farming preservation systems and strategies; (4) integrated agricultural, environmental, social, and health research; and (5) harvest management, marketing, and transportation services (Royal Project Foundation 2012).

Living by the tenets of sufficiency economy informs the local farmers on adapting their behaviors during challenging times, as Kasem in Mae Sa Mai pointed out while we were walking through the cabbage fields amidst the clouds:

> When we are running low on water from a drought and climate change, as we did this year, we have to run the water directly through a hose down to all these beds of cabbage and vegetables. In the rainy season, we grow cabbage here. If there is no rain, we have to bring water in trucks here and water the plants by hand (pointing to the hose rolled up by the edge where we were standing). We bring trucks with huge water containers to water the plants downhill. The vegetables will not be beautiful in terms of the amount and quality. We embrace it when we have a drought and sell what we can.

As captured in the narratives, especially Paw Pat's quotes earlier on mono-crops, this was not typically a profitable venture, as dependence on it can increase a family's vulnerability to market shocks. When there is an oversupply of the product, prices drop significantly, which can force families to borrow money to buy food for themselves, since they cannot eat their own cash crops. In order to achieve self-reliance, according to the principles of sufficiency economy, families are encouraged to change to integrated farming from mono-crop or cash-crop farming. This was expressed by all farmers during my fieldwork across the four villages. While the Karen specialize in rice and fruit, for instance, the non-Indigenous organic farmers are mostly focused on cash crops and agroforestry. A combination of plants, especially food plants, such as rice, vegetables, and fruit, are recommended for planting on the farm. Before the produce or value-added transformed produce is put up for sale, a sufficient quantity of it should be kept for the family's own consumption. Also, farm animals, such as cattle, play a significant role in the integrated farm, as they provide for the family's consumption needs. Measures such as this build self-reliance—doing away with that characteristic of poverty."

Paw Pat discussed the importance of early planning as a way of mitigating climate change:

> A long time ago, our ancestors had no problem with our produce. Right now when technology has been introduced, farmers have had to use chemicals. In the past, they didn't know about global warming. But now, yes, [climate change] affected my produce...If this year, I don't grow rice, I am okay because I have a crop from last year. I have only one daughter and that's why I asked her to come back.

On excessive heat and climate change adaptation, Pi Pui stated:

> We have heard what to do now. I know what to do. I will improve my soil. We have seasonal vegetables. The experiential learning made me change by going into the forest and making observations. I observed the soil around there, and changed the consistency of the soil here to match the forest. The trees survive global warming and learning about the unique qualities of forest soil is helpful for farming plants. The transference of this local knowledge (about forests being more resilient to climate change) into farming practices. By studying the difference in the soil in the forest from the soil on their farms, I believe it is useful to modify the soil of farms for adapting to climate change.

FARMER EXPRESSIONS OF LOCAL CLIMATE CHANGE RESILIENCE

The farmers mentioned the critical importance of climate change resilience as rural farmers, some of whom are Indigenous and organic farmers. For instance, in Don Jieng, the female farmer stated the importance of learning about climate change resilience from the trees and soil themselves, learning from other farmers adapting to climate extremes such as drought, in the area. The father of organic farming, Paw Pat, spoke of climate change resilience as needing to think innovatively about farming technology to adapt to climate change as follows:

> This is the worst drought I've experienced in my entire life. We have to think creatively such as doing a study of potatoes that grow on a vine on the ground rather than being rooted underground so they can grow larger, which means a greater yield of food to a family. A larger potato can feed more mouths in a family

He further stated the importance of educating other farmers on how to engage in more resilient technologies and sustainably adapt to climate change:

> We should study more about crops that tolerate the heat. We need to study the nutritional value of these crops. There's a lot of technology today that we cannot eat ... We need to teach people how to survive and adapt to their weather and ecology.

UN SUSTAINABLE DEVELOPMENT GOALS TO REDUCE INEQUALITY, ADDRESS CLIMATE CHANGE, AND PROMOTE AND PROTECT TERRESTRIAL ECOSYSTEMS

In addition to SDG 1, SDG 2, and SDG 3 noted previously, the UN SDGs that are relevant to this project that address vulnerable populations and climate change resilience, as well as sustainable development of ecosystems, include SDG 10 (Reduce inequality within and among countries); SDG 13 (Take urgent action to combat climate change and its impact); and SDG 15 (Protect, restore, and promote sustainable use of terrestrial ecosystems, sustainably manage forests, combat desertification, and halt and reverse land degradation and halt biodiversity loss) (SDG 2021). A further assessment will be considered in the Discussion and Conclusion sections.

CONCLUSIONS

In summary, this fieldwork having preceded the COVID-19 pandemic highlighted some important aspects of climate change resilient strategies among two Indigenous and two non-Indigenous villages in the Chiang Mai Province of Thailand. Recent personal correspondence with the IDSDI Director provided me with an update on how all four communities have continued to face hardships during the early strict lockdown measures by the Thai government, and some recovery efforts are currently underway in 2021.

Land is inherited intergenerationally, as are traditional beliefs and value systems for both the Karen and Hmong people in Chiang Mai Province. In contrast, non-Indigenous Thai farmers, such as organic farmers such as Pi Aun and Pi Pui, adapted to integrated agroforestry over generations and decades.

In the end, it is both their strong belief in sufficiency economy as well as their animist belief system, as well as their ongoing adaptations to climate change that are helping these communities to thrive. As Khun Sit stated:

> There is a sport where every time a baby is born in our village, a cord is tied around a tree. We do not cut down [many] trees; this is a way that in our philosophy on harmony and balance is integrated into ecological conservation.

Life, according to traditional belief systems, revolves around four pillars in their home. As described by Khun Sit:

> Everything happens around the four pillars in a home, cooking, feeding, sleeping, and implicitly, mating and birthing too. From birth to death, life begins and ends around the four pillars.

There are overarching lessons learned from this fieldwork that can be gleaned and applied to similar contexts on sustainable development for the health and well-being of local rural communities. Namely, local traditional value systems inform the ways in which rural Indigenous and non-Indigenous farmers support sustainable systems of food production. They are embedded in a larger worldview of the pillars of life that sustain local traditions and practices throughout an infinite cycle from birth to death.

RECOMMENDATIONS

- Uphold, honor, and protect cultural rights and traditional knowledge transfer of tribal Indigenous and non-Indigenous people in Thailand to help manage natural resources, combat food insecurity, and achieve proper nutrition and health status.
- Promote and support local Indigenous and non-Indigenous traditional cultural practices by the Thai government at the national, regional, and local levels.
- Promote and support participatory action research and practices for tribal and non-Indigenous that improve food security and comprehensive health status across academic institutions, nongovernmental organizations, and other relevant structures.
- Increase local knowledge of tribal and Indigenous Peoples of Thailand to enhance the creation of collaborative and cooperative solutions.
- Consider a strengths-based approach toward the relevant SDG targets, particularly related to SDG 1, SDG 2, SDG 3, SDG 10, SDG 10, SDG 13, and SDG 15 (Figure 14.14).

ACKNOWLEDGMENTS

I would like to thank Dr. Meghan Clark, Associate Professor at St. John's University, and the Catholic Relief Services for funding this global research project. I would like to give thanks to the Institute for Sustainable Development's Director, Dr. Mark Richter, and his staff for hosting me and providing me with access to their community partners in Don Jieng, Mae Sa Mai, Mae Tha, and FaMine. A very special thanks to all farmers in Chiang Mai for taking their time to show me their beautiful farms, sharing their perspectives and insights, and welcoming me into their homes, especially Kasem and his wife, and Khun Sit and his parents and sister.

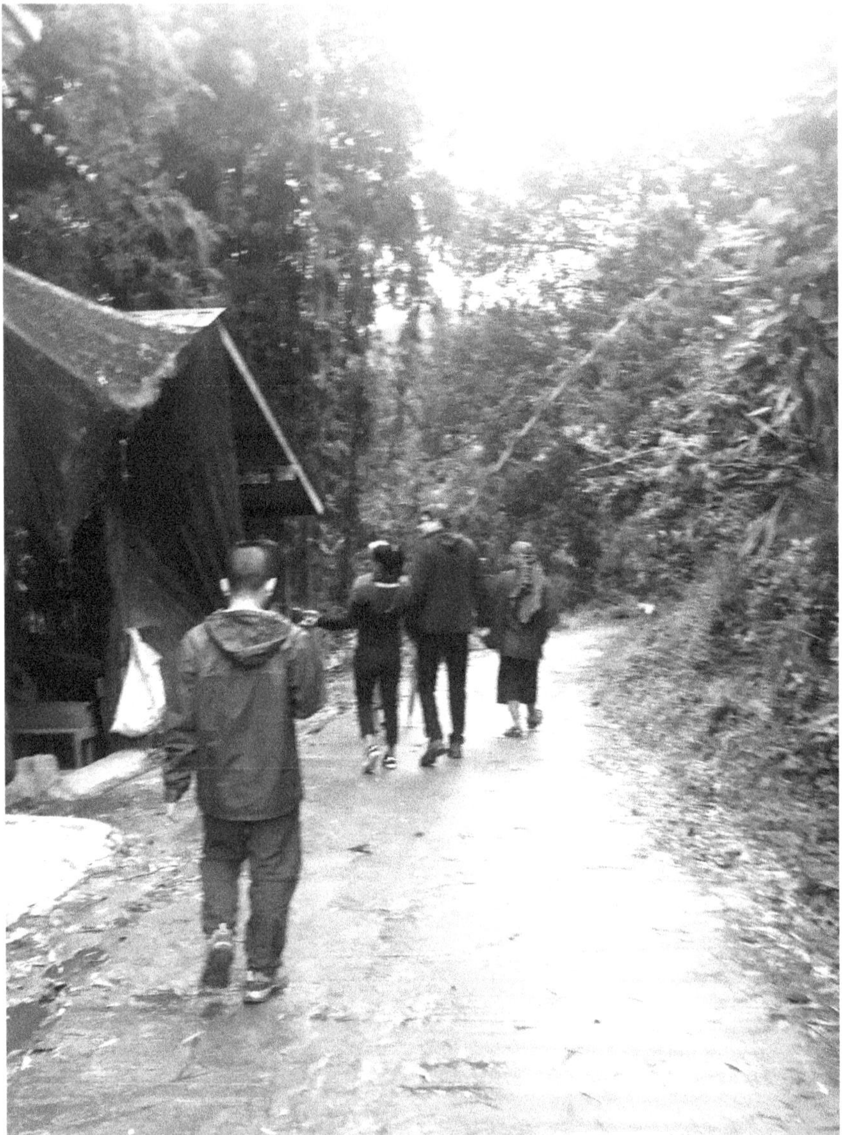

FIGURE 14.14 Eco-tourists walking in Karen Village.

REFERENCES

Chiang Mai City Life. (2022). Health & Wellness: The Thai Health Care System. https://www.chiangmaicitylife.com/clg/living/health-wellness/the-thai-health-care-system/.

Culas, Christian. (2004). Innovation and Tradition in Rituals and Cosmology: Hmong Messianism and Shamanism in Southeast Asia. In *Hmong/Miao in Asia*. Tapp Nicholas, Jean Michaud, Chiristian Culas, and Gary Yia Lee (Eds.). Pp. 97–128. Chiang Mai, Thailand: Silkworm Books.

Cultural Survival. (2020). Indigenous Peoples in Asia Battle COVID-19 on Many Fronts. https://www.culturalsurvival.org/news/Indigenous-peoples-asia-battle-covid-19-many-fronts.
Field, S. (2016). The financialization of food and the 2008–2011 food price spikes. *Environment and Planning A: Economy and Space*. 48 (11): 2272–2290. https://doi.org/10.1177/0308518X16658476.
Forest Peoples Programme (FPP). (2020). Thailand Case Study: Highland Indigenous Communities on Self-Sufficiency, Food Security and Land Tenure during COVID-19. https://www.forestpeoples.org/en/covid19-impacts-case-study-thailand.
Government Public Relations Department (PRD Thailand). Kingdom of Thailand. (n.d.). Sufficiency Economy and the Middle Path in Buddhism. https://thailand.prd.go.th/ewt_news.php?nid=131&filename=index.
International Sustainable Development Studies Institute (ISDSI). (2018). http://isdsi.org.
Isvilanonda, Somporn, and Isriya Bunyasiri. (2009). "Food Security in Thailand: Status, Rural Poor Vulnerability, and Some Policy Options," Working Papers, Kasetsart University, Department of Agricultural and Resource Economics.
Library of Congress (LOC). 2007. Country Profile: Thailand. Federal Research Division. https://www.loc.gov/rr/frd/cs/profiles/Thailand.pdf.
Mongsawad, P. (2010). The philosophy of the sufficiency economy: a contribution to the theory of development. *Asia Pacific Development Journal*. 17 (1): 123–151. http://citeseerx.ist.psu.edu/viewdoc/download?doi=10.1.1.391.2008&rep=rep1&type=pdf#page=131.
Nyeleni Declaration. 2007. https://nyeleni.org/spip.php?article290.
Royal Project Foundation. 2012. Development. http://royalprojectthailand.com/development.
United Nations (UN). Sustainable Development. 2020. Sufficiency Economy Philosophy. Thailand. https://sustainabledevelopment.un.org/partnership/?p=2126.
United Nations Development Programme (UNDP). 2019. Integrating Agriculture in National Adaptation Plans Programme. Experiences of Integrating Agriculture in Sectoral and National Adaptation Planning Processes. Thailand. Case Study. https://www.adaptation-undp.org/sites/default/files/resources/case_study2.pdf.
United Nations Development Programme (UNDP). 2020. Climate Change Adaptation. Thailand. https://www.adaptation-undp.org/explore/south-eastern-asia/thailand.
United Nations Food and Agriculture Organization (FAO). 2020. The State of Food Security and Nutrition in the World. Transforming Food Systems for Affordable Healthy Diets. http://www.fao.org/publications/sofi/2020/en/.
United Nations Food and Agriculture Organization (FAO). n.d. https://www.fao.org/right-to-food-around-the-globe/countries/THA/en/.
UN DESA. 2020. Policy Brief #70. The Impact of COVID-19 on Indigenous Peoples. https://www.un.org/development/desa/dpad/publication/un-desa-policy-brief-70-the-impact-of-covid-19-on-Indigenous-peoples/.
United Nations Sustainable Development Goals. (SDG). 2021. https://sdgs.un.org/goals.

Index

Note: **Bold** page numbers refer to tables, *italic* page numbers refer to figures, and page numbers followed by "n" denote endnotes.

For Product Safety Concerns and Information please contact our EU representative GPSR@taylorandfrancis.com
Taylor & Francis Verlag GmbH, Kaufingerstraße 24, 80331 München, Germany

www.ingramcontent.com/pod-product-compliance
Ingram Content Group UK Ltd.
Pitfield, Milton Keynes, MK11 3LW, UK
UKHW020017200926
475702UK00014B/1934

* 9 7 8 0 3 6 7 8 5 7 6 2 2 *